Respiratory Care

Respiratory Care

Edited by

Vanessa Gibson
Northumbria University
Newcastle upon Tyne, UK

David Waters
Buckinghamshire New University
Uxbridge, Middlesex, UK

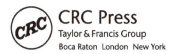

CRC Press
Taylor & Francis Group
Boca Raton   London   New York

CRC Press is an imprint of the
Taylor & Francis Group, an **informa** business

3/29/17
ww
$39.95

CRC Press
Taylor & Francis Group
6000 Broken Sound Parkway NW, Suite 300
Boca Raton, FL 33487-2742

© 2017 by Taylor & Francis Group, LLC
CRC Press is an imprint of Taylor & Francis Group, an Informa business

No claim to original U.S. Government works

Printed on acid-free paper
Version Date: 20160812

International Standard Book Number-13: 978-1-4822-4870-8 (Paperback)

Visit the Taylor & Francis Web site at
http://www.taylorandfrancis.com

and the CRC Press Web site at
http://www.crcpress.com

Printed in Great Britain by Ashford Colour Press Ltd

MIX
Paper from
responsible sources
FSC
www.fsc.org
FSC® C011748

Contents

Contents

Preface

This respiratory textbook aims to provide members of the healthcare team with a range of knowledge to inform the management of patients with respiratory disease. The book is aimed at a variety of healthcare professionals rather than one professional group; this is evidenced by the range of respiratory experts who have contributed to the text. Contributors include nurses, physiotherapists and doctors from across the United Kingdom.

The inspiration for the book originates from caring for patients with respiratory conditions, in addition to designing and delivering university-based educational programmes related to respiratory care. After teaching on these programmes for many years, it was evident that practitioners have a working knowledge of aspects of respiratory care, but that this focus was often narrow. Therefore, we identified that a straightforward, but comprehensive, text on contemporary respiratory care would be a useful addition to student texts.

This book draws on a range of current evidence including national and international guidelines and the expert opinion of authors. Not surprisingly, the book first explains the anatomy and physiology of the respiratory system, as this provides the foundation of knowledge on which to build. It is also imperative that healthcare professionals can perform a detailed respiratory assessment and examination, in addition to recording and communicating the findings; consequently, the first chapter is a key part of the text. A comprehensive review of respiratory investigations is explained over two chapters. These are followed by a range of chapters, each of which focusses on a specific respiratory condition. Each chapter provides a definition and then explains the pathogenesis, treatment, care and prevention of disease. This book differs from others because it also contains chapters on contemporary interventions such as non-invasive ventilation, pulmonary rehabilitation and cognitive behavioural therapy used in the management of respiratory disease. The wider context in which respiratory care is delivered is covered in chapters on thoracic surgery and tracheostomy care. Notably, the book finishes with a chapter on end-of-life care, which has been a neglected area in the provision of respiratory care. Information in the chapters is applied to patient care through the use of case studies. The tenet of this book is to put the patient at the centre of the learning experience.

This book has come to fruition because of the dedication and expertise of the authors who were prepared to devote their time to writing and sharing their considerable expertise. This has resulted in a contemporary, comprehensive and patient-orientated text. We are indebted to the authors and would like to formally thank them.

In addition, we would like to thank CRC Press/Taylor & Francis Group for giving us the opportunity to produce this book. The staff have been supportive, informative and helpful at every twist and turn in its production. In particular, we would like to thank Naomi Wilkinson and Jennifer Blaise for their patience and advice.

Vanessa Gibson and David Waters

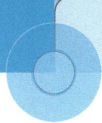

Contributors

Zoe Abel
Specialist Nurse Practitioner
Oxford Adult Cystic Fibrosis Centre
Oxford University Hospitals
    NHS Foundation Trust
Oxford, United Kingdom

Joanne Atkinson
Director of Programs
Department of Public Health and Wellbeing
Northumbria University
Newcastle upon Tyne, United Kingdom

Graham Burns
Consultant Physician
Royal Victoria Infirmary
Newcastle upon Tyne Hospitals
    NHS Foundation Trust
and
Associate Clinical Lecturer
Newcastle University
Newcastle upon Tyne, United Kingdom

Karen Corder
Senior Lecturer
Department of Public Health and Wellbeing
Northumbria University
Newcastle upon Tyne, United Kingdom

Nicola Credland
Lecturer in Critical Care and Advanced Practice
University of Hull
Hull, United Kingdom

Lee Curtis
Senior Lecturer
School of Health and Social Science
Department of Advanced Health Science
Buckinghamshire New University
High Wycombe, United Kingdom

Simon Doe
Consultant Respiratory Physician
Department of Respiratory Medicine
Royal Victoria Infirmary
Newcastle upon Tyne Hospitals
    NHS Foundation Trust
Newcastle upon Tyne, United Kingdom

Barbara Foggo
Practice Placement Facilitator
Newcastle upon Tyne Hospitals
    NHS Foundation Trust
Newcastle upon Tyne, United Kingdom

Vanessa Gibson
Teaching Fellow
Department of Healthcare
Northumbria University
Newcastle upon Tyne, United Kingdom

Cassandra Green
Specialist Nurse Practitioner Oxford Adult Cystic
    Fibrosis Centre
Oxford University Hospitals NHS Foundation
    Trust
Oxford, United Kingdom

Karen Heslop-Marshall
Nurse Consultant/National Institute of Health
    Research
Clinical Academic Research Fellow
Newcastle upon Tyne Hospitals
    NHS Foundation Trust
Newcastle upon Tyne, United Kingdom

Andrew Kerry
Senior Lecturer in Adult Nursing
Oxford Brookes University
Oxford, United Kingdom

Jane Kindred
Respiratory Nurse Specialist
Medway NHS Foundation Trust
Medway, United Kingdom

Gillian Maw
Senior Lecturer
Department of Public Health and Wellbeing
Northumbria University
Newcastle upon Tyne, United Kingdom

Jenny Mitchell
Advanced Nurse Practitioner
Thoracic Surgery
Oxford University Hospitals NHS Trust
Oxford, United Kingdom

Lorraine Mutrie
Lecturer
Department of Public Health and Wellbeing
Northumbria University
Newcastle upon Tyne, United Kingdom

Catherine Plowright
Consultant Nurse Critical Care
Medway NHS Foundation Trust
Medway, United Kingdom

Lisa Priestley
Advanced Nurse Practitioner
Oxford Adult Cystic Fibrosis Centre
Oxford University Hospitals NHS Foundation Trust
Oxford, United Kingdom

Isabel Quinn
Senior Lecturer
Department of Public Health and Wellbeing
Northumbria University
Newcastle upon Tyne, United Kingdom

Chris Stenton
Consultant Respiratory Physician
Department of Respiratory Medicine
Royal Victoria Infirmary
Newcastle upon Tyne Hospitals NHS Foundation
    Trust and Newcastle University
Newcastle upon Tyne, United Kingdom

Catherine Stoermer
Respiratory Specialist Physiotherapist
Pulmonary Rehabilitation
Oxford Health NHS Foundation Trust
Oxford, United Kingdom

Emma Tucker
Respiratory Specialist Physiotherapist
Pulmonary Rehabilitation
Oxford Health NHS Foundation Trust
Oxford, United Kingdom

Gillian Walton
Director of Programmes
Department of Public Health and Wellbeing
Northumbria University
Newcastle upon Tyne, United Kingdom

David Waters
Head of Academic Department
Faculty of Society and Health
Buckinghamshire New University
Uxbridge, United Kingdom

Abbreviations

2,3-DPG	2,3-Diphosphoglycerate
6MWT	6-minute walking test
ABG	Arterial blood gas
ABPA	Allergic bronchopulmonary aspergillosis
ACBT	Active cycle of breathing techniques
ACE	Angiotensin-converting enzyme
ACOS	Asthma COPD overlap syndrome
AD	Autogenic drainage
ADRT	Advance decision to refuse treatment
ALK	Anaplastic lymphoma kinase
AOT	Ambulatory oxygen therapy
AP	Anterior-posterior
ATP	Adenosine triphosphate
AVPU	Alert, voice, pain, unresponsive
BAL	Bronchoalveolar lavage
BCG	Bacillus Calmette–Guerin
BE	Base excess
BiPAP	Biphasic positive airway pressure
BP	Blood pressure
bpm	Beats per minute or breaths per minute
BTS	British Thoracic Society
BTS/SIGN	British Thoracic Society/Scottish Intercollegiate Guidelines Network
CA	Carbonic anhydrase
CaO_2	Arterial oxygen content
CAP	Community acquired pneumonia
CAVD	Congenital absence of the vas deferens
CBT	Cognitive behavioural therapy
CCOT	Critical care outreach team
CCQ	Clinical COPD Questionnaire
CF	Cystic fibrosis
CFRD	Cystic fibrosis related diabetes
CFTR	Cystic fibrosis transmembrane conductance regulator
cmH_2O	Centimetre of water

CNS	Clinical nurse specialist
CO_2	Carbon dioxide
COPD	Chronic obstructive pulmonary disease
COSHH	Control of substances hazardous to health
CPAP	Continuous positive airway pressure
CPET	Cardiopulmonary exercise testing
CQUIN	Commissioning for Quality and Innovation
CRB65	Confusion, raised respiratory rate, low blood pressure, age 65
CRQ	Chronic Respiratory Questionnaire
CRUK	Cancer Research United Kingdom
CSF	Cerebrospinal fluid
CT	Computed tomography
CTPA	Computed tomography pulmonary angiography
CURB65	Confusion, urea, raised respiratory rate, low blood pressure, age 65
CXR	Chest X-ray
DALY	Disability adjusted life year
DIB	Difficulty in breathing
DIOS	Distal intestinal obstructive syndrome
DNA	Deoxyribonucleic acid
DNAR	Do not attempt resuscitation
DO_2	Oxygen delivery
DOT	Directly observed therapy
DVT	Deep vein thrombosis
EBUS TBNA	Endobronchial ultrasound guided transbronchial needle aspiration
ECG	Electrocardiograph
ECMO	Extra-corporeal membrane oxygenation
ECOG	Eastern Cooperative Oncology Group
ED	Emergency department
EGFR	Epidermal growth factor receptor
EPAP	Expiratory positive airway pressure

EQ5	European Quality of Life Health Questionnaire	LABA	Long-acting β$_2$-agonists
ERV	Expiratory reserve volume	LAMA	Long-acting muscarinic antagonist
ESR	Erythrocyte sedimentation rate	LCNS	Lung cancer nurse specialist
ESWT	Endurance shuttle walk test	LTOT	Long-term oxygen therapy
EU	European Union	M. afracanum	Mycobacterium afracanum
FEF	Forced expiratory flow	M. bovis	Mycobacterium bovis
FEV$_1$	Forced expiratory volume in 1 second	mcg	Micrograms
		MCID	Minimal clinically important difference
FiO$_2$	Fraction of inspired oxygen	MDI	Metred-dose inhaler
FRC	Functional residual capacity	MDR-TB	Multi-drug-resistant tuberculosis
GCS	Glasgow Coma Score	MDT	Multidisciplinary team
GINA	Global Initiative for Asthma	mmHg	Millimetres of mercury
H$^+$	Hydrogen	mmol	milimole
HADS	Hospital anxiety and depression scale	MRC	Medical Research Council
		MRSA	Methicillin-resistant Staphylococcus aureus
HAP	Hospital-acquired pneumonia		
Hb	Haemoglobin	M. tuberculosis	Mycobacterium tuberculosis
Hb-CO$_2$	Carbaminohaemoglobin	N$_2$	Nitrogen
HCO$_3$	Bicarbonate	NCAT	National Cancer Action Team
HIV	Human immunodeficiency virus	NCIN	National Cancer Intelligence Network
H$_2$CO$_3$	Carbonic acid		
H$_2$O	Water	NEWS	National Early Warning Score
HME	Heat moisture exchanger	NHS	National Health Service
HMSO	Her Majesty's Stationary Office	NHSIC	National Health Service Information Centre
HPV	Hypoxic pulmonary vasoconstriction		
		NICE	National Institute for Health and Care Excellence
HR	Heart rate	NIV	Non-invasive ventilation
HRCT	High resolution computed tomography	NRT	Nicotine replacement therapy
		NSAID	Non-steroidal anti-inflammatory drug
HRQoL	Health related quality of life		
IASLC	International Association for the Study of Lung Cancer	NSCCG	Non-small cell cancer group
		NSCLC	Non-small cell lung cancer
ICS	Inhaled corticosteroids	O$_2$	Oxygen
IgE	Immunoglobulin E	OER	Oxygen extraction ratio
IGRA	Interferon gamma release assay	PA	Posterior-anterior
ILD	Interstitial lung disease	PAAP	Personalised asthma action plan
IPAP	Inspiratory positive airway pressure	PaCO$_2$	Partial pressure of carbon dioxide
IRV	Inspiratory reserve volume	PaO$_2$	Partial pressure of oxygen
ISWT	Incremental shuttle walk test	PCA	Patient controlled analgesia
JFC	Joint Formulary Committee	PCI	Prophylactic cranial irradiation
KCO	Transfer coefficient	PCR	Polymer chain reactions
kPa	Kilopascal	PCRS-UK	Primary Care Respiratory Society – United Kingdom
KRAS	Kirsten rat sarcoma viral oncogene homolog		
		PE	Pulmonary emboli
LA	Locally advanced	PEEP	Positive end expiratory pressure

PEF	Peak expiratory flow
PEFR	Peak expiratory flow rate
PEMax	Maximal expiratory mouth pressure
PEP	Positive expiratory pressure
PERT	Pancreatic enzyme replacement therapy
PET	Positron emission tomography
pH	A numeric scale used to specify the acidity or basicity of an aqueous solution
PHE	Public Health England
PIMax	Maximal inspiratory mouth pressure
PR	Pulmonary rehabilitation
PS	Performance status
PSI	Pneumonia severity index
PSP	Primary spontaneous pneumothorax
PsrP	Pneumococcal serine-rich repeat protein
QOF	Quality outcomes framework
RAST	Radioallergosorbent test
RCLCF	Roy Castle Lung Cancer Foundation
RCP	Royal College of Physicians
RR	Respiration rate
RV	Residual volume
SABA	Short-acting βeta_2-agonist
SaO$_2$	Arterial oxygen saturation (via an ABG)
SBRT	Stereotactic body radiotherapy
SCLC	Small cell lung cancer

SF36	Medical Outcomes Study Short Form 36
SNIP	Sniff nasal inspiratory pressure
SOB	Short of breath
S. pneumoniae	*Streptococcus pneumoniae*
SpO$_2$	Peripheral oxygen saturation (via pulse oximetry)
SPT	Skin prick test
SSP	Secondary spontaneous pneumothorax
TB	Tuberculosis
TBNA	Transbronchial nodal aspiration
TKI	Tyrosine kinase inhibitor
TLC	Total lung capacity
T$_{LCO}$	Transfer factor for carbon monoxide
TNF	Tumour necrosis factor
TNM	Tumour, node, metastases
UK	United Kingdom
US	United States
V$_A$	Alveolar minute ventilation
VAP	Ventilation acquired pneumonia
VATS	Video-assisted thoracoscopic surgery
VC	Vital capacity
V$_D$	Anatomical dead space
V$_E$	Minute volume
VO$_2$	Oxygen consumption
V/Q	Ventilation/perfusion
V$_T$	Tidal volume
WHO	World Health Organisation
XDR-TB	Extensively drug-resistant tuberculosis

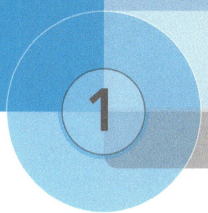

Respiratory anatomy and physiology

LEARNING OBJECTIVES

Upon completion of this chapter the reader should be able to:

- Describe the anatomical structure of the upper and lower respiratory tract
- Discuss the principles of internal and external respiration
- Explain how the body is able to control the rate and depth of breathing
- Describe oxygen and carbon dioxide transportation and diffusion

INTRODUCTION

Human cells require oxygen to survive. Oxygen concentration in the air is approximately 21% (Woodrow, 2012). As cells use the oxygen for cellular metabolism, carbon dioxide is produced as a waste product. Carbon dioxide is a respiratory acid and, if allowed to build up within the blood, will negatively affect cellular activity and disrupt haemostasis. The primary function of the respiratory system is therefore to ensure that the body extracts sufficient oxygen from inspired air and excretes the excess carbon dioxide. As oxygen is transported around the body bound to haemoglobin dissolved in plasma, effective respiration is also reliant on a fully functioning cardiovascular system.

This chapter aims to give an overview of the anatomy and physiology of the respiratory system. This will include pulmonary ventilation, external respiration, transport of gases and internal respiration. Detailed explanations of anatomy and physiology related to specific respiratory conditions will be explored further in their related chapters.

ORGANISATION

The respiratory system is divided into the upper and lower respiratory tracts. The structures found below the larynx form the lower respiratory tract. The upper respiratory tract and the uppermost portion of the lower tract are known as the conduction region where air is conducted through a series of tubes and vessels. The respiratory region (the lower respiratory tract) is the functional part of the lungs where exchange of oxygen and carbon dioxide takes place (gaseous exchange). Both the upper and lower tracts are equipped to fight off airborne bacterial or viral pathogens. These structures are microscopic, fragile and easily damaged by infection (Nair and Peate, 2013). See Chapter 10 for further details.

THE UPPER RESPIRATORY TRACT

Air enters the body via nasal and oral cavities. The nasal cavity is divided vertically into two equal sections by the nasal septum. This septum is formed from the ethmoid bones and the vomer of the skull. The space where air enters the nasal cavity is called the vestibule. Beyond each vestibule, the nasal cavities are divided into three air passages: the meatuses. These are formed by three shelf-like projections called the superior, middle and inferior nasal concha. Olfactory receptors are responsible for our sense of smell. These are contained within the superior conchae and upper septum (Clancy and McVicar, 2009). See Figure 1.1 for the structures of the upper and lower respiratory tract.

The pharynx connects the nasal and oral cavity with the larynx. The pharynx is divided into three regions known as the nasopharynx, oropharynx and laryngopharynx. The nasopharynx contains two openings that lead to the auditory (Eustachian) tubes and sits behind the nasal cavity. The oropharynx and laryngopharynx sit beneath the nasopharynx and behind the oral cavity. The oral cavity and the oropharynx are divided by the fauces (Marieb, 2012). As the oropharynx and laryngopharynx are passages for food and drink as well as air they are lined with non-keratinised stratified squamous epithelium to protect against abrasion from food particles.

The upper respiratory tract ensures that air entering the lower tract is warm, humidified and clean. The vestibule is lined with coarse hairs (cilia) that filter air and prevent large dust particles from entering the airways. The conchae are lined with a mucous membrane made from pseudostratified ciliated columnar epithelium that contains mucus-secreting goblet cells (Jenkins et al., 2010). The blood flowing through the capillaries warms the passing air, while the mucus moistens it and traps any dust particles. The mucus-covered dust particles are then propelled by the cilia towards the pharynx where they can be swallowed or expectorated. This process is sometimes referred to as the mucociliary escalator.

The upper respiratory tract is also lined with irritant receptors. When stimulated by invading particles such as dust or pollen, they force a sneeze ensuring the particles are ejected through the nose or mouth. The pharynx also contains five tonsils.

The two that are visible when the mouth is open are the palatine tonsils. Behind the tongue lie the lingual tonsils and the pharyngeal tonsil or adenoid sits on the upper back wall of the pharynx. Tonsils are lymph nodes and part of the body's defence system. Their surface epithelial lining has deep folds (crypts). These entangle invading bacteria or particles, which are then engulfed and destroyed by white blood cells (Nair and Peate, 2013).

THE LOWER RESPIRATORY TRACT

The lower respiratory tract includes the larynx, the trachea, the right and left bronchi and all the constituents of both lungs. The lungs are two cone-shaped organs that are protected by a framework of bones, the thoracic cage (the ribs, sternum and vertebrae). The tip of each lung, the apex, extends just above the clavicle and their bases sit anteriorly at the sixth intercostal space just above a concave muscle called the diaphragm (Marieb, 2012). The larynx connects the trachea and the laryngopharynx. The remainder of the lower respiratory tract divides into branches of airways and is often referred to as the bronchial tree.

LARYNX

The larynx lies in the midline of the neck anterior to the oesophagus and the fourth to sixth cervical vertebrae (C4–C6) (Tortora and Derrickson, 2013). It is made up of cartilaginous walls held in place with ligaments and skeletal muscle. There are three single pieces and three pairs of cartilage tissue. The single pieces of cartilage are the thyroid cartilage, the epiglottis and the cricoid cartilage. The thyroid and cricoid cartilages protect the vocal cords. The cricothyroid ligament, which connects the cricoid and thyroid cartilage, is the landmark for an emergency airway or tracheostomy insertion (see Chapter 15). It is connected superiorly to the cricoid cartilage and inferiorly to the first ring of the trachea (Tortora and Derrickson, 2013). The epiglottis is a piece of elastic cartilage attached to the top of the larynx that protects the airway from food and water. On swallowing, the epiglottis blocks the entry to the larynx, diverting food and fluids to the oesophagus. Inhalation of solids or liquids can block the lower respiratory tract and cut off the body's oxygen supply.

(a)

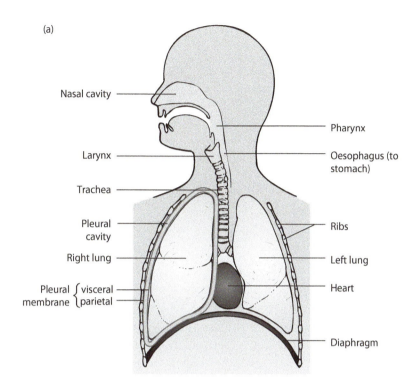

(b)

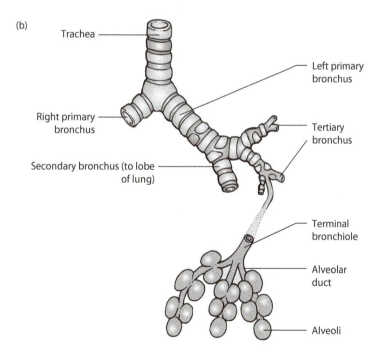

Figure 1.1 Structures of the upper and lower respiratory tract. (a) Organs of respiration and (b) the bronchial tree. (From Clancy, J. and McVicar, A. 2009. *Physiology and Anatomy for Nurses and Healthcare Practitioners: A Homeostatic Approach* [3rd ed.]. CRC Press, London. Figure 14.2. With permission.) *(Continued)*

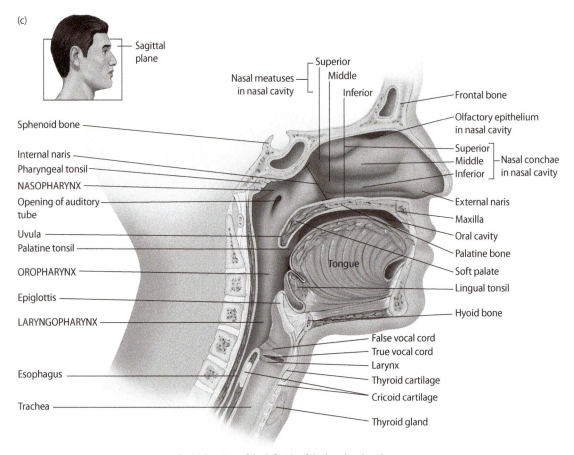

(c)

Sagittal plane

Nasal meatuses in nasal cavity — Superior / Middle / Inferior

Frontal bone

Olfactory epithelium in nasal cavity

Sphenoid bone

Superior / Middle / Inferior — Nasal conchae in nasal cavity

Internal naris

Pharyngeal tonsil

NASOPHARYNX

Opening of auditory tube

External naris

Maxilla

Uvula

Palatine tonsil

Oral cavity

Palatine bone

OROPHARYNX

Tongue

Soft palate

Lingual tonsil

Epiglottis

LARYNGOPHARYNX

Hyoid bone

False vocal cord

True vocal cord

Esophagus

Larynx

Thyroid cartilage

Trachea

Cricoid cartilage

Thyroid gland

Sagittal section of the left side of the head and neck

Figure 1.1 (Continued) Structures of the upper and lower respiratory tract. (c) Respiratory organs in the head and neck. (From Clancy, J. and McVicar, A. 2009. *Physiology and Anatomy for Nurses and Healthcare Practitioners: A Homeostatic Approach* (3rd ed.). CRC Press, London. Figure 14.2. With permission.)

The three pairs of cartilage associated with the larynx are the arytenoids, cuneiform and corniculate. The arytenoid cartilages are a pair of triangular pieces of hyaline cartilage that are located at the posterior, superior border of the cricoid cartilage (Nair and Peate, 2013). They form a synovial joint and are the most important as they influence the movement of the mucous membranes (true vocal cords) that generate voice. Speaking is reliant on a fully functioning respiratory system.

TRACHEA

The trachea is a tubular vessel approximately 12 cm long and 2.5 cm wide. It is located anterior to the oesophagus and extends from the larynx to the superior border of the fifth thoracic vertebra (T5), where it divides into the two main bronchi (Tortora and Derrickson, 2013). The trachea carries air from the larynx to the lungs and is lined with pseudostratified ciliated columnar epithelium to trap and propel debris towards the oesophagus and pharynx. The trachea and bronchi contain irritant receptors that stimulate a cough to force larger invading particles upwards. The outermost layer of the trachea contains connective tissue that is reinforced with C-shaped hyaline cartilage rings that strengthen the front and sides of the airway and prevent the trachea from collapsing during expiration. There is a lack of cartilage rings on the posterior surface of the trachea where it makes contact with the oesophagus. When a bolus of food is swallowed the oesophagus is able to expand without hindrance while the patency of the airway is maintained.

BRONCHIAL TREE

The lungs are divided into distinct regions called lobes, three lobes in the right lung and two in the left. The heart and associated major vessels sit in the cardiac notch, the space between the two lungs. Each lung is protected by two thin membranes called the parietal and visceral pleura. The parietal pleura lines the walls of the thorax and the visceral pleura adheres to the outer surface of the lungs. The vacuum between the two pleura contains a thin film of lubricating fluid. This reduces friction and allows the two layers to slide over each other during breathing (Nair and Peate, 2013).

The trachea divides into two main bronchi. These primary bronchi then divide into the secondary bronchi, three on the right and two on the left. The secondary bronchi then divide into tertiary bronchi of which there are 10 in each lung. Tertiary bronchi continue to divide into respiratory bronchioles, which eventually lead to a terminal bronchiole. The terminal bronchiole supplies a specific section of the lung, a lobule, which has its own arterial blood supply and lymph vessels. The bronchial tree continues to divide, leading to a series of bronchioles, which in turn generate alveolar ducts. The airways terminate with alveoli clustered together to form alveolar sacs. Human lungs contain an average of 480 million alveoli. The exchange of oxygen and carbon dioxide only occurs from the respiratory bronchiole onwards (Nair and Peate, 2013) (see Figure 1.2).

Deoxygenated blood is delivered to the lobules via capillaries that originate from the right and left pulmonary arteries. Once oxygenated, blood is sent back to the left side of the heart via one of the four pulmonary veins to enter the systemic circulation.

RESPIRATION

Respiration, the process where oxygen and carbon dioxide are exchanged between the atmosphere and the body cells, follows four distinct phases.

- *Pulmonary ventilation*: How air passes in and out of the lungs owing to a change in pressure.
- *External respiration*: How oxygen diffuses from the lungs to the bloodstream and how carbon dioxide diffuses from the bloodstream to the lungs.
- *Transport of gases*: How respiratory gases are moved from the lungs to the body tissues and from the tissues back to the lungs.
- *Internal respiration*: How oxygen is delivered to and carbon dioxide removed from body cells (Nair and Peate, 2013).

In order to understand these processes, it is important to appreciate a series of gas laws (Table 1.1).

PULMONARY VENTILATION

Pulmonary ventilation describes the mechanics of breathing. In order for air to pass in and out of the lungs, changes in pressure need to occur. The pressure within the lungs and the atmospheric pressure is the same prior to inspiration. During inspiration the thorax expands and intrapulmonary pressure falls below atmospheric pressure, allowing air to passively enter the lungs (Boyle's law and Dalton's law). A range of respiratory muscles are used to achieve thoracic expansion on inspiration (see Figure 1.3), the most important of which are the diaphragm and the external intercostal muscles.

The diaphragm is a dome-shaped skeletal muscle beneath the lungs at the base of the thorax. There are 11 pairs of external intercostal muscles which sit in the intercostal spaces. During inspiration, the diaphragm contracts downwards and the external intercostal muscles pull the ribcage outwards and upwards. This increases the size of the thoracic cavity and intrathoracic pressure is reduced to below atmospheric pressure as a result (see Figure 1.4). Expiration is a more passive process. The external intercostal muscles and diaphragm relax, allowing the natural elastic recoil of the lung tissue to spring back into shape and air is forced out (Marieb, 2012).

The abdominal wall muscles and internal intercostal muscles can also be used to increase the volume of air expelled on expiration (e.g. when playing a musical instrument). The sternocleidomastoids, the scalene and the pectoralis can also be used

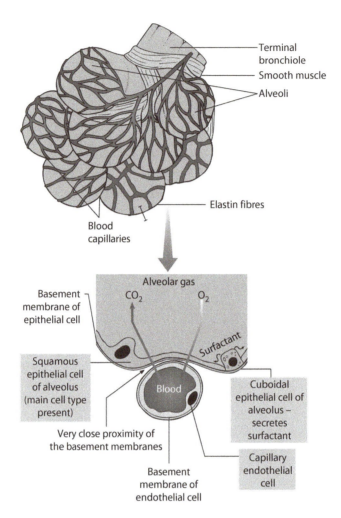

Figure 1.2 Internal and external respiration. (From Clancy, J. and McVicar, A. 2009. *Physiology and Anatomy for Nurses and Healthcare Practitioners: A Homeostatic Approach* (3rd ed.). CRC Press, London. Figure 14.4. With permission.)

to increase the volume of breath on inhalation. They are known as the accessory muscles as they are rarely used during normal, quiet breathing (Jenkins et al., 2010).

WORK OF BREATHING

The natural elastic recoil of lung tissue, the resistance to airflow through narrow airways and the surface tension forces at the liquid/air interface in the lobule all hinder thoracic expansion. The energy required to overcome these forces is known as the work of breathing. The amount of energy required is kept to a minimum by the lung compliance

(amount of stretch). Lung compliance is aided by a substance called surfactant, made in the alveoli by Type II alveolar cells (Tortora and Derrickson, 2013). Surfactant reduces the surface tension that occurs where the alveoli meet capillary blood flow in the lobule, thus reducing the amount of energy needed to inflate the alveoli. Work of breathing is also needed to overcome airway resistance. Resistance to airflow occurs as the gas molecules collide with each other within the increasingly narrow airways. Many lung diseases can affect lung compliance, airway resistance and increase work of breathing (e.g. asthma, chronic obstructive pulmonary disease [COPD]).

Table 1.1 Summary of gas laws

Gas law	Summary	Clinical application
Boyle's law	The pressure exerted by gas is inversely proportional to its volume – the higher the pressure, the lower the volume/the higher the volume, the lower the pressure	As the thorax expands, intrathoracic pressure falls below atmospheric pressure
Dalton's law	In a mixture of gases each will exert its own pressure as if no other gases are present	Differences in partial pressure control the movement of oxygen and carbon dioxide between the atmosphere, the lungs and the blood
Henry's law	The quantity of gas that will dissolve in a liquid is proportional to its pressure and its solubility	Oxygen and carbon dioxide are water soluble and carried in blood. Nitrogen is highly insoluble and, despite accounting for 79% of the atmosphere, very little is dissolved in blood
Fick's law	The rate a gas will diffuse across a membrane will depend upon pressure difference, surface area, diffusion distance and molecular weight and solubility	Exercise, respiratory diseases and altitude all influence the amount of oxygen that is diffused into the blood

Source: Information taken from Davies, A. and Moore, C. 2010. The Respiratory System (2nd ed.): *Basic Science and Clinical Conditions*. Churchill Livingstone, Edinburgh.

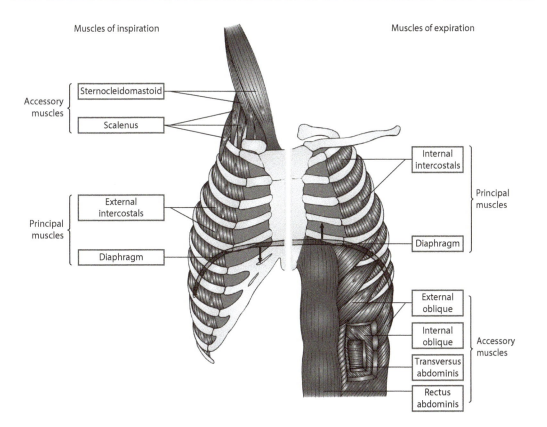

Figure 1.3 Muscles of inspiration and expiration. (From Clancy, J. and McVicar, A. 2009. *Physiology and Anatomy for Nurses and Healthcare Practitioners: A Homeostatic Approach* (3rd ed.). CRC Press, London. Figure 14.5. With permission.)

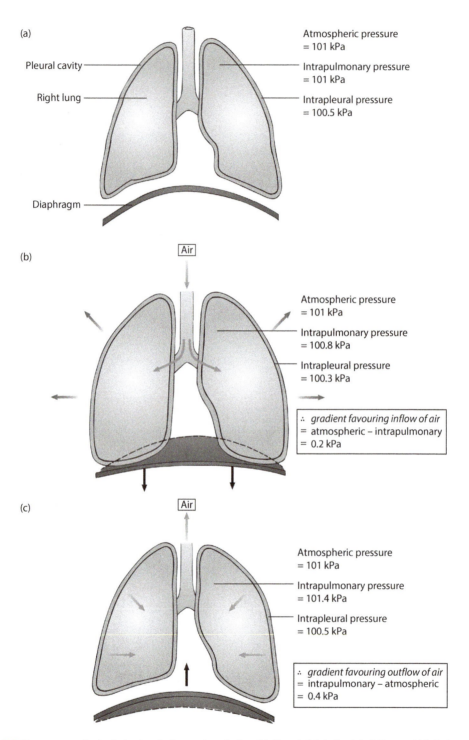

(a)

Atmospheric pressure
= 101 kPa

Pleural cavity

Intrapulmonary pressure
= 101 kPa

Right lung

Intrapleural pressure
= 100.5 kPa

Diaphragm

(b)

Air

Atmospheric pressure
= 101 kPa

Intrapulmonary pressure
= 100.8 kPa

Intrapleural pressure
= 100.3 kPa

∴ gradient favouring inflow of air
= atmospheric − intrapulmonary
= 0.2 kPa

(c)

Air

Atmospheric pressure
= 101 kPa

Intrapulmonary pressure
= 101.4 kPa

Intrapleural pressure
= 100.5 kPa

∴ gradient favouring outflow of air
= intrapulmonary − atmospheric
= 0.4 kPa

Figure 1.4 Pressure gradients during inspiration and expiration. (a) At rest, (b) during inhalation and (c) during exhalation. (From Clancy, J. and McVicar, A. 2009. *Physiology and Anatomy for Nurses and Healthcare Practitioners: A Homeostatic Approach* (3rd ed.). CRC Press, London. Figure 14.3. With permission.)

CONTROL OF RESPIRATION

Respiration is controlled by the respiratory centre in the brainstem, namely the medulla oblongata and pons (Nair and Peate, 2013). The rate of breathing is set by the medulla oblongata where there are specialised chemoreceptors that analyse carbon dioxide (CO_2) levels within cerebrospinal fluid (CSF). A rise in CO_2 instigates a message via the phrenic and intercostal nerves to the diaphragm and intercostal muscles, telling them to contract. Chemoreceptors found in the aorta and carotid arteries analyse levels of oxygen (O_2) as well as CO_2. If O_2 falls or CO_2 levels rise, messages are sent to the respiratory centres via the vagus and glossopharyngeal nerves to stimulate further contraction. The refinement of breathing occurs in the pneumotaxic and apneustic centres of the pons. The apneustic centre stimulates the inspiratory centre to lengthen inspiration, while the pneumotaxic centre sends inhibitory signals to the medulla to slow the breathing down. These actions prevent over-inflation of the lungs (Nair and Peate, 2013).

In health, a normal respiratory rate in an adult is between 12 and 20 respirations per minute. The rate and depth of breathing can be consciously controlled, although it remains largely a subconscious activity.

The inspiratory area of the respiratory centres can be stimulated by both the limbic system and the hypothalamus (Nair and Peate, 2013). These areas are both responsible for processing emotion. Therefore, pain, anxiety and stress can all cause an involuntary increase in the rate and depth of breathing. Pain and pyrexia can also affect breathing. As breathing is largely a subconscious activity, changes in respiration rate are clinically significant and are one of the first signs of a deteriorating patient (Royal College of Physicians [RCP], 2012).

LUNG VOLUMES AND CAPACITIES

Lung volumes and capacities measure the amount of air entering and leaving the lungs (see Figure 1.5). Total lung capacity (TLC) (the total amount of air the lungs can hold) is dependent on age, sex and height. TLC is then subdivided into actual and potential volumes of air:

- Tidal volume (V_T) – the amount of air that passes in and out of the lungs in one breath
- Inspiratory reserve volume (IRV) – the potential for a deeper inhalation
- Expiratory reserve volume (ERV) – the potential for a larger exhalation

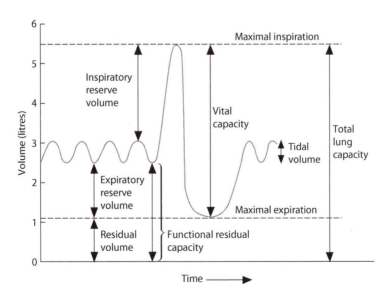

Figure 1.5 Lung volumes and capacities. (From Clancy, J. and McVicar, A. 2009. *Physiology and Anatomy for Nurses and Healthcare Practitioners: A Homeostatic Approach* (3rd ed.). CRC Press, London. Figure 14.7. With permission.)

- Residual volume (RV) – the amount of air left in the lungs after the deepest possible expiration
- Vital capacity – the largest volume of air that could possibly pass in and out of the lungs calculated by $V_T + IRV + ERV$
- Minute volume (V_E) – the amount of air inhaled in one minute and calculated by $V_T \times$ respiratory rate (in health approximately 6–8 litres per minute)
- Anatomical dead space (V_D) – the total volume of the conducting airways from the nose or mouth to the level of the terminal bronchioles
- Alveolar minute ventilation (V_A) – the amount of air available for gaseous exchange. It is calculated by subtracting anatomical dead space from minute volume × respiratory rate, which is approximately 4–6 litres per minute in health (Nair and Peate, 2013)

EXTERNAL RESPIRATION

External respiration is the diffusion of oxygen from the alveoli into the pulmonary circulation and the diffusion of carbon dioxide from the pulmonary circulation into the alveoli. Gas molecules always move from areas of high concentration to areas of low concentration (Marieb, 2012). For example, the blood within the pulmonary artery is low in oxygen, as this has already been delivered to the tissues, but high in carbon dioxide. The amount, and thus pressure, of oxygen in the alveoli is therefore greater than the arterial blood supply. Oxygen moves passively out of the alveoli and into the pulmonary circulation, which flows towards the left side of the heart. As there is more carbon dioxide within the pulmonary circulation than in the alveoli, carbon dioxide diffuses into the alveoli ready for exhalation.

There are various factors that influence the rate of gaseous exchange between the alveoli and the pulmonary circulation. These are best explained using Fick's law of diffusion (Table 1.2).

According to Fick's law, diffusion is determined by gas solubility and molecular weight, surface area, concentration difference and membrane thickness (Nair and Peate, 2013). The more water soluble a gas, the easier it is for diffusion to take place. Both O_2 and CO_2 are highly water soluble and therefore easily

Table 1.2 Fick's law of diffusion

$J = (S/wt_{mol}) \times A \times \Delta C/t$
J = rate of diffusion
S/Wt_{mol} = solubility/molecular weight
A = surface area
ΔC = concentration difference
T = membrane thickness

diffused. The most abundant gas in the atmosphere is nitrogen (N_2), which is insoluble in water. Very little nitrogen therefore diffuses into the bloodstream. The larger the surface area available for diffusion, the greater the rate of diffusion will be. Large inhalations will recruit more alveoli, thereby increasing the surface area available for the exchange of gases. The gas will diffuse faster when there is a greater gas concentration difference between the alveoli and the pulmonary circulation. As the blood travelling towards the alveoli is deoxygenated (has a low concentration of oxygen) there will always be a large concentration difference in oxygen between the alveoli and the pulmonary circulation (Marieb, 2012). The rate of diffusion can be improved if this concentration difference is increased, for example with the use of supplementary oxygen therapy. Finally, membrane thickness can affect the rate of diffusion: the further gases have to travel the slower diffusion will occur. Conditions such as pulmonary oedema result in an increased distance between the alveoli and the pulmonary circulation and therefore diffusion will be delayed.

VENTILATION AND PERFUSION

External respiration is at its most effective when there is an adequate supply of both oxygen and blood. The alveoli need to be adequately ventilated to ensure a good supply of oxygen. In health an alveolar minute ventilation (V_A) of around 4 litres is needed (Tortora and Derrickson, 2013). There also needs to be adequate pulmonary blood flow (around 5 litres per minute) to allow gaseous exchange to occur. This ideal delivery of both blood and air is known as the ventilation V_A:Perfusion Q ratio. A normal V_A:Q ratio would be 4:5. Disruption to the pulmonary blood flow or ventilation is known as a V_A:Q mismatch, resulting in reduced gaseous exchange (Nair and Peate, 2013). For example, a pulmonary embolism reduces pulmonary blood flow, and therefore less blood is available for the oxygen to diffuse into. The result would be a high V_A:Q ratio (4:3).

TRANSPORT OF OXYGEN

Haemoglobin is a substance in red blood cells consisting of the protein globin and the iron-rich red pigment haem (Jenkins et al., 2010). Approximately 98.5% of all oxygen is attached to the haemoglobin within the erythrocyte (red blood cell) for transportation. Every erythrocyte contains approximately 280 million haemoglobin (Hb) with each one able to carry oxygen molecules. Each haemoglobin can bind a maximum of four oxygen molecules (Tortora and Derrickson, 2013). The percentage of haemoglobin carrying oxygen is measured as an oxygen saturation (SaO_2). The remaining 1.5% of oxygen is dissolved in blood plasma and is measured in kilopascals (PaO_2). In health the normal reference range is 11.5–13.0 kPa (Simpson, 2004). The delivery of oxygen relies on an adequate haemoglobin and erythrocyte supply. In health the average male will have 15–18 g of haemoglobin in every 100 mL of blood. Each gram of haemoglobin has the capacity to carry approximately 1.39 mL of oxygen (Nair and Peate, 2013). This is known as the oxygen capacity. Therefore, a healthy male with a haemoglobin of 15 g/dL will have the capacity to carry 20.85 mL of oxygen in every 100 mL of blood (15 × 1.39 = 20.85). It is rare for an individual's haemoglobin to be completely saturated with oxygen. The actual amount of oxygen carried by the haemoglobin in arterial blood is called the arterial oxygen content (CaO_2). This is determined by the oxygen saturation levels, which in health are between 97% and 99%. Therefore, a healthy male with an Hb of 15 g/dL and a SaO_2 of 97% would have an oxygen content of 20.2 mL (0.97 × 20.85). Multiplying the oxygen content by cardiac output will provide the amount of oxygen being delivered to the body tissues in a minute. The volume of oxygen is called oxygen delivery (DO_2). So if cardiac output is 5000 mL per minute and the oxygen content is 20.2 mL the patient would have an oxygen delivery of 101,000 mL per minute (20.2 × 5000). A lack of oxygen within body tissues is known as hypoxia (Peate and Nair, 2011). A lack of oxygen within arterial blood is called hypoxaemia. Although hypoxaemia will lead to hypoxia within the tissues, a reduced

Table 1.3 Types and causes of hypoxia

Type of hypoxia	Cause
Circulatory	Heart failure
Histotoxic	Poisoning, e.g. carbon monoxide
Demand	When demand for oxygen is high, e.g. pyrexia
Hypoxic hypoxia	Hypoxia as a result of hypoxaemia
Haemic	Reduced circulatory volume, e.g. haemorrhage

cardiovascular function can also create a hypoxia even when the arterial blood is fully saturated with oxygen. The release of oxygen from haemoglobin can be increased by 2,3-Diphosphoglycerate (2,3-DPG). This is a substance made in red blood cells which is released during hypoxia and elevated temperatures (Tortora and Derrickson, 2013). Five major types of hypoxia and their causes can be seen in Table 1.3.

TRANSPORT OF CARBON DIOXIDE

Carbon dioxide is produced following cellular metabolism and diffuses into the blood. It is transported in the blood in three main ways (Tortora and Derrickson, 2013).

1. Around 10% of carbon dioxide is carried within plasma. When it reaches the lungs it is diffused into alveolar air and exhaled.
2. Around 20% is transported attached (bound) to haemoglobin, which has a greater affinity for carbon dioxide than oxygen. This aids the release of oxygen as carbon dioxide is being created in the tissues. As carbon dioxide levels increase (hypercapnia) the amount of oxygen binding to the haemoglobin will be reduced. Therefore, any build-up of carbon dioxide will affect the oxyhaemoglobin dissociation curve, resulting in a greater risk of hypoxaemia. The main binding sites are the proteins in the globin portion of the haemoglobin molecule. Haemoglobin that has carbon dioxide attached (bound) to it is called carbaminohaemoglobin (Hb-CO_2).
3. The remainder (~70%) is transported in blood plasma as bicarbonate ions (HCO_3^-). As carbon dioxide enters the red cells it reacts with

water in the presence of the enzyme carbonic anhydrase (CA) and forms carbonic acid. This dissociates into H^+ and HCO_3^-.

OXYGEN–HAEMOGLOBIN DISSOCIATION

The relationship between oxyhaemoglobin (SaO_2) and oxygen dissolved in plasma (PaO_2) is described by the oxyhaemoglobin dissociation curve (see Figure 1.6). As PaO_2 falls, SaO_2 decreases in a characteristic sigmoidal (S)-shaped curve. The curve is sensitive to conditions within the peripheral tissues that increase metabolic activity – acidity, increased carbon dioxide levels, temperature (Nair and Peate, 2013).

ACIDITY

The affinity of haemoglobin for oxygen decreases as acidity increases. Oxygen therefore dissociates more readily from haemoglobin. During exercise tissues are metabolically active and release lactic acid and carbonic acid. This increases acidity and promotes

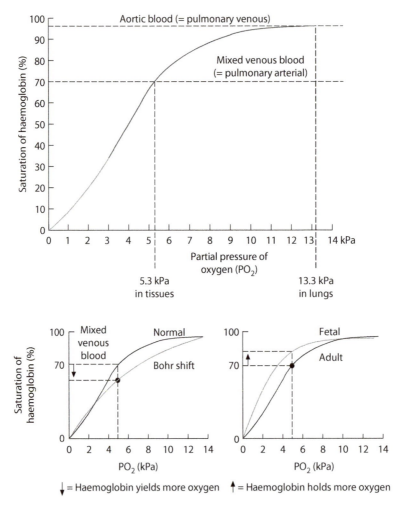

Figure 1.6 Oxygen carriage by haemoglobin. (From Clancy, J. and McVicar, A. 2009. *Physiology and Anatomy for Nurses and Healthcare Practitioners: A Homeostatic Approach* (3rd ed.). CRC Press, London. Figure 14.11. With permission.)

the release of oxygen from haemoglobin (Tortora and Derrickson, 2013).

PARTIAL PRESSURE OF CARBON DIOXIDE

As the partial pressure of carbon dioxide (P_{co2}) rises, haemoglobin releases oxygen more readily. P_{CO2} and pH are related. Low blood pH (acidity) results from high P_{CO2}. As carbon dioxide enters the blood it is temporarily converted into carbonic acid (H_2CO_3) by an enzyme in red blood cells called carbonic anhydrase. The transport of carbon dioxide as bicarbonate is summarised by the following equation. The arrow symbols indicate that the equation moves both ways. At tissue level the equation moves from left to right, whereas within the lungs it moves from right to left (Tortora and Derrickson, 2013).

$$\underset{\text{Carbon dioxide}}{CO_2} + \underset{\text{Water}}{H_2O} \rightleftharpoons \underset{\text{Carbonic acid}}{H_2CO_3} \rightleftharpoons \underset{\text{Hydrogen ion}}{H^+} + \underset{\text{Bicarbonate ion}}{HCO_3^-}$$

The carbonic acid disassociates into hydrogen ions (H^+) and bicarbonate ions $\left(HCO_3^-\right)$. As the H^+ concentration increases, the pH decreases. Therefore, an increased PCO$_2$ produces a more acidic environment, which helps to release oxygen from haemoglobin. During exercise, lactic acid (a waste product of anaerobic metabolism within muscles) also decreases the blood pH. The haemoglobin therefore releases more oxygen as the blood flows through the active tissues that are producing more carbon dioxide, such as exercising muscle tissue. CO_2 is removed from tissue cells and transported in blood plasma as HCO_3^-. As blood flows through the pulmonary capillaries in the lungs, CO_2 is exhaled (Nair and Peate, 2013).

TEMPERATURE

As the temperature increases, the amount of oxygen released from haemoglobin increases. Active tissues produce heat, which increases temperature and encourages oxygen dissociation. A similar effect will be seen in pyrexia. Conversely, in hypothermia cellular metabolism slows and the need for oxygen reduces. More oxygen therefore remains bound to the haemoglobin (Tortora and Derrickson, 2013) (see Figure 1.6 and Table 1.4).

Table 1.4 Causes of an altered oxygen dissociation curve

Curve to the left	Curve to the right
Reduced metabolic activity	Increased metabolic activity
Reduced demand for oxygen	Increased demand for oxygen
Lower levels of carbon dioxide	Increased levels of carbon dioxide
Lower levels of acidity (high blood pH)	Increased levels of acidity (low blood pH)
Lower temperature	Increased temperature

ACID–BASE BALANCE

Arterial blood pH is mainly influenced by the presence of hydrogen ions (H^+). The optimum range for blood pH is 7.35–7.45 (Nair and Peate, 2013). If the blood pH falls outside this range an acid–base disturbance may occur. The respiratory system maintains acid–base balance through the regulation of carbon dioxide levels. When the pH falls (acidosis), the respiratory rate increases in order to expel more carbon dioxide. If blood pH rises (alkalosis), respiratory rate and depth may fall and carbon dioxide is retained. Acid–base balance will be further discussed in Chapter 4.

INTERNAL RESPIRATION

Internal respiration describes the exchange of O_2 and CO_2 between the blood and the cells within the tissues. Cells use oxygen to manufacture energy in the form of adenosine triphosphate (ATP). The cells also produce water and carbon dioxide as a waste product of this process. As cells are using oxygen continuously, the concentration of oxygen is always lower within the tissues than within the blood. The level of carbon dioxide is therefore always higher within the tissue than the blood. The concentration of oxygen in venous blood flowing away from the tissues back towards the heart is described as being deoxygenated. The actual amount of oxygen used in the tissues every minute is referred to as oxygen consumption (VO_2) or oxygen extraction ratio (OER) (Nair and Peate, 2013).

SUMMARY

This chapter has explained the anatomy and physiology of the respiratory system. This system is divided into the upper and lower respiratory tracts. The upper respiratory tract ensures that air entering the lower tract is warm, humidified and clean and therefore its main role is to protect the lower respiratory tract. The lower respiratory tract includes the larynx, the trachea, the right and left bronchi and all the constituents of both lungs. Its function is to re-oxygenate arterial blood and remove excess carbon dioxide. Respiration involves four physiological processors: breathing (pulmonary ventilation), gaseous exchange (external respiration), transport of gases and internal respiration. External respiration is the diffusion of oxygen from the alveoli into the pulmonary circulation and the diffusion of carbon dioxide from the pulmonary circulation into the alveoli. Internal respiration describes the exchange of oxygen and carbon dioxide between the blood and the cells within the tissues. Effective respiration is also reliant on a fully functioning cardiovascular system.

REFERENCES

Clancy, J. and McVicar, A. 2009. *Physiology and Anatomy for Nurses and Healthcare Practitioners: A Homeostatic Approach* (3rd ed.). CRC Press, London.

Davies, A. and Moore, C. 2010. *The Respiratory System* (2nd ed.): *Basic Science and Clinical Conditions.* Churchill Livingstone, Edinburgh.

Jenkins, G., Kemnitz, C. and Tortora, G. 2010. *Anatomy and Physiology* (2nd ed.). *From Science to Life.* Wiley-Blackwell, Hoboken, New Jersey.

Marieb, E. 2012. *Essentials of Human Anatomy and Physiology.* Pearson Education, Boston, Massachusetts.

Nair, M. and Peate, I. 2013. *Fundamentals of Applied Pathophysiology* (2nd ed.). Wiley-Blackwell, Oxford.

Peate, I. and Nair, M. 2011. *Fundamentals of Anatomy and Physiology for Student Nurses.* Wiley-Blackwell, Chichester.

Royal College of Physicians. 2012. *National Early Warning Score (NEWS): Standardising the Assessment of Acute Illness Severity in the NHS.* Report of a Working Party. RCP, London.

Simpson, H. 2004. Interpretation of arterial blood gases: A clinical guide for nurses. *British Journal of Nursing* 13 (9): 522–528.

Tortora, G. and Derrickson, B. 2013. *Essentials of Anatomy and Physiology* (9th ed.). Wiley-Blackwell, Hoboken, New Jersey.

Woodrow, P. 2012. *Intensive Care Nursing: A Framework for Practice* (3rd ed.). Routledge, London.

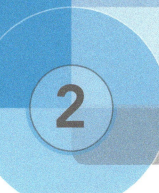

2

Respiratory history taking and physical assessment

LEE CURTIS

LEARNING OBJECTIVES

Upon completion of this chapter the reader should be able to:

- Describe the stages involved in a comprehensive respiratory assessment
- Understand the decision-making processes that are involved when conducting the initial assessment (history taking)
- Appropriately interpret the information gained from the physical assessment portion of the comprehensive respiratory assessment and link these findings to some commonly encountered respiratory conditions
- Successfully complete the respiratory assessment example at the end of this chapter

INTRODUCTION

Deterioration in respiratory function is a major cause of serious illness, emergency admissions to hospital and referral to critical care departments in the United Kingdom (UK) (Dunn, 2005; Health and Social Care Information Centre, 2014). Developing the health-care professional's ability to perform a respiratory assessment and correctly interpret the findings would assist in identifying deterioration earlier and accelerate the instigation of appropriate intervention (Hunter and Rawlings-Anderson, 2008; Higginson and Jones, 2009). Far from an extended skill, the ability to undertake a comprehensive respiratory assessment is now an essential skill (Wheeldon, 2005; Simpson, 2006; Ferns and West, 2008).

The respiratory system is responsible for a multitude of functions that are essential to human existence. Its primary role is to ensure adequate gas exchange sufficient to sustain cellular life, irrespective of the demand (Kennedy, 2007; Moore, 2007). It also has roles in the regulation of acid-base balance, musculoskeletal mobility, smell and speech (Edwards, 2007; Clifton Smith and Rowley, 2011). The complexities of this system, including all the functions the lungs perform within the context of the human body, are still under investigation (Sanderson, 2011). It is impossible to list all of the intricate interrelationships that exist and how disruption to these relationships can manifest themselves systemically in this one chapter. The aim, therefore, will be to direct the reader towards acquiring the appropriate skills to undertake a clearly structured respiratory assessment based on their solid knowledge of respiratory anatomy and physiology. It is essential that the reader understands the respiratory system in health: this is the key to understanding any abnormalities (acute or chronic) that are encountered when assessing the respiratory system in a state of ill health (Simpson, 2006; Kennedy, 2007). See Chapter 1 for a comprehensive review of the anatomy and physiology of the respiratory system.

The respiratory assessment must be a systematic and thorough investigation (Simpson, 2006) with each detail gathered being comprehensively analysed. Relevance is determined by understanding the normal (anatomy and physiology), including the established normal for the patient, and comparing this against the elicited history (Kennedy, 2007). Any findings deemed to be relevant are used to direct subsequent investigations. Seemingly irrelevant findings should be compartmentalised and ready to be drawn on again in the event that they become relevant in the future. This process continues throughout the assessment until only the truly applicable information remains. When this point is reached, an appropriate initial diagnosis can be proposed and a course of treatment planned.

There is no definitive model for undertaking a respiratory assessment (Higginson and Jones, 2009). However, for an assessment to be comprehensive it must include all the core components within two distinct but overlapping assessment sections:

1. The initial assessment (history taking) – to include all aspects of present and past history relevant to the presenting respiratory condition (direct or indirect dependent on circumstance)
2. The physical assessment – to follow the 'look, listen and feel' model (inspection, auscultation, percussion and palpation)

The quantity of information gathered for each of these sections will be dependent upon the environment where the assessment is conducted (home, walk-in clinic, Emergency Department, Critical Care Unit, etc.). It is of paramount importance that the acquisition of information is thorough, utilising all the sources available at that time. The initial diagnosis is proposed from the information gathered; any missing information will make the process of deduction more difficult.

THE INITIAL ASSESSMENT (HISTORY TAKING)

The initial assessment begins prior to any formal introductions, with the investigation starting when the patient can be seen and heard. A quick general inspection should seek to identify any obvious respiratory anomalies (Moore, 2007). Note should be taken of how the patient is walking or is positioned, whether the patient is obviously breathless, talking in full sentences, coughing, wheezing, flushed or exhibiting discomfort. This first contact should never be underestimated as a multitude of clues can be identified at this time.

Provided that the patient has the ability to recollect or recount events, they will be the preferred source for information acquisition (Kennedy, 2007). If they are unable to recollect or recount these events, then alternative sources will need to be utilised such as family, friends or other members of the healthcare team (Simpson, 2006; Hunter and Rawlings-Anderson, 2008).

The history can be subdivided into five main areas:

- History of the Presenting Condition (HPC)
- Past Medical History (PMH)
- Drug History (DH)
- Social History (SH)
- Family History (FH)

HISTORY OF PRESENTING CONDITION (HPC)

To fully explore the 'History of the Presenting Condition' in a respiratory assessment, five core areas need to be investigated: Breathing, Cough, Sputum, Wheeze and Chest Pain (Thomas, 2005; Kennedy, 2007). It is highly probable that one of these areas or indeed a combination of all five will be responsible for the patient's presenting symptoms. Each individual area should be studied, regardless of which individual area is most likely to be primarily responsible. Methodical, systematic exploration is essential as interactions can occur between each of these areas (Simpson, 2006).

The method of questioning will be dependent upon the patient and the patient's responses to these questions (Moore, 2007). To ensure a thorough assessment is conducted, information must be gathered on the onset and duration of symptoms, trajectory of the condition and the severity – including aggravating or relieving factors of the five core areas. Questioning should also seek to establish whether the patient has experienced any similar previous episodes (this is not the PMH but an attempt to identify specific information relevant to this episode).

BREATHING

Breathing is usually the first vital sign to alter in the deteriorating patient (Hunter and Rawlings-Anderson, 2008). It is imperative to understand what the patient perceives their usual breathing pattern to be in order to ensure correct identification of deterioration. Ascertaining a baseline of respiratory function will permit an accurate respiratory assessment to be carried out tailored to the individual patient (Simpson, 2006). Abnormal breathing patterns can become the normal for people with chronic respiratory conditions, e.g. pursed-lip breathing in chronic obstructive pulmonary disease (COPD) where the patient attempts to apply additional positive end expiratory pressure (PEEP) to enhance oxygenation (Thomas, 2005). These patterns, although abnormal when compared to the established 'normal', would not necessarily be perceived as an issue for that individual.

Breathing should appear effortless with an increase in effort (increased work of breathing) suggested by the employment of the accessory muscles such as the sternocleidomastoid, the scalene and the trapezium (Kennedy, 2006; Moore, 2007). Obvious increases in work of breathing will already have been identified at the time of first contact. See Table 2.1 for a summary of respiratory patterns.

Restrictive, obstructive, infective or traumatic problems associated with the respiratory system will result in respiratory dysfunction (Bennett, 2003). Shortness of breath (SOB) or difficulty in breathing (DIB) are often the symptoms reported when the body attempts to maintain/compensate for gas exchange abnormalities (Moore, 2007). Abnormalities in arterial blood gas (ABG) composition associated with respiratory and metabolic failures drive these pattern changes, although some patterns can be driven by disease and degeneration

of the respiratory control network (Nogués et al., 2002). Respiratory rate and breathing pattern are extremely important indicators of potential deterioration (Kennedy, 2007; National Institute for Health and Care Excellence [NICE], 2007; Hunter and Rawlings-Anderson, 2008).

ONSET AND DURATION

Onset and duration when combined with the nature of the presenting symptoms will provide the foundations to guide a provisional diagnosis from which further questioning can be directed (Thomas, 2005). Questioning should attempt to establish how the symptoms started: were they by direct insult, a sudden presentation or were they of insidious onset with symptoms building up over a few weeks? This information will provide the healthcare professional with essential clues to the pathogenesis of this problem. Clinical reasoning of the information gathered against known anatomy and physiology in health will direct the healthcare professional towards the processes responsible.

When discussing breathing pattern abnormalities, simultaneous observation of the pattern being demonstrated should be noted (accessory muscle involvement, the position of the patient, purse lip breathing etc.). The importance of noting these adaptations will be discussed later within this chapter (see section 'The Physical Assessment'). Establishing onset and duration can often aid in ascertaining the provisional diagnosis.

A thoracic injury will immediately affect breathing patterns. An antalgic pattern (short and shallow breaths) will be subconsciously adopted to avoid pain (Moore, 2007). Significant force is required to cause single or multiple rib fractures. Assuming the patient had normal bone density, this type of insult would usually result in pulmonary contusions (Cohn and DuBose, 2010; Arbogast et al., 2012). Further questioning and examination would be required to support this theory and exclude other possible causes (e.g. pneumothorax). If pain is not suitably managed, this pattern will eventually lead to abnormal blood gas concentrations and a different compensatory breathing pattern would be adopted.

Gradual-onset changes to breathing patterns with no known preceding event are much harder

Table 2.1 Respiratory patterns

Terminology	Pattern	Possible causes
Eupnoea (normal, relaxed, quiet)	Minimal muscle/chest wall activity seen as the diaphragm is responsible for the majority of gas movement (equal movement R + L side) Rate 12–17 breaths/minute. Inspiratory : Expiratory ratio = 1:2.	
Apnoea	Absence of breathing	Arrest (respiratory/cardiac/neurological)
Bradypnoea	Reduced respiratory rate – less than 10 breaths/minute	Drugs, increased intracranial pressure (ICP), diabetic coma
Tachypnoea	Increased respiratory rate – more than 20 breaths/minute (normal response to exercise/fear)	Pneumonia, pleurisy
Hypopnoea	Abnormally shallow breathing	Part of normal ageing process
Dyspnoea	Difficulty/laboured breathing – use of accessory muscles	Multiple respiratory causes + other body systems
Orthopnea	Dyspnoea associated with the supine position – relieved when sitting upright	Cardiac
Hyperventilation	Deep breathing associated with an increased respiratory rate – increased minute ventilation (MV) (seen in high levels of exertion and fear/anxiety)	Abnormalities in blood gas concentrations, diabetic ketoacidosis
Hypoventilation	Shallow breathing associated with a decrease in respiratory rate – decreased MV	Abnormalities in blood gas concentrations, respiratory pain avoidance, narcotics
Cheyne–Stokes	Cycles of irregular breathing patterns (increasing and decreasing rates) followed by periods of apnoea	Meningitis, increased ICP, severe heart/renal failure, end stage of life
Kussmaul's	Deep rapid breaths – 'air hunger' (centrally driven)	Diabetic ketoacidosis, acidosis
Biot's respiration	A cyclic pattern of irregular rate and depth of breath followed by a period of apnoea	Head trauma, heat stroke, encephalitis, brain abscess

Source: Adapted from Hunter, J. and Rawlings-Anderson, K. 2008. *Nursing Standard*, 22 (41): 41–43; Moore, T. 2007. *Nursing Standard*, 21 (49): 48–56; Simpson, H. 2006. *British Journal of Nursing*, 15 (9): 484–488.

to assign a provisional diagnosis. Chest infections associated with unilateral consolidation will reduce the alveoli surface area available for gas exchange, leading to ABG abnormalities. Pulmonary oedema increases the thickness of the diffusional plate where the transfer of gas takes place. This would also lead to ABG abnormalities. The patient is likely to report shortness of breath or difficulty in breathing while exhibiting a deeper/quicker breathing pattern. This pattern would be adopted to compensate for a reduced arterial blood oxygen concentration. In both these conditions it is likely that the onset would develop over a period of time with no obvious preceding event.

TRAJECTORY

The trajectory of the condition will provide additional clues related to its cause. Trajectory will also influence the treatment and any referral planning. Chest infections are projected to improve either spontaneously or following a course of treatment. They can, however, become worse or even re-establish (post treatment) in patients with chronic lung conditions or if the pathogen has not been suitably eradicated (Luks and Altemeier, 2006; Sapey and Stockley, 2006). Appropriate questioning will improve understanding of the trajectory of the symptoms and therefore the pathogenesis of the presenting condition.

SEVERITY

The severity of breathlessness is an indicator of the distress the patient personally experiences. It is how the patient perceives their symptoms and can be assessed using a simple analogue scale 0–10, with ten being the most severe. Using a Likert scale allows easy transference to other questions such as aggravating and relieving factors. Appropriate questioning in relation to severity (linked to observational findings) guides the assessment process. Severity will guide any alteration to the type and sequence of questions asked, including whether an onward referral should be considered.

If the severity is high (reported and observational), then consideration must be given to whether a comprehensive respiratory assessment is indicated. In this situation the assessment may need to be converted to the airway, breathing, circulation, disability, exposure (ABCDE) model for assessing the critically ill patient (Resuscitation Council United Kingdom [RCUK], 2010).

AGGRAVATING AND RELIEVING FACTORS

Presenting symptoms can change depending on the underlying cause and certain variables, for example patient position and day/night cycle. Understanding these changes will aid the decision-making process (Kennedy, 2007). Consolidation that affects a lobe of the lung can be improved if Ventilation : Perfusion (V:Q) matching is optimised through correct positioning. The same applies to cardiac conditions that are worse at night, especially when the patient adopts the supine position – orthopnoea (Galvin et al., 2007).

The level of improvement or deterioration of the presenting symptoms can be linked to the severity score discussed in the preceding section.

PREVIOUS EPISODES

Understanding where this specific presentation appears in relation to other previous episodes is beneficial to an overall patient assessment. Respiratory symptoms can often be unique, one-off events but they can also be part of an ongoing problem that has seen the patient present with other similar episodes. Patients may also have experienced minor

respiratory symptoms without registering that these were precursors to this present respiratory condition becoming established. Long-term deterioration in respiratory function is associated with changes in lifestyle. Patients adapt to these changes, possibly without registering them as important until they are directly questioned. Chronic lung conditions that lead to airway structural abnormalities and reduced mucociliary activity or ability leave the lungs more susceptible to pathogen colonisation and subsequent infection (Shoemark et al., 2007; Kousha et al., 2011). These conditions are often linked to repeated hospital visits with chest infections being one of the main reasons for admission.

Cough

A cough is one of the body's defence mechanisms designed to protect the lungs from inhaling foreign bodies and to aid the mucociliary escalator in the clearance of the upper airways (Chung and Pavord, 2008). The assessment of a patient's cough can provide valuable information (Moore, 2007; Hunter and Rawlings-Anderson, 2008). Ascertaining nature and duration will assist in diagnosis (Bradley, 2007) (see Table 2.2).

Sputum

Ascertaining whether a cough is productive and what it produces is extremely important information. Non-productive coughs can be due to solid consolidation or due to alternative aetiologies that do not produce sputum. Cardiac patients often experience irritation of the airways by oedema and inflammation. A cough is present but there is rarely sputum production associated with this aetiology unless there is an overlying infective element. If sputum is present, quantity and type produced should be investigated. This information can assist in condition differentiation (Moore, 2007; Hunter and Rawlings-Anderson, 2008). However, Kennedy (2007) does advise caution in this area as many exceptions to the typical have been identified (see Table 2.3).

Wheeze

Wheeze can be experienced by the patient without it being audible to the healthcare professional. It is therefore important to request this information from the patient. A wheeze is the sound made when air flows through a narrowed airway. The

Table 2.2 Cough

Acute	Chronic
Bacterial/viral – respiratory tract infection (RTI)	Chronic cardiac failure
Acute left ventricular failure (LVF)	Tuberculosis
Pulmonary embolism	COPD
Asthma	Habitual
Smoking	Lung cancer
Upper respiratory tract (URT) stimulation	Medication (angiotensin converting enzyme [ACE] inhibitors)
Idiopathic	Bronchiectasis/Cystic fibrosis
	Gastro-oesophageal reflux disease (GORD)
	Postnasal drip syndrome/Rhinitis
	Pulmonary fibrosis
	Eosinophilic bronchitis
	Idiopathic

Source: Adapted from Chung, K.F. and Pavord, I.D. 2008. *The Lancet,* 371 (9621): 1364–1374; Haque, R.A., Usmani, O.S. and Barnes P.J. 2005. *Chest,* 127 (5): 1710–1713; Lee, S.C. et al. 2013. *Archives of Physical Medicine and Rehabilitation,* 94 (8): 1580–1583; Magni, C., Chellini, E. and Zanasi, A. 2010. *Multidisciplinary Respiratory Medicine,* 5 (2): 99–103; Mazzone, S.B. 2005. *Cough,* 1 (2): 1–9.

healthcare professional must establish whether there is a condition present that causes a reduction in airway calibre, an obstructive condition either acute or chronic (King et al., 2005). It is worth noting that the presence or absence of a wheeze is a poor indicator of disease severity (Thomas, 2005). Bronchoconstriction is often seen in patients who present with asthma. Short-acting bronchodilators will alleviate this symptom quickly, but if used with airway narrowing from another cause (e.g. cardiac wheeze) the same level of symptom relief will not be seen. A severe wheeze heard on inspiration (stridor) indicates difficulty moving air into the lungs and may constitute a medical emergency (Calzavacca et al., 2008).

Chest pain

Chest pain can be caused by a multitude of differing conditions, not all of which are respiratory in nature. Some causes can be life threatening (acute cardiac events) where specialist emergency care must be sort. Other common causes are vascular, musculoskeletal or gastro-oesophageal; it is the responsibility of the healthcare professional to understand the different presentations so that the correct course of action can be followed. When a patient presents with chest pain, performing an electrocardiogram (ECG) (if available) should always be considered (see Table 2.4).

Table 2.3 Sputum

Appearance	Description	Possible causes
Normal (saliva)	Clear watery	
Mucoid	Opaque, sticky	Asthma, non-infective bronchitis/COPD
Mucopurulent	Whitish/yellowish, sticky	Cystic fibrosis (CF), pneumonia
Copious (yellow/green)	Large quantity – yellow/green	Chronic bronchitis (advanced)
Purulent	Thick, sticky, foul smelling – yellow/green/brown	Chest Infection – pseudomonas/klebsiella/haemophilus
Frothy	White or pink	Pulmonary oedema
Haemoptysis	Blood – new/old (quantity important)	Infection, trauma, lung cancer, lung abscess, tuberculosis (TB), pulmonary embolism (PE), coagulopathy
Black	Carbon deposits (black specs)	Inhaled – smoke/tar/heroin

Source: Adapted from Allegra, L. et al. 2005. *Respiratory Medicine,* 99 (6): 742–747; Day, T. 2007. *Journal of Advanced Perioperative Care,* 3 (2): 41–49; Kennedy, S. 2007. *Nursing Standard,* 21 (49): 42–46; Miravitlles, M. et al. 2012. *European Respiratory Journal,* 39 (6): 1354–1360; Moore, T. 2007. *Nursing Standard,* 21 (49): 48–56; Simpson, H. 2006. *British Journal of Nursing,* 15 (9): 484–488.

Table 2.4 Chest pain

System	Type of chest pain	Possible cause
Respiratory	Pleuritic – sharp, sudden and exacerbated by coughing, sneezing, laughing and deep breathing. Usually localised to specific area involved. Generally accompanied by shortness of breath	Chest infection URT infection Pneumothorax Pleurisy
Cardiac	Normally associated with 'pressure' pain (crushing), radiates to left arm, shoulder, neck and jaw. Often elicits a feeling of nausea and vomiting. Can be associated with shortness of breath	Myocardial infarction (MI)
Vascular	Sudden onset of central excruciating pain in anterior, posterior chest and abdomen	Aortic dissection
Musculoskeletal (MSK)	Pain specific or locally radiating that is reproducible with palpation and/or movement	Costochondral Costosternal Vertebral
Gastro-oesophageal	Burning central pain	GORD

Source: Adapted from Kennedy, S. 2007. *Nursing Standard*, 21 (49): 42–46.

PAST MEDICAL HISTORY (PMH)

Questioning in this area is aimed at opening up a narrative-based dialogue to identifying clues in the patient's past medical history that may be relevant to this current presentation (Haidet and Paterniti, 2003). Old orthopaedic surgeries are unlikely to have any relevance (unless related to the thoracic cavity and spine). However, pulmonary emboli should always be considered in sudden onset of shortness of breath after recent surgery (Agnelli, 2004; Memtsoudis et al., 2009). Recent weight loss must be quantified as any unexplained weight loss can be an indicator of a systemic pathology such as lung cancer (Khalid et al., 2007). History of tuberculosis, pneumonia and previous admissions secondary to a respiratory problem should all be included for consideration as an element of irreversible airway damage is often present (Shoemark et al., 2007).

DRUG HISTORY (DH)

The patient's prescribed and non-prescribed medications should be investigated to evaluate whether there is a causal link to the presenting symptoms. A recent study identified over 380 medications known to cause drug-induced respiratory diseases (Schwaiblmair et al., 2012); these include commonly used medications such as beta blockers.

Inhalers are a commonly prescribed delivery device for a multitude of respiratory medications. Identifying the type of inhaler, the medication for delivery and how often it is taken should be documented and the patient's delivery technique may need to be assessed. Incorrect inhaler technique will reduce the quantity of medication inhaled and therefore its overall effectiveness (Lavorini et al., 2008; Bosnic-Anticevich et al., 2010).

SOCIAL HISTORY (SH)

It is important to ascertain whether there is a possibility of exposure to respiratory irritants. Exposure can occur at work, home or even when engaged in certain hobbies/leisure pursuits. Questioning must therefore not just address the obvious such as smoking, but must also investigate moulds, paints, cleaning products etc. (Rosenman et al., 2003; Fedoruk et al., 2005; Bernard, 2007). Lifestyle should include level of alcohol consumption and recreational drug use (where appropriate) as these personal choices are important contributors to the acquisition and development of respiratory illnesses (Buster et al., 2002; Babu and Marshall, 2004; Boe et al., 2009; Kaphalia and Calhoun, 2013). Note should be taken of the patient's socio-economic status as multiple occupancy, low household income, malnutrition and low educational level have all been associated with chronic respiratory conditions (Bacon et al., 2009;

Saunders and Smith, 2010; Kanervisto et al., 2011). For more information on occupational lung disease see Chapter 9.

FAMILY HISTORY (FH)

Genetic traits and familial exposures may be important considerations in a respiratory assessment (Marshall et al., 2000; Steele et al., 2005).

It is impossible to include an exhaustive list of the questions and in what order they need to be asked when investigating individual respiratory presentations as the variations are endless. The preceding section was designed to guide the reader to develop their own systematic method of enquiry based around certain core areas of investigation. The information that is gained at each stage will direct the healthcare professional towards a likely provisional diagnosis. Subsequent questioning is directed at reinforcing this provisional diagnosis until it develops into the most likely working diagnosis. The next section in this chapter will introduce the reader to the knowledge and skills required to undertake the physical assessment portion of a comprehensive respiratory assessment.

THE PHYSICAL ASSESSMENT

The physical assessment portion of a comprehensive respiratory assessment should follow the inspection, auscultation, percussion and palpation framework (Day, 2007; Moore, 2007; Ferns and West, 2008), although there are some inevitable overlaps. These are all sophisticated skills that require education and practice (Kennedy, 2007). The breathing aspect of inspection has already been discussed in the initial assessment section as it is an easily observable activity when conducting the initial history taking assessment. However, a more detailed inspection of the chest, including breathing patterns, will be undertaken during a comprehensive physical assessment. A structured approach is good practice with general acceptance being that the peripheries are reviewed first, followed by a detailed assessment of the chest. Observations are undertaken to identify any abnormalities in skin colour, presence of lumps and swellings or any perspiration (Day, 2007).

VISUAL INSPECTION

FACE AND NECK

Central cyanosis is a late sign of hypoxaemia and is associated with a blue tinge to the oral mucosa, tongue and lips. This occurs when there is an increase in haemoglobin not bound to oxygen in the blood. This correlates to a PaO_2 of <8 kPa (Simpson, 2006; Kennedy, 2007; Hunter and Rawlings-Anderson, 2008). However, caution is advised when using the lips for cyanosis assessment in non-Caucasians, as different skin pigmentation may make assessment of oral mucosal colour difficult (Day, 2007). Purse lip breathing is often subconsciously employed to create PEEP and to maintain airway patency in exhalation. This can be an indicator of high compliance lungs associated with small airway destruction (COPD), but also in acute episodes where hypoxia is present (Thomas, 2005). Anaemia (which can lead to abnormal respiratory rates) can often be identified by reduced colouring of the conjunctivae.

Lumps and swellings around the neck must be investigated further. Structures within this area can become compressed and lead to dysphagia and dyspnoea (Frizzell et al., 2009). A bounding jugular vein is an indicator of elevated right heart pressures which can be associated with heart failure, fluid overload and cor pulmonale (Levick and Dwight, 2007).

HANDS AND FINGERS

The hands and fingers are a rich source of information for the respiratory assessor. Carbon dioxide (CO_2) retention can cause the outstretched hand to be warm, sweaty and exhibit an irregular flapping movement, and high doses of Beta 2 agonists, contained in some bronchodilator inhalers, can result in a fine tremor (Middleton and Middleton, 2002). Fingers should be inspected for nicotine staining, which is associated with chronic cigarette smoking. Peripheral cyanosis can also be seen at the tips/nail beds of the fingers and toes. Peripheral cyanosis results from vasoconstriction-reduced cardiac output or vascular occlusion (Simpson, 2006; Moore, 2007). It is seen in cardiac and respiratory conditions, but also as a result of exposure to extreme cold and therefore the situation and timing of assessments

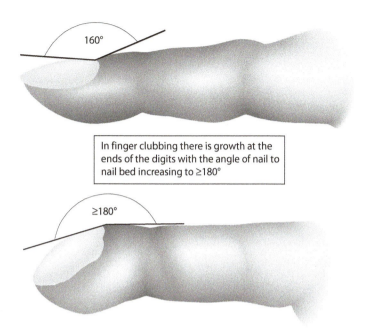

In finger clubbing there is growth at the ends of the digits with the angle of nail to nail bed increasing to ≥180°

Figure 2.1 Finger clubbing. (Image reproduced with permission of Blaize Curtis.)

must be considered. Clubbing of fingernails (see Figure 2.1) can be an indicator of chronic hypoxia associated with chronic respiratory or cardiac conditions (Hunter and Rawlings-Anderson, 2008). Further exploration of the cause will be required.

CHEST

Observation of the chest is best performed with the patient as free from clothing as possible, so a chaperon may need to be considered for this part of the assessment. Preferably the patient should be sat comfortably on a stool or plinth as this will provide 360-degree visual access (Moore, 2007). Inspection addresses normal symmetry and the overall chest should be twice as wide (shoulder to shoulder) as it is deep (front to back). Over-inflation (barrel chest) may indicate COPD or severe acute asthma. The sternum should not protrude, such as seen in pigeon chest (pectus carinatum) or be sunken, as seen in funnel chest (pectus excavatum). The spine should be straight when looked at directly from behind (no scoliosis present) and there should be a normal lumbar lordosis and thoracic kyphosis present. Abnormalities can be associated with chronic conditions that may contribute to the development of symptoms or may

be an indicator of the presenting condition itself (Higginson and Jones, 2009; Blanco et al., 2011).

Movement during the breathing cycle should be observed with decreased unilateral movements being investigated further. Common causes include pneumothorax, consolidation and pleural effusion (Kennedy, 2007; Hunter and Rawlings-Anderson, 2008). Paradoxical movements of a specific section (flail segment) would indicate rib fractures where the negative pressure within the thorax during inspiration draws the free segment inward. This is likely to be accompanied by localised intense pain and a history of direct injury. Scarring on the skin (surgical or otherwise) should be noted and their aetiology should match the history elicited during the initial assessment.

OTHER BODY AREAS

The abdomen should be observed for size, as distension can lead to dysfunction of the diaphragm affecting the effectiveness of pulmonary ventilation (Moore, 2007). Hepatomegaly will increase abdominal size and can be associated with chronic excessive alcohol intake and also right heart failure. The pattern of abdominal movement during a breathing cycle should be observed. Normal movement would see the abdomen enlarge as the diaphragm flattens down during inspiration, pushing the abdominal contents down and forwards. Paradoxical (see-saw) abdominal movements are associated with reduced control of the main respiratory muscle (diaphragm). When accompanied by the drawing in of the intercostal muscles, this is suggestive of potential life-threatening respiratory failure, requiring urgent medical intervention.

Ankle and calf areas must be visualised as bilateral swelling (pitting oedema) of this area could indicate venous insufficiency or a cardiac condition with fluid accumulating in dependent regions. If present, consideration should be given to the possibility of fluid also accumulating in the low-pressure vascular beds of the lungs (Verheij et al., 2006). Unilateral swelling may indicate lymphedema or a deep vein thrombosis (Ely et al., 2006).

AUSCULTATION

Auscultation simply means 'to listen' and has been linked to the use of a stethoscope in clinical practice (Middleton and Middleton, 2002). Breath sounds are the sounds of turbulent airflow heard at the chest wall. Turbulent airflow is predominantly generated in the trachea and main bronchi (Ferns and West, 2008). Auscultation of the chest wall identifies these sounds and if applicable the disruption to their journey from their point of generation. In practice, any pathology or anatomical irregularity along this sound pathway will ultimately alter the sound auscultated.

A clear explanation of intent is always required prior to auscultation, as the default activity for patients approached with a stethoscope is to take deep breaths prior to instruction. The patient should be asked to breathe through their mouth if possible (better sound generation) and to breathe normally. Deep breaths can be requested as need dictates. Systematic comparison from side to side and lobe to lobe should be conducted, in both inspiration and expiration (Simpson, 2006; Ferns and West, 2008). This systematic order may need to be altered for comfort and to minimise disruption for the more bed-bound patient. It is essential that the posterior lobes, and especially the posterior basal segment of the lower lobes, are not omitted as the density of the lungs and the recumbent position of the patient may distort assessment findings (Bradley, 2007; Moore, 2007). A pleural effusion is one such condition that favours a dependant position and can move in relation to the position of the patient.

A basic auscultation assessment of the chest will involve listening at 14 points distributed across the anterior and posterior chest walls (see Figure 2.2). If an abnormal breath sound is identified, then further auscultation around this point should be considered. See Table 2.5 for a summary of possible breath sounds heard on auscultation.

To support auscultation findings, the patient can be asked to speak or whisper certain words (Owen, 1998). Voice sounds are air waves vibrating at different frequencies through and across the vocal cords. Auscultation of voice is the interpretation of abnormalities in the sound pathway of these sound waves through the respiratory system. Depending on the abnormality present, voice transmission will be dulled or amplified (see Table 2.6).

PALPATION

Palpation involves the use of different parts of the hands and fingers to gather diagnostic information (Day, 2007). Palpation is an assessment skill that should never be overlooked. The findings from this assessment will support the findings from the initial visual inspection and add valuable information to the body of evidence already gathered. Palpation of the chest follows the systematic auscultation approach except it begins by ascertaining trachea centrality (Thomas, 2005; Moore, 2007). Deviation of the trachea is related to the pushing or pulling of structures within the neck, possibly due to masses on or within the thoracic cavity causing a mediastinal shift. A collapse of a lobe or a lung will see the trachea deviated towards the collapsed side (pulled) and a pleural effusion will push it away. The extent of a consolidation dictates the amount of movement, with mild consolidation usually filling the air spaces (no movement occurs). However, if the consolidation is extensive, it may cause a deviation away from the affected side (Luks and Altemeier, 2006).

Palpation of the chest starts at the top and moves downwards using both hands simultaneously providing continuous comparison of sides. The whole hand is good for the overall chest assessments

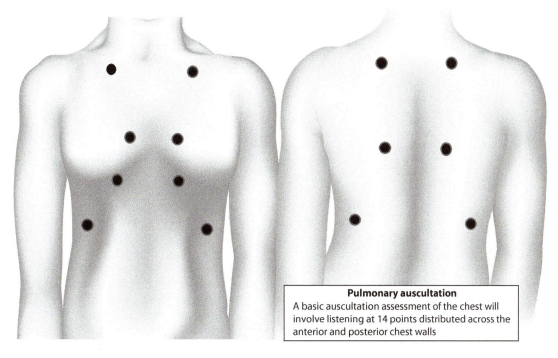

Pulmonary auscultation
A basic auscultation assessment of the chest will involve listening at 14 points distributed across the anterior and posterior chest walls

Figure 2.2 Auscultation points on the anterior and posterior chest walls. (Image reproduced with permission of Blaize Curtis.)

including bulk movements (expansion and flail segments). Fingers and thumbs are utilised to assess the 'normal' presentation and position of thoracic landmarks, whereas the ulnar aspect of the hand and fingers are adept at identifying vibrations (Moore, 2007).

Chest expansion can be measured by placing the hands laterally on the posterior aspect of the chest with the tip of the thumbs touching the spinal process (on exhalation) at the level of the tenth rib (Simpson, 2006). On inspiration the thumb tips will part as the ribs move up and out (Hunter and Rawlings-Anderson, 2008). Each thumb tip should travel equal distance with single side reduction of movement attributed to unilateral consolidation/effusion or a collapse of a lobe/lung. Bilateral reductions are experienced in asthma or pulmonary fibrosis (Moore, 2007). Tactile vocal fremitus is assessed when the patient speaks 'ninety-nine' (Day, 2007). Vibrations are more pronounced over the consolidated lung and decreased over the collapsed lung or pleural effusion.

PERCUSSION

Depending on dominance (right or left handed), the middle finger of the non-dependant hand is placed on the chest, palm down with the rest of the hand and fingers curled backwards away from the patient. The middle finger of the dominant hand is used as a tap hammer, striking the interphalangeal joint of the finger in contact with the patient. Depending on the density of the structures beneath that finger, a note will be produced (see Table 2.7). Over the air-filled lung, a very resonant note will be produced and over the consolidated lung, a more solid (dull) sound will be heard (Simpson, 2006). The points to percuss are identical to those being auscultated as each lobe must be assessed.

Further investigations such as specific blood tests, chest X-rays and arterial blood gases may all contribute to the primary assessment data and the provisionally suggested diagnosis. A full explanation of these investigations can be found in Chapters 3 and 4.

Table 2.5 Breath sounds

Breath sound	Definition	Possible causes
Normal	The correct sounds auscultated in the correct area of the chest wall.	
Abnormal	Any sounds auscultated that are: • Not in their correct areas • Not 'normal' • Absent sounds	See below
Absent	No breath sounds auscultated.	No air entry – secretion plug (main airway) Pneumothorax Severely reduced airflow to a level that cannot generate turbulence -Asthma
Vesicular	Breath sounds heard around the periphery of the lungs. Low-pitched – all of inspiration and approximately a third of expiration is heard.	Often classed as 'Normal'
Bronchial	Higher pitched, louder breath sound compared to vesicular breath sounds. All of inspiration and all of expiration can be heard. Normal only if it is heard over the trachea and main bronchi.	Consolidation (if heard where vesicular breath sounds should be present) as sound transmission of airflow has not been reduced on its journey to the chest wall.
Broncho vesicular	Mix of vesicular and bronchial – auscultated around the central part of the anterior chest, over the main airways.	Not commonly used to describe abnormal breath sounds.
Crackles	Described as course or fine (fine – previously known as crepitations). Sound generated by airways popping open and closing during the respiratory cycle. Course crackles – larger airways, more likely related to secretions/fluid etc. Fine crackles – small airways, more likely due to premature closure due to abnormalities in pressure/closing volumes.	Secretion producing infections, severe pulmonary oedema. Mild pulmonary oedema, pulmonary fibrosis, COPD, age.
Wheeze	Heard on expiration (airways narrowing and air being forced out). Monophonic – single tone, specific area Polyphonic – multiple tones, widespread	Single airway involvement – secretions Multi airway – secretions/generalised bronchoconstriction (allergic response/asthma)
Stridor	Heard on inspiration, often indicative of partial obstruction to the upper respiratory tract (acute onset = medical emergency)	Foreign body Mass Laryngeal spasm
Pleural rub	Specific to an area – heard during deeper breathing only. Rubbing sound on both inspiration and expiration (often described as the sound made when walking in new snow). Usually associated with pain and guarding. Caused by inflammation of the pleural surfaces.	Pleurisy

Source: Adapted from Day, T. 2007. *Journal of Advanced Perioperative Care*, 3 (2): 41–49; Docherty, B. 2002. *British Journal of Nursing*, 26 (11): 750–758; Ferns, T. and West, S. 2008. *British Journal of Nursing*, 17 (12): 772–777; Kennedy, S. 2007. *Nursing Standard*, 21 (49): 42–46; Owen, A. 1998. *Nursing*, 28 (4): 48–49.

Table 2.6 Vocal sounds

Spoken word or sound (terminology)	Auscultation over normal lung	Auscultation over a pathology that causes increased resonance (e.g. consolidation)
Any word/sound (Normal)	Word or sound will be heard soft, muffled and indistinct	Word or sound will be heard harder, higher and clearer
The words 'ninety-nine' (Bronchophony)	Muffled, quiet and hard to distinguish 'ninety-nine'	Higher pitched and easily distinguishable 'ninety-nine'
The letter 'E' (Egophony)	Muffled and hard to distinguish the sound – 'E'	Higher pitched and now the sound converted to - 'A'
Any word whispered (Whispering pectoriloquy)	Very hard to hear, word practically indistinguishable	Easier to hear – word relatively easy to distinguish

Source: Adapted from Greco, F.A. 2004. *American Journal of Respiratory and Critical Care Medicine*, 169 (11): 1260; Owen, A. 1998. *Nursing*, 28 (4): 48–49.

Table 2.7 Percussion note

Term for percussion note elicited	Example of percussion note	Possible pathology
Flat	Percussion note of thigh	Pleural effusion
Dull		Lobar pneumonia
Resonant	Percussion note of normal lung	Normal
Hyper-resonant		Emphysema/pneumothorax
Tympany	Percussion note of cheek	Large pneumothorax

Source: Adapted from Simpson, H. 2006. *British Journal of Nursing*, 15 (9): 484–488, 2006.

CASE STUDY

Mr Smith is a 60-year-old accountant who has presented himself to you, complaining of shortness of breath.

First contact: You note from your first contact that Mr Smith appears slightly overweight, he is obviously having an element of difficulty breathing with what you feel is a raised respiratory rate. On introducing himself he takes a big breath in between sentences and you can hear some fine but audible crackles.

Vital signs: Temp 37.6°C, SpO$_2$ 92%, HR 102 bpm (irregular), BP 150/55 mmHg, RR 20 bpm – 2 L O$_2$ via Nasal Cannula started.

The following assessment will follow the structure set out in this chapter, starting with the initial history taking assessment.

THE INITIAL ASSESSMENT

HISTORY TAKING

HPC (onset, duration, trajectory, aggravating/relieving, previous episodes)

- Shortness of breath with no known precursing event. Mr Smith reports he has had no problem with his breathing but he knows he has a problem now
- Worsening slowly over the last week – 10 days
- Better during the day (severity score of 5/10, which is reported as annoying but not disabling), worse at night (7/10) exacerbated by a cough. Last two nights unable to lay in the bed as coughing persistent and increasingly short of breath so has taken to dozing in the armchair
- No previous episodes

Cough

- Cough is problematic and can hear and feel sputum but even with a good cough, he cannot clear it and has been coughing more over the last two days. Only normally coughs when he has something to clear and can usually clear it easily. Coughs less when he sits upright

Sputum

- Not clearing anything

Wheeze

- Can feel 'inside' as he breathes out but it is not audible. Was 'off and on' but more constant now. Sitting up seems to help. Had asthma as a child but grew out of it (20s), no wheeze since then

Chest pain

- No chest pain but has funny fluttering feelings occasionally, which he has had for about four months. Mr Smith feels it is the pressure of work as 'lots going on'. He feels this is no worse
- These symptoms are the same as he had five years ago when he was under a lot of pressure because redundancy was a possibility, his GP prescribed beta blockers for stress and anxiety which were effective, and the problem fully resolved

The information reported at this stage should have led to one or more probable or provisional diagnoses.

PMH

Mr Smith reports the episode described five years previously. Further questioning on specific respiratory issues reveals that Mr Smith was a smoker with a 20-pack year history, quitting aged 38. He has had a few chest infections, the last of which was two years ago, which required antibiotics.

DH

Candersartan 8 mg
Atorvastatin 20 mg

SH

Married with three children
No hobbies, walks to the local shop to get paper at the weekends

FH

Father – Deceased at age 67, due to bowel cancer
Mother – Hypertensive, otherwise medically well

Information from this section should have supported your provisional or probable diagnosis.

PHYSICAL ASSESSMENT

VISUAL

Face and neck

- No evidence of anaemia
- Slightly clammy hands
- Faint blue tinge to the lips
- No obvious lumps or bumps
- Respiratory rate (RR) – 20 bpm (no purse lipped breathing) – audible crackles, on asked to cough, temporary resolution of crackles with nil sputum cleared

Hands

- Nil of note.

Ankle and calf

- Bilateral oedema – Mr Smith reports more than normal. He has been having this swelling off and on for a few years, generally puts feet up and it resolves. He feels it's just his work, being sedentary and his age

Abdomen

- Slightly rotund but normal breathing/ abdominal movement

Chest

- Nil of note

AUSCULTATION, PALPATION AND PERCUSSION

Auscultation

Fine crackles and wheezes throughout, decreased air entry bilateral bases with absent breath sounds in the basal segments of both lower lobes.

Palpation

Equal expansion bilaterally with widespread tactile fremitus.

Percussion

Flat percussion note at bases of lower lobes, posterior > anterior.

On completing this assessment, a working diagnosis should now be in place. Further differential tests would be requested and a treatment plan formulated and initiated.

DISCUSSION

THE INITIAL ASSESSMENT

Mr Smith presented with an altered respiratory status. Initial indications would point towards a chest infection because of the worsening of shortness of breath with audible crackles during the breathing cycle and the associated worsening cough.

Systematic and meticulous history taking revealed some interesting information which includes:

- Symptoms were of slow onset (10 days) and are a progressing or developing condition (non-acute).
- There is a day/night pattern with increase in coughing when lying down, which may indicate possible fluid shift, systemic or localised (sputum/transudate).
- Cough non-productive, which may indicate a cardiac origin or chest infection (viral).
- Wheeze (also worsening), which may indicate a cardiac origin or asthma (offered by patient). Unlikely to be sputum related as Mr Smith's cough remains non-productive.
- Chest flutters, which may indicate a cardiac origin which could be related to his current stress and anxiety.

From the initial history taking, sudden-onset causes, e.g. trauma have been excluded due to the slow progression of symptoms. The probable provisional diagnoses at this stage would include chest infection or a cardiac cause. Less likely but not for exclusion at this time would be asthma or stress related symptoms.

PMH

Questioning related to PMH must now be directed towards gathering information that supports one of these diagnoses.

Mr Smith expanded on his 'stress-related' episode, which was cardiac in origin and resolved with medication. It was possibly induced by stress and anxiety.

Extensive smoking history and therefore has resulted in possible chronic lung damage (likely as recurrent CIs) will also increase strain on heart.

On cardiac medications for BP and cholesterol.

Possible sedentary lifestyle (noted slightly overweight on initial inspection) with possible increased risk of cardiac disease.

Mother increased BP, which is possibly familial. Father had a malignancy, which cannot be excluded but unlikely from initial presenting information.

From the PMH a cardiac cause would appear to be the more likely provisional diagnosis, although a chest infection cannot be excluded. All other causes seem more remote but also should not be excluded until the full assessment has been completed.

PHYSICAL ASSESSMENT

The physical assessment identified more information to support a particular diagnosis.

Slightly clammy hands, which could support cardiac or anxiety as a cause.

Central cyanosis indicates decreased oxygen saturation, which was also noted on vital signs and supports a cardiac or chest infection as a cause.

Cough, which is non-productive and temporarily clears audible crackles would suggest a fluid shift (cardiac).

Swelling of the ankles and calf area suggests fluid retention (cardiac).

Bilateral crackles with equal and progressive decrease in breath sounds in both lower lobes suggest a systemic problem with fluid dependence (cardiac).

Percussion indicates presence of fluid or sputum and again position and bilateral nature would be more indicative of effusions (cardiac).

The weight of evidence gathered from this assessment would indicate a cardiac aetiology for Mr Smith's symptoms. A full assessment moved the diagnosis away from the originally suspected chest infection to a cardiac working diagnosis. Treatment would be started and observation of symptom response will dictate whether current treatment is continued or whether a reassessment should be considered.

SUMMARY

Ability to perform a respiratory assessment and correctly interpret the findings is an essential skill for all healthcare professionals who deal with patients with respiratory problems. Thorough respiratory assessment will assist in the early identification of deterioration and can guide appropriate treatment. A respiratory assessment must be systematic and comprehensive and there are many models seen in both the published literature and utilised by practitioners. However, for an assessment to be comprehensive it must include all the core components within two distinct but overlapping assessment phases. These are the initial assessment or history taking phase, and should include all aspects of present and past medical and social history relevant to the presenting respiratory condition. The next phase is the physical assessment which should follow the 'look, listen and feel' model of inspection, auscultation, percussion and palpation. All findings should be accurately recorded. Findings may prompt the need for further investigations but these must be justifiable as they may be uncomfortable or potentially harmful for the patient and costly to perform. Healthcare professionals not familiar with the process of history taking and physical assessment should work with, learn from and be assessed by an experienced practitioner to gain competence in this essential skill.

REFERENCES

Agnelli, G. 2004. Prevention of venous thromboembolism in surgical patients. *Circulation* 110 (suppl 4): 4–12.

Allegra, L., Blasi, F., Diano, P.L., Cosentini, R., Tarsia, P., Confalonieri, M., Dimakou, K. and Valenti, V. 2005. Sputum colour as a marker of acute bacterial exacerbations of chronic obstructive pulmonary disease. *Respiratory Medicine,* 99 (6): 742–747.

Arbogast, K.B., Locey, C.M. and Zonfrillo, M.R. 2012. Differences in thoracic injury causation patterns between seat belt restrained children and adults. *Annals of Advanced Automotive Medicine* 56: 213–221.

Babu, K.S. and Marshall, B.G. 2004. Drug induced airway disease. *Clinics in Chest Medicine* 25 (1): 113–122.

Bacon, S.L., Bouchard, A., Loucks, E.B. and Lavoie, K.L. 2009. Individual-level socioeconomic status is associated with worse asthma morbidity in patients with asthma. *Respiratory Research* 17 (10): 125.

Bennett, C. 2003. Nursing the breathless patient. *Nursing Standard* 17 (17): 45–51.

Bernard, A. 2007. Chlorination products: Emerging links with allergic diseases. *Current Medicinal Chemistry* 14 (16): 1771–1782.

Blanco, F.C., Elliot, S.T. and Sandler A.D. 2011. Management of congenital chest wall deformities. *Seminars in Plastic Surgery* 25 (1): 107–116.

Boe, D.M., Vandivier, R.W., Burnham, E.L. and Moss, M. 2009. Alcohol abuse and pulmonary disease. *Journal of Leukocyte Biology* 86 (5): 1097–1104.

Bosnic-Anticevich, S.Z., Sinha, H., So, S. and Reddel, H.K. 2010. Metered-dose inhaler technique: The effect of two educational interventions delivered in community pharmacy over time. *Journal of Asthma* 47 (3): 251–256.

Bradley, B. 2007. Improving respiratory skills. Diagnostic tips. *The Journal for Nurse Practitioners* 3 (4): 276–277.

Buster, M., Rook, L., van Brussel, G.H., van Ree, J. and van den Brink, W. 2002. Chasing the dragon, related to the impaired lung function among heroin users. *Drug and Alcohol Dependence* 68 (2): 221–228.

Calzavacca, P., Licari, E., Tee, A., Egi, M., Haase, M., Haase-Fielitz, A. and Bellomo, R. 2008. A prospective study of factors influencing the outcome of patients after a Medical Emergency Team review. *Intensive Care Medicine* 34 (11): 2112–2116.

Chung, K.F. and Pavord, I.D. 2008. Prevalence, pathogenesis, and causes of chronic cough. *The Lancet* 371 (9621): 1364–1374.

Clifton Smith, T. and Rowley, J. 2011. Breathing pattern disorders and physiotherapy: Inspiration for our profession. *Physical Therapy Reviews* 16 (1): 75–86.

Cohn, S.M. and DuBose, J.J. 2010. Pulmonary contusion: An update on recent advances in clinical management. *World Journal of Surgery* 34 (8): 1959–1970.

Day, T. 2007. Respiratory assessment in the recovery unit: Essential skills for the perioperative practitioner. *Journal of Advanced Perioperative Care* 3 (2): 41–49.

Docherty, B. 2002. Cardiorespiratory physical assessment for the acutely ill. *British Journal of Nursing* 26 (11): 750–758.

Dunn, L. 2005. Pneumonia: Classification, diagnosis and nursing management. *Nursing Standard* 19 (42): 50–54.

Edwards, S.L. 2007. Pathophysiology of acid base balance: The theory practice relationship. *Intensive and Critical Care Nursing* 24 (1): 28–40.

Ely, J.W., Osheroff, J.A., Chambliss, M.L. and Ebell, M.H. 2006. Approach to leg edema of unclear etiology. *Journal of the American Board of Family Medicine* 19 (2): 148–160.

Fedoruk, M.J., Bronstein, R. and Kerger, B.D. 2005. Ammonia exposure and hazard assessment for selected household cleaning product uses. *Journal of Exposure Analysis and Environmental Epidemiology* 15 (6): 534–544.

Ferns, T. and West, S. 2008. The art of auscultation: Evaluating a patient's respiratory pathology. *British Journal of Nursing* 17 (12): 772–777.

Frizzell, J.D., Perkins, B.J. and Morehead, R.S. 2009. Case report: Thyroid lymphoma as a cause of dysphagia and dyspnea in a patient without palpable nodules or goiter. *Case Reports in Medicine* 2009: 1–2. DOI: 10.1155/2009/385461.

Galvin, I., Drummond, G.B. and Nirmalan, M. 2007. Distribution of blood flow and ventilation in the lung: Gravity is not the only factor. *British Journal of Anaesthesia* 98 (4): 420–428.

Greco, F.A. 2004. Interpretation of breath sounds. *American Journal of Respiratory and Critical Care Medicine* 169 (11): 1260.

Haidet, P. and Paterniti, D.A. 2003. 'Building' a history rather than 'Taking' one. A perspective on information sharing during the medical interview. *Archives of Internal Medicine* 163 (10): 1134–1140.

Haque, R.A., Usmani, O.S. and Barnes P.J. 2005. Chronic idiopathic cough: A discrete clinical entity? *Chest* 127 (5): 1710–1713.

Health and Social Care Information Centre. 2014. Hospital Episode Statistics–Adult Critical Care Data (April 2012–March 2013). Available at: http://www.hscic.gov.uk/article/2021/Website-Search?productid=14501&q=title%3a+%22Adult+Critical+Care+Data+in+England%22&sort=Most+recent&size=10&page=1&area=both#top. Accessed 20 March 2015.

Higginson, R. and Jones, B. 2009. Respiratory assessment in critically ill patients: Airway and breathing. *British Journal of Nursing* 18 (8): 456–461.

Hunter, J. and Rawlings-Anderson, K. 2008. Respiratory assessment. *Nursing Standard* 22 (41): 41–43.

Kanervisto, M., Vasankari, T., Laitinen, T., Heliovaara, M., Jousilahti, P. and Saarelainen, S. 2011. Low socioeconomic status is associated with chronic obstructive airway disease. *Respiratory Medicine* 105 (8): 1140–1146.

Kaphalia, L. and Calhoun, W.J. 2013. Alcoholic lung injury: Metabolic, biochemical and immunological aspects. *Toxicology Letters* 222 (2): 171–179.

Kennedy, S. 2006. Assessment of a patient with an acute exacerbation of asthma. *Nursing Standard* 21 (4): 35–38.

Kennedy, S. 2007. Detecting changes in the respiratory status of ward patients. *Nursing Standard* 21 (49): 42–46.

Khalid, U., Spiro, A., Baldwin, C., Sharma, B., McGough, C., Norman, A.R., Eisen, T., O'Brien, M.E., Cunningham, D. and Andreyev, H.J. 2007. Symptoms and weight loss in patients with gastrointestinal and lung cancer at presentation. *Support Care in Cancer* 15 (1): 39–46.

King, G.G., Brown, N.J., Diba, C., Thorpe, C.W., Muñoz, P., Marks, G.B., Toelle, B. et al. 2005. The effects of body weight on airway calibre. *European Respiratory Journal* 25 (5): 896–901.

Kousha, M., Tadi, R. and Soubani, A.O. 2011. Pulmonary aspergillosis: A clinical review. *European Respiratory Review* 20 (121): 156–174.

Lavorini, F., Magnan, A., Dubus, J.C., Voshaar, T., Corbetta, L., Broeders, M., Dekhuijzen, R. et al. 2008. Effect of incorrect use of dry powder inhalers on management of patients with asthma and COPD. *Respiratory Medicine* 102 (4): 593–604.

Lee, S.C., Kang, S.-W., Kim, M.T., Kim, Y.K., Chang, W.H. and Im, S.H. 2013. Correlation between voluntary cough and laryngeal cough reflex flows in patients with traumatic brain injury. *Archives of Physical Medicine and Rehabilitation* 94 (8): 1580–1583.

Levick, C. and Dwight, J. 2007. Examination of the cardiovascular system. *Journal of Clinical Examination* 3: 8–14.

Luks, A.M. and Altemeier, W.A. 2006. Typical symptoms and atypical radiographic findings in a case of chronic eosinophilic pneumonia. *Respiratory Care* 51 (7): 764–767.

Magni, C., Chellini, E. and Zanasi, A. 2010. Cough variant asthma and atopic cough. *Multidisciplinary Respiratory Medicine*, 5 (2): 99–103.

Marshall, R.P., Puddicombe, A., Cookson, W.O.C. and Laurent, G.J. 2000. Adult familial cryptogenic fibrosing alveolitis in the United Kingdom. *Thorax* 55 (2): 143–146.

Mazzone, S.B. 2005. An overview of the sensory receptors regulating cough. *Cough*, 1 (2): 1–9.

Memtsoudis, S.G., Besculides, M.C., Gaber, L., Liu, S. and Valle, A.G.D. 2009. Risk factors for pulmonary embolism after hip and knee arthroplasty: A population-based study. *International Orthopaedics* 33 (6): 1739–1745.

Middleton, S. and Middleton, P.G. 2002. Assessment and investigations of patient perceptions. In: Prior, J.A. and Praesd, S.A. (eds.). *Physiotherapy for Respiratory Care and Cardiac Problems* (3rd ed.). Churchill Livingstone, London.

Miravitlles, M., Kruesmann, F., Haverstock, D., Perroncel, R., Choudhri, S.H. and Arvis, P. 2012. Sputum colour and bacteria in chronic bronchitis exacerbations: A pooled analysis. *European Respiratory Journal*, 39 (6): 1354–1360.

Moore, T. 2007. Respiratory assessment in adults. *Nursing Standard* 21 (49): 48–56.

National Institute for Health and Clinical Excellence. 2007. A*cutely Ill Patients in Hospital; Recognition of and Response to Acute Illness in Adults in Hospital*. NICE, London.

Nogués, M.A., Roncoroni, A.J. and Benarroch, E. 2002. Breathing control in neurological diseases. *Clinical Autonomic Research* 12 (6): 440–449.

Owen, A. 1998. Respiratory assessment revisited: Refresh your technique for spotting pulmonary problems. *Nursing* 28 (4): 48–49.

Resuscitation Council United Kingdom. 2010. *Resuscitation Guidelines*. Resuscitation Council, London.

Rosenman, K.D., Reilly, M.J., Schill, D.P., Valiante, D., Flattery, J., Harrison, R., Reinisch, F. et al. 2003. Cleaning products and work-related asthma. *Journal of Occupational & Environmental Medicine* 45 (5): 556–563.

Sanderson, M.J. 2011. Exploring lung physiology in health and disease with lung slices. *Pulmonary Pharmacological Therapy* 24 (5): 452–465.

Sapey, E. and Stockley, R.A. 2006. COPD exacerbations – 2: Aetiology. *Thorax* 61 (3): 250–258.

Saunders, J. and Smith, T. 2010. Malnutrition: Causes and consequences. *Clinical Medicine* 10 (6): 624–627.

Schwaiblmair, M., Behr, W., Haeckel, T., Märkl, B., Foerg, W. and Berghaus, T. 2012. Drug induced interstitial lung disease. *Open Respiratory Medical Journal* 6: 63–74.

Shoemark, A., Ozerovitch, L. and Wilson, R. 2007. Aetiology in adult patients with bronchiectasis. *Respiratory Medicine* 101 (6): 1163–1170.

Simpson, H. 2006. Respiratory assessment. *British Journal of Nursing* 15 (9): 484–488.

Steele, M.P., Speer, M.C., Loyd, J.E., Brown, K.K., Herron, A., Slifer, S.H., Burch, L.H. et al. 2005. Clinical and pathologic features of familial interstitial pneumonia. *American Journal of Respiratory and Critical Care Medicine* 172 (9): 1146–1152.

Thomas, P. 2005. 'I can't breathe' assessment and emergency management of acute dyspnoea. *Australian Family Physician* 34 (7): 523–529.

Verheij, J., van Lingen, A., Raijmakers, P.G., Rijnsburger, E.R., Veerman, D.P., Wisselink, W., Girbes, A.R. and Groeneveld, A.B. 2006. Effect of fluid loading with saline or colloids on pulmonary permeability, oedema and lung injury score after cardiac and major vascular surgery. *British Journal of Anaesthesia* 96 (1): 21–30.

Wheeldon, A. 2005. Exploring nursing roles: Using physical assessment in the respiratory unit. *British Journal of Nursing* 14 (10) 571–574.

Respiratory investigations

3

SIMON DOE

LEARNING OBJECTIVES

Upon completion of this chapter the reader should be able to:

- Identify the basic investigations used in respiratory medicine
- Describe tests of pulmonary function
- Identify methods of thoracic imaging
- Consider the appropriate clinical context for each investigation

INTRODUCTION

A starting point for reaching an accurate diagnosis is taking a detailed history followed by a comprehensive examination. This should help ideas form, to allow a differential diagnosis to be produced. In order to come to a firm diagnosis, it is usual to instigate a series of appropriate investigations which help confirm or refute initial suspicions. Investigations in respiratory care are important tools in differentiating diseases, but can also play a key role in monitoring disease progression and response to treatment.

This chapter will introduce some of the key investigations that are used in respiratory care and will demonstrate their utility in the diagnostic and monitoring process. However, it is vital to consider the patient experience and provide adequate explanation and support during the investigation and diagnostic process. Although investigations are unquestionably useful, they should not be performed without justification, as they may be uncomfortable and potentially harmful to the patient, and costly to the health service.

TESTS OF PULMONARY FUNCTION

There are many tests of pulmonary and ventilatory function and it can seem somewhat overwhelming for the uninitiated to overcome the numerous acronyms and technical data that healthcare professionals can be presented with. A simple understanding of each test and its relevance to clinical practice is all that is needed for most practitioners.

One concept that it is important to consider is what constitutes a 'normal' result. Any result is best considered in terms of 'Z scores', i.e. numbers of standard deviations from the mean that any individual result lies. As we are predominantly interested in values that are lower than 'normal', it is accepted that values of greater than 1.64 standard deviations below the mean are abnormal, this encompasses the lowest 5% of results.

SPIROMETRY

This is the most commonly used test of pulmonary function. Simply it is a test of the speed and amount (volume and flow) of air that can be exhaled from the lungs (Miller et al., 2005). Measurement of spirometry should be undertaken by persons trained to do so as technical deficiencies in the acquisition of the data can lead to significant misinterpretation of the results. Spirometry allows measurements such as the following to be made:

- Vital Capacity (VC)
- Forced Expiratory Volume in 1 Second (FEV$_1$)
- FEV$_1$/VC Ratio
- Forced Expiratory Flow in middle half of expiration (FEF 25-75)

VITAL CAPACITY

To measure vital capacity, from full inspiration a subject is asked to exhale fully. This volume of air is known as the vital capacity. In most cases the subject will be asked to do this with maximal effort with the term applied to this value known as the forced vital capacity (FVC) (Davies and Moores, 2010). If a slow, relaxed exhalation is used, this is sometimes termed the slow VC. The relevance of this is that in health the FVC and slow VC should be very similar. In the setting of airway obstruction with associated gas trapping this abnormality is amplified by the manoeuvre undertaken for a FVC, thus limiting the result compared with what may be achieved in a slow VC. This is a common pitfall encountered by the uninitiated and illustrates the importance of viewing the curve on a spirogram so that one can be certain that vital capacity has been reached (a flat line is seen for at least one second.)

Table 3.1 Causes of ventilatory defects on spirometry

Obstructive	Restrictive
COPD	Pulmonary fibrosis
Asthma (spirometry may be normal)	Neuromuscular abnormalities
Bronchiectasis	Thoracic cage abnormalities
	Obesity

Reduction in VC can be seen in association with any condition that limits full inspiration including:

- Thoracic cage abnormalities such as kyphoscoliosis
- Muscle weakness such as myasthenia gravis
- Decreased lung compliance such as pulmonary fibrosis
- Air trapping and hyperinflation such as chronic obstructive pulmonary disease (COPD) (Davies and Moores, 2010) (see Table 3.1)

FORCED EXPIRATORY VOLUME IN ONE SECOND (FEV$_1$) AND RATIO OF FEV$_1$/VC

To measure forced expiratory volume in 1 second (FEV$_1$), from full inspiration a subject is asked to exhale forcefully. The volume of air expired in the first second is known as the forced expiratory volume in one second (FEV$_1$). Any condition affecting the lungs will cause a reduction in the FEV$_1$, but this is particularly marked in the setting of airway obstruction. An important calculation is to derive the ratio of FEV$_1$ to VC – the FEV$_1$/VC. If this figure is below 0.7, airway obstruction is likely present and is known as an *obstructive defect*. If there is equal diminution of FEV$_1$ and VC, the FEV$_1$/VC is maintained and a *restrictive defect* is termed. See Figure 3.1 for an illustration of how FEV$_1$ and FVC may appear in health and how they might be changed by respiratory disease.

FORCED EXPIRATORY FLOW IN MIDDLE HALF OF EXPIRATION (FEF 25-75)

Many spirometers will give figures reflecting the airflow during the middle half of expiration. Diminution in these figures can reflect changes in the small

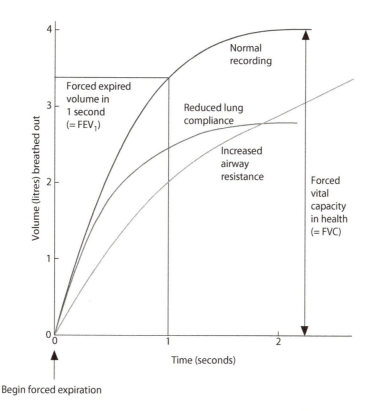

Figure 3.1 Example of spirogram showing normal, obstructive and restrictive curves. (From Clancy, J. and McVicar, A. 2009. *Physiology and Anatomy for Nurses and Healthcare Practitioners: A Homeostatic Approach* (3rd ed.). CRC Press, London. Figure 14.8. With permission.)

peripheral airways (for example in obliterative bron-chiolitis) before more diffuse changes develop; on such occasions the FEV_1 and VC may be normal.

OTHER TESTS OF PULMONARY FUNCTION

More detailed pulmonary function testing involves testing with more complex equipment using either helium dilution or body plethysmography (also known as a 'body box') (Borg and Thompson, 2012). A detailed understanding of these techniques is not required, but readers should be aware of the potential limitations of testing methods, e.g. morbid obesity or other mobility issues can prevent a patient entering plethysmography equipment. Similarly, tests utilis-ing helium dilution can involve breath holding that may not be achievable by the very breathless patient.

Other measurements that can be obtained in this way include:

- Total Lung Capacity (TLC)
- Residual Volume (RV)
- Transfer Factor (TLCO)
- Transfer Coefficient (KCO)

Total lung capacity is the volume of gas in the lungs after full inspiration. Generally speaking, this will be reduced in a restrictive disorder and can be increased in the setting of airway obstruction (secondary to gas trapping and hyperinflation). Individual methods for measuring TLC can be subject to some specific prob-lems causing misinterpretation.

Residual volume is the name given to the volume of air that remains in the lung after a full expiration. This volume commonly increases with chronic air-way disease owing to small airway collapse during expiration and subsequent gas trapping.

Transfer factor or TLCO is the correct name for a measurement that gives some information on the functionality of the alveolar-capillary membrane. The test uses carbon monoxide (the CO part of the acronym) to measure the ability of the body to transfer a gas to the bloodstream from the lung. The most commonly used technique to measure this is the single-breath method. A patient is asked to inspire a mix of gas containing helium and carbon monoxide and then hold their breath for 10 seconds, hence not all patients are able to complete this measurement (Davies and Moores, 2010). The concentration of gases is measured in the expired air and a formula applied to calculate a value for the TLCO. Many factors can influence the TLCO and include:

- Ventilation perfusion mismatch, which is common in many lung diseases
- Reduction in the area of alveolar-capillary membrane, for example emphysema
- Increased thickness of alveolar-capillary membrane, for example pulmonary fibrosis
- Pulmonary blood flow, for example pulmonary hypertension
- Haemoglobin concentration, for example anaemia leads to a decrease in TLCO

The transfer coefficient (KCO) is a value that is calculated by dividing the TLCO by the alveolar volume (VA). It is a useful measurement to give information on functionality 'per unit volume' of lung. The simplest example to consider would be a patient who undergoes a pneumonectomy, leaving behind a perfectly normally functioning single lung. In this case the TLCO would be reduced by 50% because simply there is less lung available. However, the lung that remains is normal, with a normal alveolar-capillary membrane; thus the KCO would be at 100%. In practical terms the measurement of TLCO/KCO can help differentiate disease states (see Table 3.2).

FLOW VOLUME LOOP

Flow volume loops can be another useful test to help differentiate the site of airway obstruction. It is particularly useful if concerns regarding large airway obstruction are apparent. Simply a flow volume loop plots flow (on the y axis) against volume (x axis)

Table 3.2 Patterns of transfer factor and coefficient in different respiratory diseases

	TLCO	KCO
Obstructive defect		
Asthma	Normal	Normal
COPD	Decreased	Decreased
Restrictive defect		
Intrapulmonary (e.g. IPF)	Decreased	Decreased
Extrapulmonary (e.g. obesity, thoracic cage abnormalities, etc.)	Decreased	Increased
Normal ventilation		
Pulmonary hypertension	Decreased	Decreased

(see Figure 3.2a). A forced expiration from TLC is the starting point. The nature of the airways is such that peak flow is reached quickly and can be measured. At full inspiration, airways are fully dilated with minimal airway resistance. Flow diminishes as expiration continues. The inspiratory limb is not a mirror image; a more symmetrical loop is produced owing to a larger contribution by the muscles of inspiration.

The flow volume loop has a typical appearance in the setting of diffuse airway obstruction as in COPD and is often said to have a 'church and steeple' appearance (see Figure 3.2c). Large airway obstruction (e.g. tracheal stenosis) also causes a recognisable appearance on the flow volume loop, termed the 'hamburger box' (see Figure 3.2c).

PEAK EXPIRATORY FLOW RATE

Peak expiratory flow rate (PEFR) can be derived from the flow volume loop, but is more commonly measured separately with a simple handheld device. The best of three attempts should be taken. It provides a measurement of diffuse airway obstruction and has a key role in the diagnosis and assessment of asthma. Variability noted on serial monitoring can help make the diagnosis in the correct circumstances. In an acute attack, PEFR can help clarify the severity of an attack and help monitor improvement with treatment. Changes in PEFR can be used by patients in a self-management plan to help them know when to seek medical attention (British Thoracic Society/Scottish Intercollegiate Guideline Network [BTS/SIGN, 2014]).

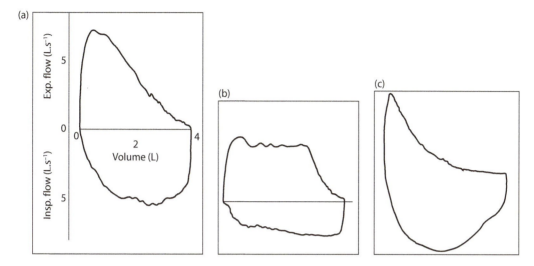

Figure 3.2 Examples of flow volume loops: (a) normal, (b) large airway obstruction ('hamburger box'), (c) diffuse small airway obstruction ('church and steeple').

TESTS OF BRONCHIAL HYPER RESPONSIVENESS

When the diagnosis of asthma is being considered:

1. *Bronchodilator reversibility:* If airway obstruction (FEV_1/VC <70%) is noted on spirometry, repeat testing after the administration of a bronchodilator such as nebulised salbutamol can help to determine if the obstruction is fixed and irreversible (e.g. COPD) or reversible (e.g. asthma). An improvement in FEV_1 of greater than 12% and 200 mL is taken as a positive test.
2. *Airways response:* Methacholine challenge is where increasing doses of a bronchoconstrictor agent, usually methacholine or histamine, can be administered and serial spirometry performed. If a greater than 20% fall in FEV_1 is noted, the likelihood of diagnosis of asthma can be inferred, depending on the concentration needed to elicit this fall.

RESPIRATORY MUSCLE TESTING

1. Erect and supine forced vital capacity is where weakness of the diaphragm typical leads to a decrease in VC of approximately 30% when the test is performed supine.

2. Mouth pressures is maximal inspiratory mouth pressure (PIMax) and maximal expiratory mouth pressure (PEMax) can be measured. Sniff nasal inspiratory pressure (SNIP) can also be measured. These values tend to fall globally with generalised muscle weakness. Inspiratory values are preferentially reduced with pure diaphragmatic weakness.

TESTS OF EXERCISE CAPACITY

1. Cardiopulmonary exercise testing (CPET) is a non-invasive test that simultaneously measures cardiorespiratory function. It has no real practical role in clinical respiratory medicine, but is utilised in helping assess risk for patients scheduled to undergo major surgery.
2. Six-minute walk test (6MWT) is a simple measurement of the distance walked in 6 minutes and oxygen saturation during this period, and can be a useful measure of functional status in patients with respiratory disease. It is often used as part of lung transplant assessment protocols (see Chapter 19).

THORACIC IMAGING

Imaging of the thorax is a key component in the investigation of likely respiratory disease. Some techniques are widely available, whereas others are more specialised and hospital based.

CHEST RADIOGRAPH (X-RAY)

The chest radiograph or X-ray is the most widely available and performed investigation into potential respiratory disease. Although a chest X-ray uses ionising radiation and consideration of risk should be given to all requests, the actual dose of radiation that a routine chest X-ray subjects a patient to is very low: on average it is 0.1 mSv, which is the equivalent to 10 days' exposure to background radiation in the atmosphere. This means that it is an accessible and appropriate investigation for most patients presenting with respiratory symptoms to help provide further information and/or guide further investigation.

Ideally films should be taken with the posterior–anterior (PA) view with the patient in the erect position. This minimises problems with interpretation caused by either over-magnification, for example when assessing cardiac size, or by artefacts produced by multiple structures overlying one another because a patient is asked to move their arms in such a way that the scapula are drawn from view. If a patient is very unwell, it may be necessary to perform an anterior–posterior (AP) or supine film. Ideally a lateral chest X-ray should also be taken as this aids interpretation and localisation of potential abnormalities (Ash-Miles and Callaway, 2008).

The viewer of a chest X-ray should have a structured approach to interpreting the film so that the chance of missing subtle abnormalities is minimised. Specific abnormalities can be seen on a chest X-ray including lobar collapse, consolidation, hyperinflation, abnormal masses, interstitial shadowing, cavitation and pleural effusions. Some of these abnormalities are so clear-cut and associated with the appropriate clinical context that no further imaging is required. The best example is of lobar consolidation on a chest X-ray of a patient presenting with a short history of fever, malaise, cough and sputum product providing a diagnosis of community-acquired pneumonia. Other abnormalities, once seen, may trigger further investigations, for example a smoker presenting with a new cough and lobar collapse on a chest X-ray will require a CT scan and bronchoscopy to look for a diagnosis of lung cancer.

COMPUTED TOMOGRAPHY (CT)

Computed tomography or CT scanning allows for cross-sectional imaging of the thorax. Developed in 1967 by Godfrey Hounsfield, images are generated by computer re-synthesis of data obtained from multiple X-ray beams that are shone at the patient and picked up by multiple X-ray detectors that rotate around them. Intravenous administration of radio-contrast material can be used to help define structures and interrogate blood vessels.

Technological developments have meant that the capability and resolution of CT scanners has dramatically increased in the last few years and this ability to acquire more and more detailed images is likely to progress. Such advances have meant that it is possible to acquire these images while administering a much smaller dose of ionising radiation than previously. However, the dose is still significantly greater than with a chest X-ray and should be considered with all patients. Special focus should be given to either pregnant or post-partum females as maternal breast tissue is very sensitive.

At the moment CT scanning can allow diagnosis and definition of many lung diseases, but it is important to be aware of the different techniques of undertaking the scan to ensure that the appropriate question is asked/answered.

CT THORAX WITH CONTRAST

This classical technique allows for cross-sectional imaging of the thorax and is used when initially assessing patients with undifferentiated disease. A staging CT of thorax and upper abdominal structures in the setting of likely lung cancer allows assessment of nodal status and inspection for possible metastatic disease in the liver, bones and adrenal glands. A delayed acquisition of images following contrast administration allows assessment of the pleura when worried about the potential of pleural malignancy and/or pleural infection such as empyema, a so-called pleural protocol CT.

HIGH-RESOLUTION CT SCANS (HRCT)

High-resolution CT is the term given to an acquisition process that leads to the production of highly detailed images. Its difference from 'normal' CT is that much thinner slices/images are reconstructed, typically 0.5–1 mm compared with 3–5 mm, with algorithms applied to increase detail. Typically, contrast is not administered. These images have traditionally been provided at 10 mm intervals of the lungs so that large areas are not directly imaged; therefore, small nodules or even tumours could be missed by this technique. It is designed to provide detail on processes that diffusely affect the lung so as not to require entire coverage. Principally this is used when assessing interstitial lung disease (ILD) or possible bronchiectasis. Accurate HRCT combined with expert interpretation can help multidisciplinary discussion of patients with suspected ILD and prevent the need for unnecessary tests such as biopsy. It is useful to obtain these images with the patient in the prone position so that subtle basal fibrotic changes can be seen and not mistaken for gravity-dependent changes that are commonly seen in the lung bases. If there is a good clinical suspicion of a hypersensitivity pneumonitis, images should be captured during inspiration and expiration so as to accentuate the typical findings of air trapping and mosaicism.

CT PULMONARY ANGIOGRAM (CTPA)

This investigation has evolved into the first-line investigation for suspected pulmonary embolism (PE), having been introduced in the 1990s as an alternative to ventilation/perfusion scanning. Intravenous contrast is used and image acquisition timed to allow optimal viewing of the pulmonary arteries with pulmonary emboli showing as a so-called 'filling defect' within them. Although CTPA has a high sensitivity and specificity, many scans are performed with a negative result, i.e. no PE is seen. They should only be requested when a full clinical assessment of the patient has been performed, ideally with reference to a clinical probability tool such as the Wells score (Wells et al., 1998, 2000; NICE, 2012).

CT GUIDED BIOPSY

CT can also be used to perform percutaneous sampling of a lung mass lesion allowing the operator to accurately localise this (NICE, 2011). Both fine needle aspirate for cytology and formal trucut biopsy for histology can be performed. There is a small but potentially serious risk of pneumothorax, so patient selection for the procedure is important.

OTHER IMAGING MODALITIES

VENTILATION PERFUSION SCANNING (V/Q SCAN)

This imaging technique utilises radionuclide imaging to gain information on both ventilation and perfusion in the lungs such that the scan is performed in two parts. V/Q scanning has largely been superseded by CTPA in recent times as the investigation of choice for diagnosing PE. It is still a useful test in some settings, including:

- Diagnosing PE in special circumstances such as first-line investigation in pregnant female alongside Doppler ultrasound of the legs (Royal College of Obstetricians and Gynaecologists [RCOG], 2015).
- Assessment of chronic thromboembolic disease.
- In assessing suitability for surgery in patients with borderline fitness, a differential perfusion scan may prove that a certain lobe of lung contributes little to overall function and could safely be removed.

POSITRON EMISSION TOMOGRAPHY CT (PET-CT)

A PET-CT scan uses two different forms of imaging at the same time and in respiratory medicine is commonly used to aid staging of lung cancer (NICE,

2011) and in the assessment of a solitary pulmonary nodule.

The PET component of the scan involves intravenous administration of radioactive glucose known as fluorodeoxyglucose or FDG. Metabolically active cells such as in cancerous tumours or inflammatory conditions such as sarcoidosis take up this compound preferentially. Given the radioactive nature of the compound a gamma camera is used to localise the site of the emission. Unenhanced CT images are then taken to provide more detailed anatomical information such as pinpointing the emission to a single lymph node or potential unexpected metastasis in an adrenal gland.

ULTRASOUND

Normal lung tissue filled with air does not transmit high-frequency sound waves such that ultrasound is not a routine investigation used in the assessment of lung disease. Where it is a very useful technique is in the assessment of pleural disease and pleural fluid. Bedside ultrasound can be used to localise pleural fluid for sampling. Following an alert issued by the National Patient Safety Agency (NPSA) (2008), it is recommended that ultrasound is used for all pleural procedures. Ultrasound can also be used to guide biopsy of pleural-based or chest wall masses.

BRONCHOSCOPY AND ENDOBRONCHIAL ULTRASOUND (EBUS)

Bronchoscopy is a procedure that allows direct access, visualisation and potential sampling of the bronchial tree. Flexible bronchoscopy is more commonly performed and can be done with topical anaesthesia and/or conscious sedation. A flexible bronchoscope allows access to segmental bronchi and sampling from these small airways. The usual indications to consider this investigation would be if a patient presented with symptoms of haemoptysis or if a potential lung cancer is suspected by findings on a chest X-ray.

Rigid bronchoscopy tends to be performed under general anaesthesia and can only visualise large airways. It may be more appropriate to perform in situations such as when concern exists about potential large volume haemoptysis as its greater diameter can allow for a greater degree of intervention.

BRONCHOSCOPIC SAMPLING AND INTERVENTIONS

There are many different types of samples that can be taken during a bronchoscopy and these are discussed below. Increasingly, bronchoscopy can be used for a potential therapeutic intervention and this is discussed briefly too.

- Bronchoalveolar lavage (BAL) allows up to 60 millilitres of normal saline to be instilled into the airway. This can usually be directly inserted into a specific segment of the lung. This fluid is then aspirated from the lung and can be sent to the laboratory where it can undergo cytological analysis for possible malignancy and microbiological analysis.
- Bronchial brush is a small brush that can be directed through the bronchoscope to take samples from an abnormal-looking area of mucosa. This can then be sent for cytological analysis. A bronchial brush is usually performed when malignancy is suspected.
- Endobronchial biopsy under direct-vision forceps can sample visualised abnormalities with samples able to undergo histological analysis.
- Transbronchial biopsy can be taken from the alveolar spaces when the forceps are directed into a specific segmental airway. The procedure is performed when considering a diagnosis of interstitial lung disease. It should be undertaken with caution. It can be complicated by the development of a pneumothorax.
- Transbronchial nodal aspiration (TBNA) attempts to sample lymph nodes lying beyond the airway. A needle can be passed through the wall with samples adequate for cytological analysis. It requires an excellent appreciation of normal anatomy and more recently has been superseded by TBNA performed during endobronchial ultrasound (EBUS).
- Insertion of airway stents means airways that have been narrowed, usually by tumours, can be mechanically opened by the insertion of a stent.

- Endobronchial laser is often used as an adjunct to stenting to debulk bulky obstructing tumours.
- Removal of foreign body is best achieved with a rigid bronchoscope. It most commonly takes the form of vegetable matter such as a pea.
- Insertion of endobronchial valve is an emerging technique in patients with significant emphysema. A one-way valve is inserted to attempt a form of lung volume reduction surgery. Data are still emerging on their effectiveness.

Within the last 10 years, EBUS has been developed and it is now a vital part of the investigation of respiratory disease. In this setting, a modified bronchoscope is used with an ultrasound probe mounted onto the distal end. This allows the operator to localise mediastinal lymph nodes and aspirate samples under direct vision. It is a very useful investigation in staging the mediastinum in lung cancer, but can also be used in non-malignant disease such as sarcoidosis and TB lymphadenitis.

Bronchoscopy and EBUS are generally safe procedures to undergo. Caution should be exercised in those with low levels of lung function, particularly if sedation is to be used.

USEFUL INVESTIGATIONS

BLOOD TESTS

There are several blood tests that can be useful in investigating potential respiratory disease, although no test in itself is diagnostic. These include:

- Full blood count as the white blood cell count can be a useful marker of acute infection/ inflammation. The differential count can be useful as serum eosinophils can be raised in some cases of asthma.
- Erythrocyte sedimentation rate (ESR) can be raised with a diagnosis of cryptogenic organising pneumonia, among other conditions.
- Auto antibodies: it is necessary to check auto antibodies when faced with a new diagnosis of interstitial lung disease, particularly if there

are extra-pulmonary features that may indicate connective tissue disease.
- Immunoglobulins as hypogammaglobulinemia can be associated with bronchiectasis.
- Serum angiotensin converting enzyme (ACE) can be raised in sarcoidosis, although it is not specific. This is more useful as a serial marker of disease activity over time than a diagnostic test based on a single figure.
- Immunoglobulin E (IgE): In uncontrolled asthma a raised level of IgE can suggest treatment benefit from anti-IgE treatment such as Omalizumab.
- Anti-nuclear cytoplasmic antibody (ANCA) is used if a diagnosis of vasculitis is being considered.
- D-Dimer if used appropriately has a role in the diagnosis of DVT/PE. Combined with a clinical probability score suggesting a low probability of PE, a low D-Dimer means further investigation does not need to be pursued. If the clinical probability of PE is high, further investigation is needed irrespective of D-Dimer level.
- Arterial blood gases: Interpretation of ABGs is covered in detail in Chapter 4.

SPUTUM CULTURE AND SENSITIVITY

Sputum culture and sensitivity is a very important test in patients with bronchiectasis or presenting with acute cough and sputum production where diagnosis of pneumonia is considered. If pneumonia is confirmed, urine for pneumococcal and legionella antigen should be sent if the CURB-65 score is greater than 1 (NICE, 2014) (see Chapter 10). If TB is a differential diagnosis, sputum should be sent specifically for smear testing: ideally three samples and prolonged TB culture, which can take up to 6 weeks.

SKIN PRICK TESTS (SPTs)

SPTs are an inexpensive test that rely upon immediate type hypersensitivity. A small amount of diluted antigen is placed under the skin alongside histamine as a positive control, and an inert solution to act as a negative control. Local reaction is then looked for. Common tests included in the panel are: house dust mite, grasses, pollen, cats, dogs and Aspergillus. They should be considered in patients with uncontrolled asthma to allow identification of potential allergens. If considering Omalizumab therapy, allergy to a common aero-allergen needs to be demonstrated (NICE, 2013).

SWEAT TEST

This test is performed if a diagnosis of cystic fibrosis (CF) is being considered. A value of sweat chloride of more than 60 mmol/L is diagnostic of CF in the appropriate clinical setting. A value of less than 30 mmol/L is normal. Results between 30 and 60 mmol/L should be considered indeterminate with interpretation alongside clinical information on CF genotyping (Farrell et al., 2008).

SUMMARY

There are many and varied investigations that can be considered when reviewing a patient with possible respiratory disease. To help summarise it could be useful to consider things differently by listing the most appropriate investigations to consider in specific situations:

1. *Chronic Obstructive Pulmonary Disease*
   Diagnosis is aided by performing spirometry demonstrating an FEV_1/VC ratio of <0.7. TLCO/KCO low will suggest emphysema. A chest X-ray will demonstrate signs of hyperinflation.
2. *Asthma*
   A chest X-ray may be normal or show signs of hyperinflation. Spirometry may be normal or show significant bronchodilator reversibility. A bronchial hyper responsiveness test may be performed. A full blood count may demonstrate an eosinophilia. SPTs and IgE may be positive.
3. *Interstitial Lung Disease (including sarcoidosis)*
   A chest X-ray will show reduced lung volumes and reticular-nodular infiltrate prompting a high-resolution CT scan. Spirometry will show a restrictive defect and TLCO/KCO will be reduced. Auto antibodies should be checked. On occasions bronchoscopy and transbronchial biopsy may be considered.
4. *Lung Cancer*
   A chest X-ray will prompt further investigation. A staging CT thorax should be performed. A biopsy will need to be undertaken and this may need a CT guided approach, bronchoscopy or EBUS. PET-CT may be needed to complete staging. Spirometry and TLCO/KCO will help assess patient suitability for treatment.
5. *Bronchiectasis*
   Chest X-ray and spirometry should be performed but diagnosis will be made on HRCT chest. Sputum culture should be performed and thought given to the potential cause of bronchiectasis such that some blood tests, auto antibodies and immunoglobulins including IgE, and investigating for CF such as a sweat test may be considered.
6. *Pleural Effusion*
   A chest X-ray will show an effusion. If appropriate, a pleural protocol CT thorax should be done. Ultrasound guided aspiration of fluid will allow sampling to be undertaken.

The above represents a good introduction to the common investigations that are performed when assessing a patient with potential respiratory disease. More detailed understanding of the pathophysiological processes of these diseases, covered in the later chapters of this book, should enable a more comprehensive understanding of when and where each test should be performed and how it should be interpreted.

REFERENCES

Ash-Miles, J. and Callaway, M. 2008. Understanding and interpretating a chest x-ray. *British Journal of Cardiac Nursing* 3 (11): 500–505.

Borg, B.M. and Thompson, B.R. 2012. The measurement of lung volumes using body plethysmography: A comparison of methodologies. *Respiratory Care* 57 (7): 1067–1083.

British Thoracic Society/Scottish Intercollegiate Guidelines Network. 2014. *British Guideline on the Management of Asthma: Revised 2014.* Available at: https://www.brit-thoracic.org.uk/document-library/clinical-information/asthma/btssign-asthma-guideline-2014/

Davies, A. and Moores, C. 2010. *The Respiratory System* (2nd ed.). *Basic Science and Clinical Conditions.* Churchill Livingstone, Edinburgh.

Farrell, P.M., Rosenstein, B.J., White, T.B., Accurso, F.J., Castellani, C., Cutting, G.R., Durie, P.R. et al. 2008. Guidelines for diagnosis of cystic fibrosis in newborns through older adults: Cystic Fibrosis Foundation Consensus Report. *Journal of Pediatrics* 153 (2): S4–S14.

Miller, M.R., Hankinson, J., Brusasco, V., Burgos, F., Casaburi, R., Coates, A., Crapo, R. et al. 2005. Standardisation of spirometry. *European Respiratory Journal* 6 (20): 319–338.

National Institute of Health and Care Excellence. 2011. *Lung Cancer: The Diagnosis and Treatment of Lung Cancer.* Clinical Guideline 121. NICE, London.

National Institute of Health and Care Excellence. 2012. *Venous Thromboembolic Diseases: The Management of Venous Thromboembolic Diseases and the Role of Thrombophilia Testing.* Clinical Guideline 144. NICE, London.

National Institute of Health and Care Excellence. 2013. *Omalizumab for Treating Severe Persistent Allergic Asthma (Review of Technology Appraisal Guidance 133 and 201) Technology Appraisal Guidance.* Technology Appraisal Guidance 278. NICE, London.

National Institute for Health and Care Excellence. 2014. *Pneumonia. Diagnosis and Management of Community and Hospital Acquired Pneumonia in Adults.* Clinical Guideline 191. NICE, London.

National Patient Safety Agency. 2008. Rapid Response Report. Chest drains: Risks of chest drain insertion. NPSA/2008/RRR003.

Royal College of Obstetricians and Gynaecologists. 2015. *Thromboembolic Disease in Pregnancy and the Puerperium: Acute Management.* Green Top Guideline No. 37b. RCOG.

Wells, P.S., Anderson, D.R., Rodger, M., Ginsberg, J.S., Kearon, C., Gent, M., Turpie, A.G. et al. 2000. Derivation of a simple clinical model to categorize patients probability of pulmonary embolism: Increasing the models utility with the SimpliRED D-dimer. *Journal of Thrombosis and Haemostasis* 83 (3): 416–420.

Wells, P.S., Ginsberg, J.S., Anderson, D.R., Kearon, C., Gent, M., Turpie, A.G., Bormanis, J. et al. 1998. Use of a clinical model for safe management of patients with suspected pulmonary embolism. *Annals of Internal Medicine* 129 (12): 997–1005.

FURTHER READING

Gibson, G.J. 2009. *Clinical Tests of Respiratory Function.* Oxford University Press, Oxford.

Hansell, D.M. 2003. Thoracic imaging. In: Gibson, G.J., Geddes, D.M., Costabel, U., Sterk, P.J., Corrin, B. (eds.). *Respiratory Medicine.* WB Saunders Co, London, 316–351.

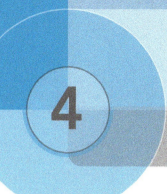

Pulse oximetry and arterial blood gas analysis

4

VANESSA GIBSON

LEARNING OBJECTIVES

Upon completion of this chapter the reader should be able to:

- Differentiate between Type 1 and Type 2 respiratory failure
- Differentiate between SpO_2 and PaO_2
- Discuss the indications and limitations of pulse oximetry
- Describe the key factors that affect acid-base balance
- Identify the components of arterial blood gases and understand their significance
- Demonstrate an ability to interpret arterial blood gases correctly

INTRODUCTION

Both pulse oximetry and arterial blood gas (ABG) measurement provide important information in the assessment of patients with respiratory disease. Pulse oximetry is a simple, non-invasive measure of arterial oxygen saturation (SpO_2), but does have limitations regarding the amount of information it provides. In contrast, an ABG measurement provides much more information concerning the patient's physiological status, such as their respiratory and metabolic function, in addition to other parameters such as electrolytes and haemoglobin measurements. However, obtaining an ABG sample can be a painful procedure for the patient, owing to either cannulation of an artery to insert an arterial line, or by the 'arterial stab' method (Crawford, 2004). Capillary blood gases may provide an easier and less painful alternative to sampling arterial blood and this method is now used by a number of respiratory services (Zavorsky et al., 2006). Whether arterial or capillary blood is used in the sample, it is vital that healthcare staff have the knowledge and skills to interpret the results.

This chapter will cover the relevant physiology in relation to oxygen (O_2) and carbon dioxide (CO_2) transport. The section on pulse oximetry will discuss how it works, what it measures and its uses and

45

limitations. Normal values for ABGs will be discussed and the importance of each component will be explained in turn. A five-step framework will be explained to aid in the interpretation of ABGs and some examples will be given so that the reader can practice interpretation.

PULSE OXIMETRY

The British Thoracic Society (BTS) recommends that oxygen saturation should be checked by trained staff using pulse oximetry in all breathless and acutely unwell patients (O'Driscoll et al., 2008). This should be recorded on the patient's observation chart, along with the inspired oxygen concentration if the patient is receiving oxygen therapy. If the patient is breathing air this should also be documented. A normal oxygen saturation does not confirm that a patient is not in a dangerous situation; an oxygen saturation may be normal in a patient, but they may have dangerously altered pH or CO_2 levels. In this situation an ABG will be invaluable and O'Driscoll et al. (2008) give advice as to when ABG sampling is necessary (see later in this chapter). Pulse oximetry must be available in all locations where emergency oxygen is being used and the BTS makes reference to the fact that emergency oxygen should be available in primary care settings and that pulse oximetry should be continuously in use until the patient arrives at hospital and has a full assessment (O'Driscoll et al., 2008).

The pulse oximeter measures and displays the pulse rate and the saturation of haemoglobin in arterial blood. It uses a combination of red and infrared light together with a sensor and photo detector to determine the oxygen saturation. The probe must be placed over a pulsating vascular bed such as the index finger or earlobe. Toes may be used but are likely to produce a poor signal because of decreased perfusion. Pulse oximeters do not require calibration. Pulse oximetry is a useful tool in the evaluation of a patient's oxygenation as it is simple to use, reliable, non-invasive, continuous and accurate when used appropriately. However, there are a number of limitations that the user should be aware of (Demeulenaere, 2007).

The pulse oximeter is obviously more sensitive than the human eye in detecting hypoxemia, but there is a short time delay between the reading and the patient's condition. There will be an interval of approximately 8 seconds after the patient's oxygen saturation starts to fall before it is detected by the device (Demeulenaere, 2007).

Poor perfusion is the most common cause of failure in obtaining an adequate signal. Poor peripheral perfusion may be caused by hypotension, cold extremities, vasoconstriction, low cardiac output or vasoactive drugs such as norepinephrine (noradrenaline). Poor waveforms indicate poor blood flow making the readings spurious. Warming the peripheries if possible or repositioning the probe may help (Woodrow, 2012).

Motion caused by the patient continually moving about, shivering or seizures will cause inaccurate readings. Other conditions that may affect the reading include venous congestion of the limb, oedema and cardiac arrhythmias. Because the pulse oximeter relies on light detection to calculate oxygen saturation, high-intensity lighting may affect the accuracy of the reading. There has been some debate as to whether or not skin pigmentation, bilirubinaemia and nail polish affect readings (Booker, 2008; Woodrow, 2012). Demeulenaere (2007) suggests that only black, green or blue polish will affect the signal.

Demeulenaere (2007) also suggests that pulse oximeters may be inaccurate in the presence of abnormal haemoglobin levels. Pulse oximeters measure the percentage saturation of haemoglobin, not the quantity of haemoglobin or oxygen available, and should always be interpreted in relation to haemoglobin levels (Woodrow, 2012). Carbon monoxide poisoning will result in inaccurate SpO_2 readings, owing to the presence of carboxyhaemoglobin, which will produce falsely high levels. Smokers will often have falsely high SpO_2 owing to increased carboxyhaemoglobin levels.

The pulse oximeter provides useful, but limited, information. SpO_2 is the percentage measure of oxygen-saturated haemoglobin in a person's circulating bloodstream. The measurement, however, does not provide information about the delivery or consumption of oxygen. Tissue oxygen supply is affected by the amount of haemoglobin, haemoglobin saturation, oxygen dissociation and perfusion pressure (Woodrow, 2012). It provides no indication of pH or CO_2 levels. Pulse oximetry is thought to be reliable at readings that range between 70% and 100% SpO_2.

Presumably a decreasing SpO_2 would alert clinical staff to conduct further tests and intervene with the patient long before saturation levels reach 70%. Super saturation levels of 199% have also been reported and were thought to be a technical problem with the monitor (Bhatia, 2012). Because of the limitations discussed above, clinical staff should not be complacent about the pulse oximeter reading and it should never replace careful clinical assessment of the patient.

A small audit by Howell (2002) demonstrated deficits in knowledge among nurses and doctors regarding the correct use and interpretation of pulse oximetry. Therefore, clinical staff should always ensure that:

- The chosen area for the probe is warm and has good circulation.
- The pulse oximeter is given five minutes to settle before the reading is recorded.
- The probe is the correct size and type for the chosen area, e.g. finger probes should not be used on the earlobe.
- The light emitter and photo detector are correctly aligned opposite each other.
- Self-adhesive probes are not applied too tightly.
- The probe is repositioned every one to two hours and the skin is checked for pressure damage and burns.
- The pulse oximeter is recording a pulse wave that corresponds to the radial pulse or ECG recording.
- Pulse oximeters are serviced regularly.

(Howell, 2002; Booker, 2008; Woodrow, 2012).

ARTERIAL BLOOD GASES

Analysis of arterial blood gases will provide clinical staff with a range of information about the respiratory and metabolic status of the patient. It will also indicate the severity of the problem and whether or not the condition is acute or chronic. However, in order to determine this information staff must have an understanding of the underlying physiological mechanisms which maintain oxygenation, CO_2 and acid–base balance. This information should always be interpreted alongside the patient's clinical history and current condition.

The BTS recommend that ABGs should be measured in the following situations:

- All critically ill patients.
- Unexpected or inappropriate hypoxemia (SpO_2 <94%) or any patient requiring oxygen to achieve this target saturation.
- Deteriorating oxygen saturation or increased breathlessness in a patient with previously stable hypoxemia, e.g. chronic obstructive pulmonary disease (COPD).
- Any previously stable patient who deteriorates and requires increased inspired oxygen concentration.
- Any patient with risk factors for hypercapnic respiratory failure who develops acute breathlessness, deteriorating SpO_2, drowsiness, or other symptoms of CO_2 retention.
- Breathless patients who are at risk of metabolic conditions such as diabetic ketoacidosis.
- Acutely breathless or critically ill patients with poor peripheral circulation where pulse oximetry may be unreliable due to a poor signal.
- Any other evidence from the patient's medical condition that would indicate ABGs would be useful (e.g. an unexpected change in the patient's early warning score [EWS] or a fall in SpO_2 by 3%).

(O'Driscoll et al., 2008)

THE COMPONENTS OF ARTERIAL BLOOD GASES

Although contemporary blood gas analysers can provide a number of blood results such as blood glucose, sodium and potassium (Woodrow, 2012), the components of ABGs have traditionally included the following:

- Hydrogen ion concentration (pH).
- Partial pressure of oxygen dissolved in arterial blood (PaO_2).
- Partial pressure of CO_2 dissolved in arterial blood ($PaCO_2$).
- Bicarbonate (HCO_3) (this may be both actual and standard bicarbonate).
- Base excess/Base deficit (BE) (the estimate of the degree of metabolic acidosis or alkalosis;

refers to the amount of acid or base that is needed to restore the pH to normal).

- Saturation of haemoglobin by oxygen in arterial blood (SaO_2).

(Simpson, 2004).

Each of these will be discussed in turn, together with their normal values (see Table 4.1). Normal values may differ slightly in different texts and in different departments, but for the purposes of this chapter the values given by Simpson (2004) will be used as a reference point. It should also be remembered that the normal range of PaO_2, and SaO_2 will differ with age and whether the person is in an upright or supine position (O'Driscoll et al., 2008). In the United Kingdom (UK) blood gases are measured in kilopascals (kPa), whereas in other countries such as the United States (US) millimetres of mercury (mmHg) are used (Simpson, 2004). For purposes of conversion (Woodrow, 2012), 1 kPa equals 7.4 mmHg.

In order to analyse arterial blood gases a sample of arterial blood will be taken. This may be taken as a one-off procedure known as an 'arterial stab' or an arterial catheter may be inserted if the patient is in a critical care unit. The arterial catheter will allow continuous measurement of blood pressure and regular arterial blood sampling without the need to repeatedly puncture the patient. Crawford (2004) reports that during an 'arterial stab' procedure, patients recorded a pain level of 5 or above using a visual analogue scale; O'Driscoll et al. (2008) therefore recommend that local anaesthesia should always be used, except in emergencies or if the patient is unconscious or anaesthetised. An arterial stab may have other complications such as arteriospasm and haematoma formation and should only be performed by competent staff that are

aware of these potential complications. In addition, the sample requires careful handling so that sampling errors do not occur. All air bubbles should be expelled from the sample, it should not be shaken and it should be transported to the laboratory immediately if a blood gas analyser is not available in the clinical area (Casey, 2013). Arterial lines are associated with a number of very significant risks including haemorrhage, thrombus formation, air emboli, ischaemia and inappropriate fluid use leading to hypoglycaemia and therefore should only be utilised in the critical care unit by staff who have been trained in their use (Kaur, 2006; Leslie et al., 2013). Capillary sampling offers a safer and more convenient alternative for clinical areas that do not commonly use arterial lines or when staff are unfamiliar with their use.

ACID–BASE BALANCE

In order to interpret ABGs and understand acid–base balance, some terminology must be understood and this is given in Table 4.2. Acid–base balance maintains the body's pH within normal limits by a number of compensatory mechanisms, the most important ones being buffers and the respiratory and renal systems.

pH refers to the number of hydrogen (H^+) ions present in a solution. The pH scale ranges from 0 (very acidic, lots of hydrogen ions) to 14 (very alkalotic). Water has a pH of 7 and is therefore neutral. The normal pH of arterial blood is 7.35–7.45, whereas the normal H^+ concentration is 36–44 mmol/L. Hydrogen ion concentration and pH have an inverse relationship to each other, that is, as H^+ ion concentration in the blood increases, pH will decrease, indicating an acidosis (Davies and Moores, 2010). Therefore, in relation to arterial blood, a pH of less than 7.35 (low) would indicate an acidosis, whereas a pH of above 7.45 (high) would indicate an alkalosis. It has been suggested that a pH of below 7 or above 7.8 would make survival unlikely (Davies and Moores, 2010). However, that will depend on the cause of the acid–base disturbance and the swiftness and effectiveness of treatment.

A number of potentially life-threatening changes may take place in the body because of an abnormal pH. The biochemistry of the body is very tightly controlled to maintain homeostasis. Several biochemical processes are conducted by enzymes, which will

Table 4.1 Normal values for arterial blood gases

Parameter	Normal value
PaO_2	11.5–13 kPa
pH	7.35–7.45
$PaCO_2$	4.5–6.0 kPa
HCO_3 (Standard)	22–26
BE	–2 to +2 mmol/L
SaO_2	94%–98% (O'Driscoll et al., 2008)

Source: Adapted from Simpson, H. 2004. *British Journal of Nursing*, 13 (9); 522–528.

Table 4.2 Explanations of terminology

Acid	A hydrogen ion donor. In solution strong acids will dissociate, releasing hydrogen ions and lowering pH and therefore contribute to acidosis
Base	A hydrogen ion acceptor. Bases are substances that will accept a free hydrogen ion and therefore reduce the hydrogen ion concentration of a solution and increase pH (alkalines)
Acidaemia	Arterial blood pH of less than 7.35
Alkalaemia	Arterial blood pH of greater than 7.45
Acidosis	An abnormal process that lowers pH
Alkalosis	An abnormal process that increases pH
Mixed disorder	Where two or more primary acid–base abnormalities co-exist. For instance, very sick patients may have both a respiratory and a metabolic cause for their acidosis or alkalosis
Compensation	These are normal body functions (respiratory or renal) that will endeavour to return the pH to normal and therefore maintain acid–base balance
Buffer	These are substances that can combine with acids or bases to help return the pH to normal
Hypoxia	Reduced oxygen content of the tissues
Hypoxaemia	Reduced oxygen content in arterial blood
Hypercapnia	Abnormally high levels of CO_2 in the blood

Source: Adapted from Tortora, G.J. and Derrickson, B. 2012. *Principles of Anatomy and Physiology* (13th ed.). John Wiley and Sons Inc, Hoboken, NJ; Marieb, E.N. 2012. *Essentials of Human Anatomy and Physiology* (10th ed.). Benjamin Cummings, Boston, MA; Hennessey, I.A.M. and Japp, A.G. 2016. *Arterial Blood Gases Made Easy* (2nd ed.). Elsevier, Edinburgh.

only function correctly within the normal pH range. Abnormal pH will affect the oxygen dissociation curve (see Chapter 1) and therefore oxygen delivery to, and consumption by vital organs. Abnormal pH can affect blood vessels, cell membranes and electrolyte balance. Because H+ is positively charged it effects the concentration of other positively charged ions including potassium, sodium and calcium. Potassium, sodium and calcium are all important in electrical impulse production and muscle function. See Table 4.3 for further signs and symptoms.

OXYGENATION

During normal cellular metabolism all cells utilise oxygen and produce CO_2 as a waste product, and therefore cells require a constant supply of oxygen. As oxygen is inhaled into the lungs the concentration gradient between the lungs and the pulmonary capillaries means that oxygen diffuses into the blood. The oxygen molecules are then transported around the body, either reversibly bound to haemoglobin (97%), or dissolved in plasma (3%). PaO_2 measured in ABGs represents the partial pressure of oxygen in arterial blood and is the small percentage of oxygen that is

dissolved in plasma. Because of the concentration gradient between oxygen in the blood and oxygen in the cells, oxygen diffuses into the cells where it is utilised to produce adenosine triphosphate (ATP). As with SpO_2, PaO_2 should always be interpreted in the context of the amount of oxygen the patient was receiving when the ABGs were taken. A PaO_2 of 12 kPa on room air provides a different picture than a PaO_2 of 12 kPa for a patient breathing 80% oxygen (Simpson, 2004).

Although pH is an important indicator of respiratory efficiency, hypoxemia is life threatening and therefore it has been used as Step 1 in the framework given below. Because of the limitations of pulse oximetry, PaO_2 should always be assessed if there are concerns about the patient. In interpreting the PaO_2, if the value is lower than the normal range (11.5–13 kPa) then the patient has hypoxemia and should result in treatment to correct this. The patient's PaO_2 may also be above the upper limit, indicating hyper-oxygenation. This situation is equally undesirable and should result in strategies to reduce the patient's oxygen level to normal (Woodrow, 2012). In some cases, people with chronic disease such as COPD may function with a lower than normal PaO_2. It is therefore vitally important when interpreting ABGs to know what is 'normal' for the patient and consult previous ABG results.

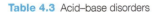

Table 4.3 Acid–base disorders

Respiratory acidosis	Respiratory alkalosis
Potential sources may be inadequate ventilation resulting in an increase in CO_2 levels. Under ventilation might be as a result of respiratory disease, neurological disease, neuromuscular weakness, drug-induced (opiates) or inappropriate mechanical ventilation.	**Potential sources** may be over ventilation resulting in a decrease in CO_2 levels. Over ventilation might be the result of anxiety, respiratory disease such as early COPD, drug-induced (salicylates) or inappropriate mechanical ventilation.
Signs and symptoms include: Flushing, vasodilation and warm peripheries, headache and raised intracranial pressure, drowsiness, confusion, coma, flapping tremor and muscle weakness.	**Signs and symptom include**: Increased heart rate, angina, arrhythmias, anxiety, sweating, dizziness and tingling to the extremities.
Metabolic acidosis	**Metabolic alkalosis**
Potential sources may be excess production of hydrogen ions. This may include diabetic ketoacidosis, starvation, alcohol abuse, lactic acidosis (shock), renal failure, excessive loss of alkaline secretions such as diarrhoea or ingestion (methanol, salicylates).	**Potential sources** may be excessive loss of acids from the body such as severe prolonged vomiting or gastric drainage, diuretic therapy or alkaline ingestion or administration.
Signs and symptoms include: Deep rapid respiration (Kussmaul's breathing), headache, lethargy, nausea and vomiting, arrhythmias, hypotension and coma. Acidosis will result in hyperkalaemia, which is life threatening.	**Signs and symptoms include**: Decreased respiration, confusion, convulsions, muscle cramps, tetany and arrhythmias. Alkalosis will result in hypokalaemia, which is life threatening.

Source: Adapted from Simpson, H. 2004. *British Journal of Nursing*, 13 (9): 522–528; Rogers, K. and McCutcheon, K. 2013. *The Journal of Perioperative Practice*, 23 (9): 191–197.

CARBON DIOXIDE

Air contains virtually no CO_2, but during normal cellular metabolism the body produces around 200 mL per minute. Because of the concentration gradient between the cells and the blood, CO_2 diffuses into the blood where it is transported to the lungs either bound to haemoglobin (20%), dissolved in plasma (10%) or as bicarbonate (70%). The haemoglobin of the red blood cells produces bicarbonate from CO_2 and this is released into the blood. In solution, CO_2 combines with water to produce carbonic acid (H_2CO_3) (see Chapter 1).

$$CO_2 + H_2O = H_2CO_3$$

In the lungs carbonic acid converts back into water and CO_2 and is excreted (Woodrow, 2012). Normally an increase in $PaCO_2$ would stimulate an increased respiratory rate until the $PaCO_2$ returns to normal. Therefore, a normal $PaCO_2$ is an indication of efficient breathing. Any circumstances that result in increased levels of CO_2 in the blood will result in an acidosis. This is normally a result of decreased tidal volume or decreased respiratory rate (see Table 4.3).

When interpreting the $PaCO_2$, if the value is higher than the normal range (5.5–6 kPa) then the patient has hypercapnia, which may require an intervention to correct this. This will almost certainly require the use of non-invasive ventilation (NIV) or mechanical ventilation (see Chapter 17). The patient's $PaCO_2$ may also be lower than normal and this situation is equally undesirable and should result in strategies to bring the patient's $PaCO_2$ up to normal levels. In some cases, people with chronic disease such as COPD may function with a higher than normal $PaCO_2$, it is therefore vitally important when interpreting ABGs to know what is 'normal' for the patient and consult previous ABG results.

BUFFERS

Put simply, buffers can either release or extract (mop up) H^+ ions, depending on the H^+ ion concentration in the blood (Casey, 2013). By donating or binding a H^+ ion, buffers are able to maintain the pH within normal limits. Buffers include the bicarbonate and carbonic acid chain (represented by the equation in Chapter 1), haemoglobin, plasma proteins, phosphates, respiratory and renal systems. Buffers keep the H^+ ions 'mopped up' until they can be excreted by either the respiratory or the renal system. As previously discussed the lungs maintain pH via the excretion of CO_2, whereas the kidneys maintain pH via the excretion of H^+ ions into the urine and the reabsorption of bicarbonate. The kidneys can adjust the excretion of H^+ and bicarbonate in response to the pH of the blood (Hennessey and Japp, 2016). The respiratory system responds very quickly to changes in pH (seconds), whereas the renal system is much slower and can take hours to days (Burns, 2014).

BASE EXCESS/BASE DEFICIT

The base excess or base deficit is indicative of metabolic alkalosis (excess) or metabolic acidosis (deficit). However, this is usually referred to as just base excess (BE). This is given as a calculated figure with the normal range being: –2 to +2. A figure more positive than +2 would indicate an excess of bases (metabolic alkalosis), whereas a figure more negative than –2 would indicate a deficit of bases (metabolic acidosis). BE measures metabolic acid-base balance and is used to indicate moles of acid or base needed to restore one litre of blood to pH 7.4 (Woodrow, 2012). BE indicates the amount of all bases, not just bicarbonate. Bicarbonate is the biggest component of the base buffers and therefore, in terms of practical purposes and simplicity, BE provides principally the same information as bicarbonate (HCO_3) (Burns, 2014). BE and HCO_3 follow the same direction, so in effect if the bicarbonate is high the BE will be positive. Indeed, Simpson (2004) suggests that clinical staff do not need to use BE to interpret blood gas readings correctly.

COMPENSATION

Every day the body will produce acid as a by-product of metabolism. As previously discussed these acids or H^+ ions will be buffered until they are excreted by either the respiratory or renal systems. If, for example, during illness an excess of H^+ ions are produced (e.g. during shock) the body will attempt to compensate for this and maintain the pH within the normal range. This involves the respiratory and metabolic (renal) systems working collaboratively. So if there is a metabolic problem (e.g. shock/lactic acidosis) the respiratory system will increase the respiratory rate and compensate by 'blowing off' CO_2. On the other hand, if there is a respiratory problem (retention of CO_2) the renal system will increase reabsorption of bicarbonate to neutralise the excess acid created by the CO_2. It is when the compensation mechanisms fail that an abnormal pH is seen and an acid-base disturbance is created. When reviewing blood gases there are several types of compensation which can occur and this can lead to confusion in interpreting ABGs. These are:

- An uncompensated condition. This indicates an acute illness where the normal compensatory mechanisms have been quickly overwhelmed. An example of this might be acute, severe pneumonia where respiration has started to fail and the patient retains CO_2. The retained CO_2 will produce carbonic acid, which eventually lowers the pH leading to an acidosis. So in this situation the pH is low, the $PaCO_2$ is high but the HCO_3 will be normal. Remember in an uncompensated condition the pH will always be abnormal. This is probably the easiest situation to interpret.
- A partially compensated condition. This may be seen in acute/sub-acute and in chronic or acute on chronic conditions. For example, the primary problem may be hypoventilation, leading to an increased $PaCO_2$ and therefore low pH. However, because the condition develops slowly, the body begins to compensate by increasing the HCO_3 to 'neutralise' the acid produced by the CO_2. In this case the pH is low, the $PaCO_2$ is high and the HCO_3 is rising above normal.
- A fully compensated condition. This is usually seen in chronic conditions of gradual onset, giving the body time to fully compensate. An example of this might be in COPD. Over time, the patient's respiratory system fails, leading to increased CO_2 retention, which would cause a respiratory acidosis. In response to this the body compensates by increasing bicarbonate,

which 'neutralises' the acid and returns the pH to normal. Remember, in a fully compensated condition the pH will be normal, but both the $PaCO_2$ and HCO_3 will be abnormal.

The purpose of compensation is to return the pH to normal.

RESPIRATORY FAILURE

Respiratory failure can be caused by problems with the airways, lungs, pulmonary vessels, nervous system, muscles and the chest wall. Respiratory failure results in inadequate gas exchange and resultant abnormalities in ABGs. ABG analysis will help determine the type of respiratory failure, whereas the patient's clinical history will help determine the cause. Traditionally, respiratory failure has been classified into Type 1 and Type 2 (British Thoracic Society Standards of Care Committee, 2002).

Type 1 respiratory failure is also known as hypoxic respiratory failure and is defined as a PaO_2 of < 8 kPa with a normal or low $PaCO_2$.

Type 2 respiratory failure is also known as hypercapnic respiratory failure (see Table 4.4) and is defined as a PaO_2 of <8 kPa and a $PaCO_2$ of >6 kPa.

Type 2 respiratory failure can also be classified as acute, acute on chronic and chronic. It is important to distinguish which type of respiratory failure the patient has so that they are given the correct treatment in the correct location.

- Acute hypercapnic respiratory failure will result in low pH, high $PaCO_2$ and normal HCO_3. The patient will have no history, or only minor history, of pre-existing lung disease.

- Acute on chronic hypercapnic respiratory failure will result in a low pH, high $PaCO_2$ and high HCO_3. The patient will have a significant history of chronic respiratory disease accompanied by an acute illness (British Thoracic Society Standards of Care Committee, 2002).
- Chronic hypercapnic respiratory failure will result in a normal pH, high $PaCO_2$ and high HCO_3 (see discussion of compensation earlier in this chapter). The patient will have a significant history of chronic respiratory disease.

In assessing the patient with respiratory failure, a detailed clinical history and examination are vital (see Chapter 2) and should also include pulse oximetry, ABG measurement and a chest X-ray. For Type 2 respiratory failure, Suh and Hart (2012) recommend detailed cardiopulmonary, neurological and musculoskeletal assessments as well because dysfunction of these systems can be the cause of the Type 2 respiratory failure. The main treatment for Type 1 respiratory failure is oxygen therapy with a target saturation of 94%–98% or 88%–92% for patients at risk of hypercapnic respiratory failure (O'Driscoll et al., 2008) (see Chapter 16 for further information). Type 2 respiratory failure will almost always require NIV and this may be available on some emergency departments, respiratory wards or indeed at home, but it may also require the patient to be transferred to a critical care unit (see Chapter 17 for further information regarding NIV). Causes of Type 1 and Type 2 respiratory failure are summarised in Table 4.5. It is

Table 4.4 Summary of hypercapnic respiratory failure

Classification of respiratory failure	pH	$PaCO_2$	HCO_3
Acute hypercapnic (Type 2) respiratory failure	Low	High	Normal
Acute on chronic hypercapnic respiratory failure	Low	High	High
Chronic hypercapnic respiratory failure	Normal	High	High

Source: Adapted from Hennessey, I.A.M. and Japp, A.G. 2016. *Arterial Blood Gases Made Easy* (2nd ed.). Elsevier, Edinburgh.

Table 4.5 Summary of causes of respiratory failure

Type 1	Type 2
Usually related to impaired V/Q mismatch	Usually related to inadequate ventilation
Pneumonia	Depression of the respiratory centre, i.e. due to opiate usage
Asthma	Neurological disorders
Pulmonary embolism	Neuromuscular disorders
Pulmonary oedema	Obesity
COPD	COPD

Source: Adapted from Hennessey, I.A.M. and Japp, A.G. 2016. *Arterial Blood Gases Made Easy* (2nd ed.). Elsevier, Edinburgh.

Table 4.6 Five-step blood gas analysis

Normal range for ABGs

pH: 7.35–7.45

PaO_2: 11.5–13 kPa (80–100 mmHg)

$PaCO_2$: 4.5–6 kPa (35–45 mmHg)

HCO_3: 22–26 mmols/L

BE: – 2– + 2

SpO_2: 94%–98%

Step one

Look at PaO_2 – Does this indicate hypoxaemia?

When analysing the results always check how much oxygen the patient was receiving when the blood sample was taken (Referred to as FiO_2).

Remember: The PaO_2 represents the amount of free oxygen molecules dissolved in plasma (not bound to haemoglobin) and as such represents only a tiny proportion of the total amount of oxygen in the arterial blood. PaO_2 gives a more accurate estimation of oxygenation than SpO_2.

Step two

Look at the pH – Is it normal?

Is it low = ACIDOSIS

Is it high = ALKALOSIS

Step three

Look at the $PaCO_2$ – Is it normal?

Is it high = a $PaCO_2$ of greater than 6 together with a low pH would indicate a respiratory acidosis

Is it low = a $PaCO_2$ of less than 4.5 together with a high pH would indicate a respiratory alkalosis

Remember: $PaCO_2$ is a measure of respiratory efficiency. If patients are moving sufficient amounts of air in and out of their lungs, they will excrete CO_2 efficiently.

Step four

Look at the HCO_3 – Is it normal?

Is it low = a HCO_3 of less than 22 together with a low pH would indicate a metabolic acidosis

Is it high = a HCO_3 of more than 26 together with a high pH would indicate a metabolic alkalosis

Remember that a normal level of bicarbonate is a measure of metabolic efficiency.

Step five

Does the pH show if compensation has taken place?

An uncompensated condition is when the pH is abnormal. Either the PCO_2 or the HCO_3 may be normal, indicating an uncompensated condition. This is usually an acute or an acute on chronic episode of illness and may be life threatening.

A compensated condition is when the pH has returned to normal but both the PCO_2 and HCO_3 will be abnormal. This represents a chronic condition because compensation takes time to happen. This usually represents a stable condition.

Remember that compensation can also be partial and this often causes confusion when trying to interpret ABGs.

Source: Adapted from Burns, G.P. 2014. *Clinical Medicine* 14(1): 66–68; Rogers, K. and McCutcheon, K. 2013. *The Journal of Perioperative Practice*, 23(9): 191–197; Simpson, H. 2004. *British Journal of Nursing*, 13(9): 522–528.

important to remember that a patient can have both Type 1 and Type 2 respiratory failure (e.g. COPD) or that Type 1 respiratory failure can develop into Type 2 respiratory failure (e.g. severe pneumonia) (Burns, 2014).

INTERPRETING ARTERIAL BLOOD GASES: A FIVE STEP FRAMEWORK

A review of the literature reveals numerous approaches to ABG interpretation using a step-wise approach and the reader must find their own preferred method (Simpson, 2004; Rogers and McCutcheon, 2013; Burns, 2014). For the purposes of this chapter, a five-step framework is used (see Table 4.6). It is recommended that inexperienced clinical staff always use a framework to guide them, as ABG interpretation can be very difficult. Examples of respiratory disorders are given in the case studies below, but remember that an acid-base disorder may also be metabolic in origin and indeed a patient may have both a metabolic and respiratory disorder, in which case the patient will be very ill and require admission to a critical care unit. Try analysing the ABGs in the case studies given below. Draw your own conclusions before you read the explanation.

CASE STUDIES

CASE STUDY ONE

Jenny Pearce is a 17 year old who is having difficulty coming to terms with her asthma. She is particularly concerned about body image and taking inhaled cortico-steroids (ICS), despite being reassured that the dose is very small. She has been admitted to the emergency department and on examination is anxious, sweaty, hyperventilating, dizzy and has tingling in her fingers and toes. RR 32 bpm, HR 110 bpm, BP 110/60 mmHg, Temperature 36.9°C, SpO_2 is 97% on room air. ABGs are as follows:

	Jenny's ABGs	Normal values	Your comments
pH	7.52	7.35–7.45	
PaO_2	13	11.5–13 kPa	
$PaCO_2$	3.0	4.5–6 kPa	
HCO_3	22	22–26	
BE	+1	−2–+2	
SpO_2	97%	94%–98%	

Using the five-step framework above, answer the following questions about Jenny.

1. Does Jenny have hypoxemia and require oxygen therapy?
2. Does Jenny have an acid-base disturbance?
3. What will you do about her acid-base disturbance?

Discussion

Step 1 Jenny's PaO_2 is normal and therefore she does not have hypoxemia and does not require oxygen therapy.

Step 2 Jenny's pH is not normal, it is high and therefore indicates an alkalosis.

Step 3 Jenny's $PaCO_2$ is not normal, it is low, indicating a respiratory problem.

Step 4 Jenny's HCO_3 is normal, indicating that this is not a metabolic problem.

Step 5 Jenny's pH is abnormal, indicating that this is an uncompensated and acute condition.

Jenny has a respiratory alkalosis precipitated by an anxiety attack. Her hyperventilation means that she is excreting too much CO_2, which has led to an increase in her pH. Respiratory alkalosis is a common acid-base disturbance and one that can be easily corrected. Jenny needs to relax and breathe into a bag. This way she will rebreathe her own CO_2 and the disturbance will quickly correct itself.

A week later Jenny is readmitted to the emergency department accompanied by her very anxious mother. Audible wheezing is present on inspiration and expiration. Jenny has a headache and is quite restless and has a dusky look to her skin. RR 17 bpm, HR 100 bpm, BP 110/60 mmHg, Temp 36.9°C, SpO_2 is 92% on room air.

	Jenny's ABGs	Normal values	Your comments
pH	7.29	7.35–7.45	
PaO_2	9	11.5–13 kPa	
$PaCO_2$	7.1	4.5–6 kPa	
HCO_3	22	22–26	
BE	–1	–2–+2	
SpO_2	92%	94%–98%	

Using the five-step framework above, answer the following questions about Jenny.

1. Does Jenny have hypoxemia and require oxygen therapy?
2. Does Jenny have an acid-base disturbance?
3. What will you do about her acid-base disturbance?

Discussion

Step 1: Jenny's PaO_2 is not normal, it is low and therefore she does have hypoxemia and does require oxygen therapy.

Step 2: Jenny's pH is not normal, it is low and therefore indicates an acidosis.

Step 3: Jenny's $PaCO_2$ is not normal, it is high, indicating a respiratory problem.

Step 4: Jenny's HCO_3 is normal, indicating that this is not a metabolic problem.

Step 5: Jenny's pH is abnormal, indicating that this is an uncompensated and acute condition.

Jenny has a respiratory acidosis precipitated by an asthma attack. The ABGs give an entirely different picture from her admission the week before. Jenny's asthma attack may have been triggered by her reluctance to take her inhaled medication. She has audible wheezes on inspiration and expiration, indicating that she has bronchospasm. She is having difficulty getting air into her chest and therefore has hypoxemia, but she is also having difficulty getting air out of her chest and therefore has hypercapnia. In someone with hypoxia and hypercapnia you would expect to see an increased respiratory rate, but Jenny's is only 17, indicating that she is exhausted. Although oxygen therapy might correct her hypoxemia, it will not alter her $PaCO_2$. Jenny needs to be reviewed by a senior doctor or the critical care outreach team and possible commencement of NIV or mechanical ventilation if standard drug therapy does not bring about a rapid improvement. Jenny's condition is extremely urgent.

CASE STUDY TWO

Bob Howie is a 74-year-old gentleman with a 2-day history of fever and a productive cough. He is flushed and restless and complaining of a headache on admission to the ward. Bob is receiving 50% oxygen via a simple facemask and his SpO$_2$ is 96%. RR 10 bpm, HR 115 bpm, BP 110/60 mmHg, Temp 38.0°C. Sometime later ABGs are taken and are as follows:

	Bob's ABGs	Normal values	Your comments
pH	7.24	7.35–7.45	
PaO$_2$	12	11.5–13 kPa	
PaCO$_2$	8	4.5–6 kPa	
HCO$_3$	22	22–26	
BE	+1	–2–+2	
SpO$_2$	96%	94%–98%	

Using the five-step framework above, answer the following questions about Bob.

1. Does Bob have hypoxemia and require oxygen therapy?
2. Does Bob have an acid-base disturbance?
3. What will you do about his acid-base disturbance?

Discussion

Step 1: Bob's PaO$_2$ is normal, but he is receiving 50% oxygen therapy and this needs to continue.
Step 2: Bob's pH is not normal, it is low, and therefore indicates an acidosis.
Step 3: Bob's PaCO$_2$ is not normal, it is high, indicating a respiratory problem.
Step 4: Bob's HCO$_3$ is normal, indicating this is not a metabolic problem.
Step 5: Bob's pH is abnormal, indicating that this is an uncompensated and acute condition.

Bob has a respiratory acidosis triggered by a severe chest infection. On admission to the ward his SpO$_2$ was 96%. Oxygen saturation readings should never be taken in isolation. This example demonstrates that, although this patient has an adequate oxygen saturation, he is in an extremely dangerous condition and his ABGs should have been checked sooner. His supplementary oxygen is maintaining his SpO$_2$, but remember that SpO$_2$ tells you nothing about the patient's pH or PaCO$_2$ but only about the percentage of haemoglobin saturated by oxygen. His chest infection means that he has a ventilation/perfusion (V/Q) mismatch and in addition he is elderly and exhausted, as indicated by his low respiratory rate. Bob is having difficulty getting oxygen in and CO$_2$ out of his lungs. The CO$_2$ has produced the respiratory acidosis because of conversion to carbonic acid. If this situation continues Bob will have a respiratory arrest because of the narcotic effect of CO$_2$ on the brainstem or he may have a cardiac arrest because the pH acts as a negative inotrope and will also have disturbed Bob's potassium causing him to have hyperkalaemia. Bob has a high PaCO$_2$ but there is no history of pre-existing lung disease and the normal HCO$_3$ indicates this is an acute condition. The abnormal pH suggests that this is an uncompensated, acute condition of rapid onset. Bob requires a senior review urgently and NIV or even mechanical ventilation.

CASE STUDY THREE

Jack Stevenson is a 69-year-old gentleman and has been admitted to the ward following a minor surgical procedure undertaken with local anaesthetic. He is known to have COPD and he is receiving 24% oxygen via a Venturi mask. Jack is responsive to voice, but is lying with his eyes closed. He is sat upright in the bed. RR 22 bpm, HR 90 bpm, BP 150/80 mmHg, Temp 37.0°C and SpO$_2$ is 90% on 24% oxygen therapy. Because of Jack's COPD the anaesthetist checks his ABGs.

	Jack's ABGs	Normal values	Your comments
pH	7.35	7.35–7.45	
PaO$_2$	9.4	11.5–13 kPa	
PaCO$_2$	8.5	4.5–6 kPa	
HCO$_3$	30	22–26	
BE	+5	−2–+2	
SpO$_2$	90%	94%–98%	

Using the Five -Step Framework above answer the following questions about Jack.

1. Does Jack have hypoxemia and require oxygen therapy?
2. Does Jack have an acid-base disturbance?
3. What will you do about his acid-base disturbance?

Discussion

Step 1 Jack's PaO$_2$ is low and he is receiving 24% oxygen therapy post-operatively.

Step 2 Jack's pH is normal and therefore this suggests he does not have an acid-base disturbance. However, you need to carry on and review the rest of the ABGs to get a full picture.

Step 3 Jack's PaCO$_2$ is not normal, it is high, indicating a respiratory problem.

Step 4 Jack's HCO$_3$ is high, indicating this condition has a metabolic element to it.

Step 5 Jack's pH is normal, indicating that this is a compensated and chronic condition. The pH is normal but both the PaCO$_2$ and HCO$_3$ are abnormal.

These ABGs show a compensated respiratory acidosis. Jack has COPD and over the years this has led to poor lung function, which means Jack is both hypoxic and hypercapnic. Retention of CO$_2$ will usually cause an acidosis and a low pH. However, because deterioration has been slow, Jack's body has compensated by retaining HCO$_3$ and 'neutralising' the acid. This process explains why the HCO$_3$ is so high and has returned the pH to normal. The high PaCO$_2$ and high HCO$_3$ represent a chronic problem and therefore caution with oxygen therapy is required. This is in contrast to Bob, who had a high PaCO$_2$ but normal HCO$_3$, indicating an acute problem. Jack's current oxygen therapy is maintaining his SpO$_2$ within the stated BTS recommended SpO$_2$ of 88%–92% (O'Driscoll et al., 2008) for someone with hypercapnic respiratory failure. Jack requires careful monitoring until he is discharged. His normal pH suggests that he is stable from a respiratory perspective. It would be very useful to consult Jack's medical notes and compare his current ABG with previous ones. Jack should discontinue his oxygen therapy as soon as the anaesthetist states that it is safe to do so and clinical staff should consult with the anaesthetist promptly if there are any changes.

SUMMARY

Pulse oximetry is a useful, non-invasive tool for giving an indication of oxygenation. However, it should never be used in isolation or replace careful clinical assessment. Pulse oximetry does not provide any information about a patient's pH or CO$_2$ levels. ABGs provide detailed information about the patient's respiratory and metabolic status, whether the condition is acute or chronic and how severe/urgent it is. However, ABGs are difficult to interpret and it is vital they are interpreted correctly and acted upon promptly. Inexperienced staff should always use a framework to guide ABG interpretation until they are confident. A five-step framework is provided in this chapter, but many alternatives exist. Both hypoxemia and acid-base disturbance can be life threatening and it does not matter which framework is used if it results in the correct interpretation and prompt treatment for the patient.

REFERENCES

Bhatia, P. 2012. Oxygen (Super) saturation. Indian *Journal of Anaesthesia* 56 (6): 592–593.

Booker, R. 2008. Pulse oximetry. *Nursing Standard* 22 (30): 39–41.

British Thoracic Society Standards of Care Committee. 2002. BTS Guideline: Non-invasive ventilation in acute respiratory failure. *Thorax* 57 (3): 192–211.

Burns, G.P. 2014. Arterial blood gases made easy. *Clinical Medicine* 14 (1): 66–68.

Casey, G. 2013. Interpreting arterial blood gases. *Kai Tiaki Nursing New Zealand* 19 (6): 20–24.

Crawford, A. 2004. An audit of the patient's experience of arterial blood gas testing. *British Journal of Nursing* 13 (9): 529–532.

Davies, A. and Moores, C. 2010. *The Respiratory System* (2nd ed.). Churchill Livingstone, Edinburgh.

DeMeulenaere, S. 2007. Pulse oximetry: Uses and limitations. *The Journal for Nurse Practitioners* 3 (5): 312–317.

Hennessey, I.A.M. and Japp, A.G. 2016. *Arterial Blood Gases Made Easy* (2nd ed.). Elsevier, Edinburgh.

Howell, M. 2002. Pulse oximetry: An audit of nursing and medical staff understanding. *British Journal of Nursing* 11 (3): 191–197.

Kaur, A. 2006. Caring for a patient with an arterial line. *Nursing* 36 (4): 64cc1–64cc3.

Leslie, R.A., Gouldson, S., Habib, N., Harris, N., Murray, H., Wells, V. and Cook, T.M. 2013. Management of arterial lines and arterial blood sampling in intensive care: A threat to patient safety. *Anaesthesia* 68: 1114–1119.

Marieb, E.N. 2012. *Essentials of Human Anatomy and Physiology* (10th ed.). Benjamin Cummings, Boston, MA.

O'Driscoll, B.R., Howard, L.S. and Davison, A.G. 2008. British thoracic society guideline for emergency oxygen use in adult patients. *Thorax* 63 (Suppl 6): vi1–vi73.

Rogers, K. and McCutcheon, K. 2013. Understanding arterial blood gases. *The Journal of Perioperative Practice* 23 (9): 191–197.

Simpson, H. 2004. Interpretation of arterial blood gases: A clinical guide for nurses. *British Journal of Nursing* 13 (9): 522–528.

Suh, E.S. and Hart, N. 2012. Respiratory failure. *Medicine* 40 (6): 293–297.

Tortora, G.J. and Derrickson, B. 2012. *Principles of Anatomy and Physiology* (13th ed.). John Wiley and Sons Inc, Hoboken, NJ.

Woodrow, P. 2012. *Intensive Care Nursing: A Framework for Practice* (3rd ed.). Routledge, London.

Zavorsky, G.S., Cao, J., Mayo, N.E., Gabby, R. Murias, J.M. 2006. Arterial versus capillary blood gases: A meta-analysis. *Respiratory Physiology and Neurobiology* 155: 268–279.

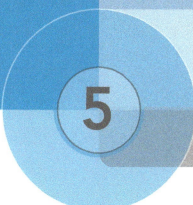

Chronic obstructive pulmonary disease

5

GRAHAM BURNS

LEARNING OBJECTIVES

Upon completion of this chapter the reader should be able to:

- Discuss the pathology of chronic obstructive pulmonary disease and the meaning of the terms: emphysema, chronic bronchitis and airway obstruction
- Describe how the diagnosis of chronic obstructive pulmonary disease is made
- Discuss the impact that appropriate treatment can have on a patient's quality and quantity of life
- Identify the importance of smoking cessation on prognosis
- Discuss the place of oxygen therapy in management of chronic obstructive pulmonary disease
- Develop an understanding of the difference between treatment aimed at symptomatic relief and that given for prognostic benefit

INTRODUCTION

Chronic obstructive pulmonary disease (COPD) is a major disease on a global scale. It not only shortens life, but has a devastating impact on quality of life. In the United Kingdom (UK) an estimated 3 million people have COPD yet more than 2 million of these remain undiagnosed (National Institute for Health and Care Excellence [NICE], 2010). There are 11,000 admissions to hospital with exacerbations of COPD and 30,000 people die of the disease each year. Mortality rates have fallen in men but continue to rise in women, reflecting smoking patterns over the second half of the twentieth century (see Chapter 18). Although in the UK and the United States (US)

smoking prevalence has slowly declined since its peak in the 1970s, worldwide the epidemic of smoking continues to grow. With increasing numbers smoking in China, Africa and Asia, COPD is now the third most common cause of death worldwide. There is an urgent need to improve awareness, prevention and treatment of this disease.

This chapter aims to discuss the pathophysiology of the disease and describe the individual components that contribute to COPD. Making a diagnosis will be discussed with reference to distinguishing between COPD and asthma. An overview of the management of COPD is provided, including emergency care and oxygen therapy. Finally, a case study will be used to consider the management of this respiratory condition.

PATHOPHYSIOLOGY

COPD is defined as a chronic, slowly progressive disorder characterised by airflow obstruction that does not change markedly over several months (NICE, 2010). Although there is some overlap in the features of COPD and asthma, they are separate disorders with different aetiologies, pathologies, natural history and responses to treatment. It is therefore important to be clear when establishing a diagnosis. In asthma, the principal feature is airway inflammation. In COPD, structural and histological changes occur that give rise to the various facets of the condition: chronic bronchitis, emphysema and airway obstruction.

CHRONIC BRONCHITIS

Cigarette smoke irritates the airways of the lung, causing inflammation. In an attempt to form a protective barrier, the airways produce excess mucus. Unfortunately smoking also leads to an impairment of the normal ability of the lungs to clear mucus. The airways of patients with COPD are therefore always full of sputum, resulting in what patients recognise as 'smoker's cough'. Formally chronic bronchitis is defined as: a cough productive of mucus on most days, for at least three months, in at least two consecutive years (Kim et al., 2015).

EMPHYSEMA

Emphysema is a disease of the alveoli rather than the airways. In susceptible smokers there is progressive destruction of alveolar walls. The fine sponge-like network of air pockets is gradually destroyed, leaving bigger and bigger holes in the lung. Very large holes are known as bullae. This facet of COPD does not improve with smoking cessation. The loss of surface area for gas transfer is one important consequence. It is reflected in a reduction in the transfer factor for carbon monoxide (T_{LCO}) and transfer coefficient (K_{CO}), (see later under Section 'Diagnosis of COPD'). These lung function tests are one of the ways in which COPD can be distinguished from asthma (Bourke and Burns, 2015).

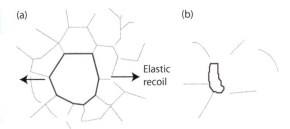

Figure 5.1 Emphysema consists of dilatation of the terminal air spaces of the lungs, distal to the terminal bronchiole with destruction of their walls. (a) Small peripheral airways lack cartilage and depend on the support of the surrounding alveoli to maintain their patency. (b) Alveolar destruction in emphysema results in a loss of elastic recoil and a loss of outward traction on the small airways such that they collapse on expiration contributing to the observed airway obstruction.

AIRWAY OBSTRUCTION

Airway obstruction is an increased resistance to airflow caused by diffuse airway narrowing. The presence of airway obstruction is detected by spirometry (The Primary Care Respiratory Society UK [PCRS-UK], 2010). A number of factors contribute to airway obstruction in COPD and include destruction of alveoli by emphysema, leading to loss of the supporting structures that hold the small airways open, thereby leaving them prone to collapse on expiration (Figure 5.1). Airway inflammation with thickening of the airway wall and accumulation of mucous secretions obstructs the airway lumen.

SIGNS AND SYMPTOMS

COPD has a wide spectrum of severity. The cardinal symptom is breathlessness. This responds, although only partially, to treatment with inhalers. It also progresses gradually but relentlessly over years, particularly in those who continue to smoke. Humans possess pulmonary reserve ('spare lung capacity') and therefore patients often do not notice, or at least do not report, breathlessness until a great deal of lung function has been lost. Unfortunately, emphysema is permanent; once the damage is done it can never be reversed. Many people are in their 50s at the time of diagnosis and may have been smoking since their teens. Figure 5.2 illustrates the insidious progressive way in which lung function is lost in COPD. The graph also demonstrates the benefits of smoking cessation.

Chronic cough and sputum production result from the overproduction of mucus in the airways – chronic bronchitis. Unlike emphysema, this aspect of COPD usually improves with smoking cessation. When cigarette smoke is no longer irritating the airways, the hypersecretion of mucus is reduced. The mucus clearance system becomes active and clears out the residual phlegm. After a brief period when the cough may be reported to be worse, the cough and sputum can resolve entirely in those who remain ex-smokers.

Exacerbations of COPD are common and decrease the quality of life of many patients with the condition (PCRS-UK, 2010). These episodes, which are usually referred to as 'chest infections' by patients themselves, are characterised by worsening breathlessness and increased cough with purulent sputum. Severe episodes may result in hospital admission.

DIAGNOSIS OF COPD

There is no single diagnostic test for COPD. Diagnosis relies on clinical judgement based on a combination of history, physical examination and confirmation of the presence of airflow obstruction using spirometry (Celli and MacNee, 2004).

Spirometry is the most accurate measure of airflow obstruction and is therefore crucial in the diagnosis of COPD. In the context of COPD, the diagnosis of airflow obstruction and the assessment of severity are based on post-bronchodilator spirometry. The forced expiratory volume in 1 second/vital capacity (FEV_1/VC) ratio declines naturally with age and the definition of airway obstruction should more correctly be defined by the lower limit of the normal range for the patient's age, but for convenience a ratio FEV_1/VC < 0.7 is generally taken to define airway obstruction irrespective of age. Once airway obstruction is determined to be present (by this ratio), its severity is usually classified by comparing FEV_1 to the predicted value: **mild** (FEV_1 ≥80% predicted), **moderate** (FEV_1 79%–50% predicted), **severe** (FEV_1 49%–30% predicted) and **very severe** (FEV_1 <30% predicted).

ASTHMA OR COPD?

Airway obstruction is a feature of both asthma and COPD, so distinguishing between the two is not always straightforward. Because of uncertainty, some clinicians fail to make the distinction and then simply manage the patient with a random selection of inhalers. Asthma and COPD are very different conditions; they respond differently to treatments. Establishing the correct diagnosis right at the start is critically important. See Chapter 6 for a detailed discussion of asthma.

Making the diagnosis begins with a careful history. When a patient presents, for example in their 50s with breathlessness, there are a number of important questions to ask. When asked about duration of symptoms, many patients will date their breathlessness from some recent event, such as a severe chest infection. Careful questioning, however, will usually reveal that their breathing 'hasn't been right' for a substantial period of time, usually years on reflection. Childhood symptoms are not usually volunteered without a direct question: 'Did you have any chest trouble while at school?' It is surprising how often this question will reveal a history which, in retrospect, clearly indicates asthma, even if it was not diagnosed at the time. If asthma was present in childhood, it is likely that it is at least a component of the problem now.

In patients labelled and treated as COPD, the question too obvious to ask: 'have you ever had asthma?' will surprisingly frequently yield the reply: 'I've had it all my life'. One of the cardinal features of asthma is its variability; this is often manifest as a variation in symptoms with the time of the day. While many patients with COPD will report their cough to be worse in the mornings, a history of a tight, wheezy chest and breathlessness in the mornings, easing considerably in the afternoon should prompt consideration of asthma. Asthma also typically causes patients to wake from sleep in the early hours owing to breathlessness or cough. This is not the same as the patient who wakes to go to the toilet and finds themselves breathless after walking back to bed.

Establishing the patient's smoking history is important for many reasons, including diagnosis. On a global scale, exposure to biomass fuels is an important risk factor, rare genetic conditions can also lead to COPD without cigarette smoking, but in the UK unless a patient has smoked it is extremely unlikely they have COPD.

Although a single episode of spirometry cannot distinguish COPD from asthma, measurement of spirometry pre- and post-bronchodilator (or course of steroids) can be used to assess the degree of reversibility of the airway obstruction. When the reversibility is particularly marked, it can help to identify asthma. However, this is a complex area. There is considerable variability in the change in FEV_1 in response to the same stimulus from day to day and there is no universally agreed threshold for reversibility that defines asthma.

In secondary care further pulmonary function can be carried out, which can help clarify the diagnosis. The transfer factor for carbon monoxide (T_{LCO}) and the transfer coefficient (K_{CO} = the T_{LCO} corrected for lung volume) are measurements of the lungs' ability to transfer gas (oxygen is of course the gas of most interest). With the loss of surface area for gas transfer in emphysema, these values are typically reduced in emphysema. In asthma, K_{CO} tends to be elevated.

As COPD and asthma are two different conditions it is, of course, entirely possible that a patient could have both. This has long been recognised and patients may, after specialist assessment, have a problem list that carefully documents the presence of both conditions and reflects the relative balance between the two, e.g. 'COPD with an asthmatic component' or 'Asthma – minor element of COPD'. It is currently fashionable to label these conditions as asthma COPD overlap syndrome (ACOS). When both conditions are present, treatment should cover both. In particular, if asthma is present, it is almost always necessary to include an inhaled corticosteroid.

COPD AS A MULTISYSTEM DISEASE

It is common for patients with COPD to have a number of co-morbidities. Some of these are the result of a common aetiological factor (e.g. smoking and ischaemic heart disease), some are a direct consequence of the lung condition itself. COPD can lead to patho-physiological changes outside of the lung in a number of ways including: mechanistic effects

(such as pulmonary hypertension and right heart failure owing to hypoxia) and inflammatory overspill, where inflammatory mediators from the lung may contribute to problems elsewhere in the body including cachexia, loss of muscle mass, osteoporosis, cardiac failure and diabetes (PCRS-UK, 2010).

Depression and anxiety are very common accompaniments to COPD, reported in up to 50% of all patients. Breathlessness is not just unpleasant; at times it is very frightening. It is not surprising therefore that frequent though unpredictable attacks of breathlessness may ultimately lead to a persistently anxious state. The general debility and potential for social isolation that COPD can bring are obvious risk factors for depression. Despite their prevalence, these debilitating conditions are usually entirely overlooked by doctors. Screening (e.g. Hospital Anxiety and Depression questionnaire) is necessary to identify cases.

TREATMENT, INTERVENTIONS AND THERAPY

For years COPD has suffered from a rather negative image. It seemed to compare unfavourably with asthma. In COPD airway obstruction is generally regarded as 'non-reversible'. 'Non-reversible' is too easily confused with 'non-treatable'. COPD was therefore regarded as the disease for which little could be done. In the past decade there has been a revolution in the approach to COPD. With the development of new treatments, and indeed a fresh look at some of the old, opinion has moved beyond the old nihilistic mind-set. In COPD it is now recognised that it is possible to have a very positive impact on a great number of clinically important outcomes, including: breathlessness, cough, sputum, exacerbation rate, hospital admission rate, disability, exercise endurance, quality of life, anxiety, depression, rate of progression of the disease and even mortality. The interventions that achieve these outcomes still do not have a great short-term impact on FEV_1, but it would be difficult to continue to view COPD as an 'untreatable' condition.

In managing patients with COPD there are now a number of tools at the disposal of healthcare professionals, including pharmacological, physical

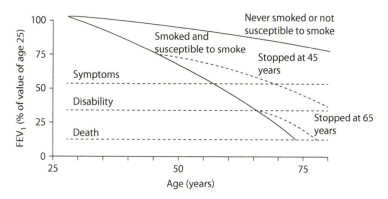

Figure 5.2 Change in FEV₁ with age: effect of smoking and stopping smoking. Non-smokers show a small progressive decline in function with age. Many smokers are unaffected by smoking and show the same decline as non-smokers. Some smokers are affected and show a steeper decline. By the time disability is noted, ventilatory function is seriously reduced to about one-third of predicted normal values. Those affected by smoking can be detected by measurement of FEV₁ many years before they become disabled. Stopping smoking slows the rate of decline. (Adapted from Fletcher, C. and Peto, R. 1977. *British Medical Journal* 1 (6077): 1645–1648.)

and psychological interventions. The application of each needs to be considered carefully for every patient and integrated into an overall comprehensive individualised management plan. The overwhelming priority in any patient still smoking is smoking cessation (NICE, 2010). If this can be achieved, it will have a far greater impact on long-term prognosis than any other intervention (see Chapter 18).

SMOKING CESSATION

Figure 5.2 illustrates the decline in lung function seen in smokers with COPD. Many patients have well-recognised disease before the diagnosis is made. The graph also demonstrates the effect of smoking cessation on disease progression. Although it is clear that the lung function lost is never regained (emphysema is permanent damage), smoking cessation changes the course of the disease. Indeed, despite the vast sums of money spent on drug development, smoking cessation remains the only proven disease-modifying intervention for COPD (West et al., 2000). If smoking cessation occurs early enough in the course of the disease, then the rate of decline in FEV₁ returns (approximately) to what it would have been had the patient never smoked – a natural age-related decline. Clearly the earlier smoking cessation can be achieved, the better the preservation of lung function. Although lung function never returns to

normal, it is clear that the patient will be far better off than if they had continued to smoke. Year on year they will experience fewer symptoms and a better quality of life as well as living longer. All patients still smoking, regardless of age, should be encouraged to stop, and offered help to do so, at every opportunity (NICE, 2010).

GETTING THE INDIVIDUAL TO WANT TO STOP

The risk of lung cancer is an important issue to discuss, but many patients are well aware of this increased 'risk' and have already rationalised the issue in their own mind. What many COPD patients are not aware of is the startling decline in quality of life that will happen if they continue to smoke. Progression can be surprisingly rapid once symptoms become apparent; from stopping occasionally for breath when walking around town, to struggling to get to the corner shop, to breathless at the garden gate to being entirely housebound. A description of the practical implication of declining lung function can have a powerful impact on a patient's determination to quit. Without a firm commitment by the individual, smoking cessations aid will achieve little. When used in conjunction with willpower, pharmacotherapy can improve quit rates (Alberg and Carpenter, 2012).

PHARMACOTHERAPY FOR SMOKING CESSATION

A number of pharmacotherapies exist to aid smoking cessation: Nicotine replacement (in a variety of forms), Bupropion (amfebutamone) and Varenicline. In the context of an individual determined to quit and with the support of a smoking cessation service, they can increase the chances of a successful quit attempt (Ferguson et al., 2005).

Electronic cigarettes (e-cigarettes) are battery-powered devices, which contain a heating element that vaporises a liquid solution containing nicotine and a mixture of other chemicals (e.g. propylene glycol, vegetable glycerine and flavourings). The vapour is inhaled in a manner that mimics cigarette smoking. They remain controversial. Although some health-care professionals argue that they are significantly safer than smoking cigarettes, they are not without problems. At present they remain unregulated; therefore there is no control on what other chemicals are inhaled along with the nicotine. Regulation would restrict the use of chemicals to a prescribed 'safe list', but even if benign in the short term, the long-term effects of inhaling foreign substances into the lung may take time to emerge. It is also difficult to see how the use of flavours such as *bubble gum* can do anything other than attract children to the market and increase nicotine addiction.

SHORT-ACTING BRONCHODILATORS

Short-acting βeta_2-agonists (SABAs), such as salbutamol and terbutaline, relax bronchial smooth muscle by stimulation of β-adrenoreceptors. Short-acting anti-cholinergic drugs, such as ipratropium, produce bronchodilatation by blocking the bronchoconstrictor effect of vagal nerve stimulation of bronchial smooth muscle. The bronchodilatation is associated with some short-term alleviation of breathlessness. β_2-agonists remain first-line drugs, particularly in mild COPD (NICE, 2010).

LONG-ACTING BRONCHODILATORS

Tiotropium and Glycopyrronium are long-acting muscarinic antagonists (LAMAs); they have a duration of action that is at least 24 hours and therefore a convenient once-daily dosage. Aclidinium has a shorter duration of action and needs to be delivered twice daily, but has the advantage of fewer anti-cholinergic side effects (e.g. dry mouth). LAMAs are often used as a first-line maintenance therapy when SABAs are not sufficient to control symptoms.

Long-acting β_2-agonists (LABAs), such as salmeterol and formoterol, with a 12 hours' duration of action and Indacaterol (24 hours) also offer prolonged relief of symptoms and would seem a reasonable additional maintenance therapy, though cost (if used in addition to a LAMA) has probably limited their use.

Dual bronchodilator (LAMA/LABA) combinations (e.g. Duaklir®, Anoro®, Ultibro®, Spiriva/Striverdi®) are now available. These are generally more efficacious than either a LAMA or LABA alone. For patients not adequately controlled on LAMAs, but who don't need inhaled corticosteroids (see below), they offer a second-line maintenance therapy.

PROGNOSTIC TREATMENT

Although symptomatic relief of breathlessness is an important aim of treatment, COPD is a multifaceted disease and modern, comprehensive treatment strategies must therefore offer more than just short-term relief from this symptom. In many other areas of medicine, drugs are employed that offer prognostic benefit. Statins for example do not improve symptoms in ischaemic heart disease, but they have measurable impact on the frequency of future adverse events: 'prognostic benefit'.

INHALED CORTICOSTEROIDS

In certain patients with COPD, inhaled corticosteroids (ICS) reduce the risk of exacerbations and hospital admissions. A reduction in the frequency of these adverse events represents real prognostic benefit. This effect is greatest when ICS are combined with a long-acting β_2-agonists in a ICS/LABA combination inhaler (e.g. Symbicort®, Seretide®, Relvar® and Fostair®). The combination typically produces a 30% reduction in exacerbation frequency with a beneficial effect on hospital admission rates. These important benefits are seen principally in patients with an $FEV_1 < 60\%$ predicted (and probably in those just above that threshold who have a history of exacerbations).

LONG-ACTING MUSCARINIC ANTAGONISTS (PROGNOSTIC BENEFITS)

The symptomatic relief of breathlessness offered by LAMAs has already been discussed. In this sense they are effective in all grades of severity. In addition, as with the ICS/LABA combination inhalers, in moderate to severe disease LAMAs have a beneficial impact on both exacerbation frequency and hospital admission rates.

TREATMENT STRATEGY

In relation to the inhaled therapies, the treatment strategy differs depending on the severity of the disease. In patients with an $FEV_1 > 60\%$ predicted and no history of exacerbations, treatment (other than smoking cessation) offers only short-term symptomatic control of breathlessness. SABAs, LAMAs and LAMA/LABA combinations can be trialled in turn. They are usually effective but if any specific drug is not effective, it will be evident and should be stopped.

In patients with FEV < 60% predicted (or a history of recurrent exacerbations) the situation is very different. Although symptom control remains important there is, in addition, evidence of prognostic benefit from the use of both an (ICS/LABA) combination inhaler and a LAMA (Calverley et al., 2007; Tashkin et al., 2008). Given together, this 'triple therapy' will have maximum impact on reducing the frequency of both exacerbations and hospital admissions. In contrast to the symptom controllers in milder disease, prognostic treatments should not be stopped if the patient reports no immediate benefit. This is comparable to not stopping blood pressure medication when a patient tells us they feel no different.

INHALER TECHNIQUE

It is often assumed that most people who have inhalers do not use them properly. This is not usually the fault of the patient, but of the prescriber who failed to spend time teaching and checking inhaler technique. Sub-optimal inhaler technique results in poor or even zero delivery of the drug to the lung. Whenever an inhaler is prescribed, care must be taken to coach (and then test) inhaler technique. This should, of course, be done by a healthcare professional who understands it themselves. Technique should then be tested every time the patient is reviewed (Halpin et al., 2015).

VACCINATION

Pneumococcal vaccination and annual influenza vaccination are recommended for patients with COPD (PCRS-UK, 2010).

MUCOLYTICS

These drugs increase the expectoration of sputum by reducing its viscosity. Although mucolytics do not have an impact on FEV_1, they can improve cough symptoms in some patients with COPD who have a chronic productive cough (PCRS-UK, 2010).

PSYCHOLOGICAL TREATMENT

Anxiety and depression are common in COPD of all grades of severity and not just confined to severe disease. Cognitive behavioural therapy (CBT) is proven to reduce both anxiety and depression and appears to be effective in the context of COPD (Heslop et al., 2009). The impact on the general well-being of the patient can be striking (see Chapter 20). A study is currently underway in the UK to determine if a reduction in the level of anxiety would lead to a reduction in the frequency of hospital admission (Heslop et al., 2013).

PULMONARY REHABILITATION

Pulmonary rehabilitation is a multidisciplinary programme of care for patients with COPD that is individually tailored and designed to optimise the patient's physical and social performance and autonomy (see Chapter 19). Pulmonary rehabilitation involves the skills of a truly multidisciplinary team. Many patients with COPD are in a vicious cycle of breathlessness, reduced physical activity and deconditioning of skeletal muscles, with resultant loss of social contact and autonomy. Pulmonary rehabilitation can break this vicious cycle and can reduce dyspnoea, improve exercise tolerance and quality of life. When delivered early after an admission it can reduce the chance of future admission.

The key components of a rehabilitation programme need to be adjusted to meet the needs of the individual patient, but typically include the following:

- Exercise training
- Smoking cessation support
- Optimisation of drug treatment
- Education about the nature of the disease and its management
- Breathing control techniques
- Social and occupational therapy support
- Psychological support
- Nutritional advice

Pulmonary rehabilitation is an enormously valuable intervention, but the benefits can eventually be lost unless the patient continues regular exercise; many such opportunities exist in local sports centres and gyms. Patients also benefit in this context from being on appropriate inhaled medication. The right medication will amplify the initial benefit from the programme and help maintain the improvement longer.

OXYGEN THERAPY IN STABLE DISEASE

'Short of breath' does not imply 'short of oxygen'. It is important to understand that it is quite possible to experience breathlessness without being hypoxic. If a patient is not hypoxic, breathing supplemental oxygen will achieve nothing (O'Driscoll et al., 2008). Many breathless patients ask their doctor for oxygen therapy, and many well-meaning doctors duly prescribe it. These prescriptions are costly and many are of no benefit to the patient whatsoever. There are, nevertheless, a number of circumstances when oxygen therapy can not only improve symptoms but also extend life. Proper (specialist) assessment is required to ensure that the patients who need oxygen therapy receive it and those that do not, do not (O'Driscoll et al., 2008; NHS, 2011) (see Chapter 16).

LONG-TERM OXYGEN THERAPY

Hypoxia within the lung leads to constriction of the blood vessels running through the lungs (pulmonary vasoconstriction). The increased vascular resistance puts a strain on the right heart. The right heart may struggle for a while, but eventually fails. Right heart failure caused by lung disease is known as cor pulmonale. The first sign is often ankle swelling, but ultimately cor pulmonale can be fatal. Patients with COPD and chronic hypoxia have a poor prognosis with a mortality rate of about 50% within 3 years. The administration of oxygen for at least 15 hours/day (preferably longer) improves survival in patients with hypoxia (Medical Research Council, 1981; NICE, 2010). Oxygen therapy has no impact on the progression of COPD (rate of decline of FEV_1); the improvement in survival is due to the easing of the strain on the right heart, which prevents premature death from cor pulmonale.

AMBULATORY OXYGEN

Ambulatory oxygen may be appropriate for patients who are active enough to leave the home regularly, who demonstrate a fall in oxygen saturation to below 90% on exercise and who show symptomatic benefit from oxygen in terms of walking distance. It is given using a refillable portable container of liquid oxygen. The aim of this treatment is to improve quality of life rather than extend it.

HYPOXIA DURING AIR TRAVEL

Commercial aircraft routinely fly at about 38,000 feet and are pressurised to a cabin altitude of 8000 feet. The reduced partial pressure of oxygen at this altitude is equivalent to breathing 15% oxygen at sea level, and causes the PaO_2 of a healthy passenger to fall to between 7.0 and 8.5 kPa. Although this does not usually cause symptoms or problems for most passengers, it can produce critical hypoxia for patients with lung disease. Most patients with COPD (even severe disease) are not precluded from flying, but a specialist pre-flight assessment may be needed to determine if supplementary in-flight oxygen is necessary (Ahmedzai et al., 2011).

SURGERY

A very small number of patients with COPD may benefit from surgery. Lung transplantation is an option, although lack of donor organs severely limits the utilisation of this procedure. Bullectomy may be appropriate where a large bulla is compressing surrounding viable lung. Lung volume reduction surgery is an option for selected patients with severe disability. Such procedures can only be considered after optimisation of all medical therapy under the direction of a respiratory specialist. See Chapter 14 for further details.

EMERGENCY TREATMENT

Exacerbations of COPD are characterised by an acute worsening of symptoms with increased breathlessness, sputum volume and sputum purulence. They may occur spontaneously or as a result of infections. Patients can be taught to recognise the onset of an exacerbation and to start a self-management plan whereby they increase the dose and frequency of bronchodilator medication and start a course of oral prednisolone and an antibiotic, according to a predetermined plan. Mild exacerbations can be managed at home, but patients with severe exacerbations require admission to hospital. Deciding whether a patient can be managed at home requires an overall assessment of the severity of the COPD (e.g. baseline FEV_1, oxygen saturation, exercise capacity), the home circumstances (e.g. family support, able to cope) and key adverse features that indicate a severe exacerbation (e.g. confusion, cyanosis, severe respiratory distress) (BTS, 2007). Patients admitted to hospital should have a chest X-ray, oximetry, arterial blood gas measurement, an ECG, full blood count and urea and electrolyte measurements. Culture of sputum is often performed, but rarely produces a result in time to influence antibiotic prescribing. Bronchodilator therapy is usually given by nebuliser using a combination of salbutamol 2.5–5 mg and ipratropium 500 mcg with prednisolone 30 mg/day for 7–14 days (NICE, 2010).

ANTIBIOTICS

Not all exacerbations are associated with bacterial infection. From a practical perspective, antibiotics should be used when there is a history of more purulent sputum. Resistance to amoxicillin is rising in the bacteria commonly associated with exacerbations. Doxycycline is more commonly used first line now with other antibiotics such as co-amoxiclav as a second line.

EMERGENCY OXYGEN

Oxygen is delivered in most emergency situations with the aim of achieving a near normal saturation of 94%–98% (O'Driscoll et al., 2008). However, for some patients such levels are dangerous and may be life threatening. Uncontrolled oxygen therapy poses a risk to this subset of patients with COPD; however, the risk, of course, must be balanced against the threat of hypoxia. Debate exists over the 'hypoxic drive' theory in association with the administration of oxygen therapy. Regardless of the underlying physiology, it is important that patients with hypercapnia receive an adequate oxygen supply. In patients at risk of hypercapnic respiratory failure (which unless proven otherwise includes any patient with an exacerbation of COPD) treatment should be commenced using controlled oxygen with an initial target saturation of 88%–92% pending urgent blood gas assessment. In this 'Goldilocks' zone the patient will not die of hypoxia and it is very unlikely there will be any appreciable respiratory depression (O'Driscoll et al., 2008).

VENTILATORY SUPPORT

Occasionally acute respiratory acidosis complicates an exacerbation of COPD, despite the best efforts of doctors and nurses. It is crucially important to recognise respiratory acidosis when it is present; therefore, blood gas analysis is essential to the management of acute exacerbations of COPD in hospital (see Chapter 4). After initial management with nebulised bronchodilators and appropriate oxygen therapy, if the pH is below the normal range (<7.35) then non-invasive ventilation (NIV) should be employed. It should be delivered in a dedicated setting with staff who have been trained in its application and there should be a clear plan covering what to do in the event of deterioration. When used in this context, NIV not only reduces the likelihood that the patient will progress to need invasive ventilation, it has also been demonstrated to reduce inpatient mortality by 50% (Royal College of Physicians [RCP] et al., 2008). See Chapter 17 for a more detailed discussion of NIV.

ADMISSION AVOIDANCE AND EARLY SUPPORTED DISCHARGE FOR COPD

Novel ways of managing patients with acute exacerbations of COPD are being developed. In some cases, admission to hospital can be avoided by undertaking an initial assessment, in the patient's home, usually by a specialist nurse according to an agreed protocol with the backup of a respiratory specialist (and the option of admission if needed). Easy access to such a reassuring review can often prevent patients calling an ambulance unnecessarily. Such schemes are being increasingly adopted and in the hands of appropriately skilled and experienced healthcare professionals appear to be safe. For other patients, early supported discharge is more appropriate whereby after initial treatment and stabilisation in hospital ongoing care is provided to the patient in their own home. This model of care is now well established. It is safe, effective and very popular with patients (BTS, 2007).

CASE STUDY

Mr Wilson, a 62-year-old man, was brought to the emergency department (ED). He was severely breathless and said he'd thought he was 'breathing his last' when his wife called the ambulance. On arrival at the hospital his oxygen saturation was 95% (breathing room air), he had a cough, productive of clear sputum, though he said this was no different to usual. His chest X-ray showed no signs of pneumonia. He was given nebulised salbutamol and ipratropium and within an hour or so said he felt better. He was keen to go home because he knew 'the doctors and nurses were very busy'. He was given a short course of oral prednisolone and because this had been his third attendance at the ED in the past 4 months he was given an outpatient appointment for the chest clinic.

When he was reviewed by the specialist in clinic three weeks later, Mr Wilson explained that his breathing had been a problem for about six months. With careful questioning, however, it was clear he had been struggling over several years. Mr Wilson worked all of his life in labouring jobs, but three years ago found himself having to give up work entirely. Since giving up work things had really declined and apart from his three trips to ED he had not been out of the house for 5 months. Mr Wilson said he had been given a blue and a brown inhaler by his GP; he found the blue one very useful and was going though one every two weeks. He admitted that he did not use the brown one as 'it didn't do anything.' Mr Wilson admitted that he had smoked since the age of 15 (about 20 cigarettes per day), he knew it was not good for him, but it was 'the only pleasure he had left'. Since he had stopped going to his local social club, he no longer saw anyone apart from his wife. Even his activity around the house was curtailed, and he worried that if he did too much he would not be able to catch his breath at all. Exploring this, Mr Wilson said he found episodes of breathlessness frightening and that they made him panic. He reported a cough productive of clear sputum on a daily basis, although he had had a number of chest infections where his sputum turned green and he had needed antibiotics from his GP about once a month.

Lung function testing in the chest clinic revealed obstructive spirometry with FEV_1/VC ratio 49% and his FEV_1 was only 53% of the predicted value. Gas transfer was diminished with the transfer coefficient (K_{CO}) only 72% of the predicted value. His oxygen saturation was 94%. When the doctor walked him along the corridor, although Mr Wilson quickly became quite breathless, his saturation actually picked up a little to 95%. A Hospital Anxiety and Depression questionnaire suggested Mr Wilson had a high level of anxiety.

When his inhaler technique was checked it was found that he was not really co-ordinating 'the press and the breathe in' very well and the nurse suspected most of the drug was probably getting no further than the back of his throat. The doctor explained to Mr Wilson that he had a condition called 'COPD', which stood for chronic obstructive pulmonary disease. Mr Wilson had not heard of it but when the doctor explained that it was what used to be called 'chronic bronchitis and emphysema', Mr Wilson explained that his mother had had that and that he did not want 'to go the way she'd gone in the end'. The doctor explained that there was only one way he could avoid that and that was to stop smoking. The memory of his mother frightened Mr Wilson and he made a firm commitment to quit. He accepted referral to the smoking cessation clinic for support.

Mr Wilson asked the doctor if he could have oxygen at home to help his breathing. The doctor took time to explain why he did not need home oxygen and that it would not help.

Mr Wilson was started on an ICS/LABA combination inhaler and a separate LAMA inhaler in addition to his old salbutamol. The nurse carefully coached and then tested his inhaler technique. She also explained that the inhalers were not just to help him feel less breathless, but to stop him getting so many 'chest infections'. He should therefore stick with them even if he was not sure at first how much they were helping.

Mr Wilson was offered a place on the pulmonary rehabilitation (PR) course, but said it was not really for him. When the issue of panic and anxiety was discussed, however, Mr Wilson agreed to see the specialist nurse for cognitive behavioural therapy (CBT). It was explained that he would be taught special techniques and 'breathing exercises' that would stop him panicking and help him keep control of his breathing when he felt it was getting out of hand.

When seen back in clinic 3 months later Mr Wilson showed significant improvement. He said the new inhalers really worked and that he was rarely using his blue inhaler now. Since seeing the CBT nurse, he had only had one 'panic attack' but felt he had been able to get things back under control with what the nurse had taught him. When the doctor offered him pulmonary rehabilitation he was very keen to accept referral this time.

When seen back in clinic after his rehabilitation course, Mr Wilson said he was now able to walk much further without stopping for breath. This had enabled him to get back out to see his friends at the club twice a week, he felt he was no longer 'under his wife's feet' all of the time and although he had had a course of antibiotics for a chest infection a month ago, this was the first in about 6 months.

CASE STUDY DISCUSSION

Mr Wilson's case demonstrates that COPD is a multifaceted disease, not only was it affecting Mr Wilson's physical health, but he had been forced to give up employment (affecting his income), he was anxious and depressed (affecting his mental health), he had become socially isolated (affecting his quality of life) and had become dependent on his wife (affecting their relationship). Mr Wilson's frequent attendance at the ED prompted referral to a specialist, who with careful history taking and spirometry was able to prescribe appropriate medication to improve Mr Wilson's condition and quality of life. Despite the enhanced medication, giving up smoking was the single greatest factor that would improve disease progression for Mr Wilson (NICE 2010).

The case study also demonstrates how a multidisciplinary approach to the management of COPD is vital. A number of healthcare professionals were involved in the care of Mr Wilson. Accurate diagnosis and appropriate prescription by a specialist physician are vital, but it was also vital that Mr Wilson was taught how to use the inhalers by the nurse. Inhaler technique should be checked at every review (Halpin et al., 2015). Other specialist nurses and services also contributed to Mr Wilson's care in the form of CBT, PR and smoking cessation. Mr Wilson was not given oxygen despite being very breathless as his saturation at 95% was above the target of 88%–92% (O'Driscoll et al., 2008). This demonstrates the point that 'short of breath' does not imply 'short of oxygen'. Similarly, Mr Wilson's chest X-ray was clear, which suggested that this exacerbation was not due to infection and therefore antibiotics were not prescribed.

SUMMARY

COPD is an umbrella term encompassing the inter-related entities of emphysema, chronic bronchitis and airway obstruction. Getting the diagnosis right is critical: it relies on a careful history and quality-assured, correctly interpreted spirometry. In COPD appropriate treatment can now offer improvements in breathlessness, cough, quality of life, anxiety, depression, exercise capacity, exacerbation rate, hospitalisation rate, disease progression and even survival. Smoking cessation does not allow the lungs to return to normal, but it prevents further damage occurring. Over time this will have a dramatic impact on a patient's quality as well as quantity of life. Oxygen therapy is of no use to patients who are not hypoxic. In patients who desaturate significantly on exertion ambulatory oxygen may help them do more. In patients permanently and significantly hypoxic at rest oxygen therapy can prolong life.

Some treatments in COPD offer more than just short-term alleviation of breathlessness. When a treatment is given for prognostic benefit (e.g. to reduce the risk of exacerbations) it should be continued whether or not a patient notices any immediate improvement in symptoms.

REFERENCES

Ahmedzai, S., Balfour-Lynn, I.M., Bewick, T., Buchdahl, R., Coker, R.K., Cummin, A.R., Gradwell, D.P. et al. 2011. Managing passengers with stable respiratory disease planning air travel: British Thoracic Society recommendations. *Thorax* 66 (Suppl 1): i1–i30.

Alberg, A.J. and Carpenter, M.J. 2012. Enhancing the effectiveness of smoking cessation interventions: A cancer prevention imperative. *Journal of the National Cancer Institute* 104 (4): 260–262.

Bourke, S.J. and Burns, G.P. 2015. *Respiratory Medicine Lecture Notes* (9th Ed.). Wiley Blackwell, Oxford.

British Thoracic Society (BTS). 2007. Intermediate care: Hospital at Home in chronic obstructive pulmonary disease: British Thoracic Society Guideline. *Thorax* 62 (suppl 3): 200–210.

Calverley, P.M.A., Anderson, J.A., Celli, B., Ferguson, G.T., Jenkins, C., Jones, P.W., Yates, J.C. and Vestbo, J. for the TORCH investigators 2007. Salmeterol and fluticasone propionate and survival in chronic obstructive pulmonary disease. *New England Journal of Medicine* 356: 775–789.

Celli, B.R. and MacNee, W. 2004. Standards for the diagnosis and treatment of patients with COPD: A summary of the ATS/ERS position paper. *European Respiratory Journal* 23 (6): 932–946.

Ferguson, J., Bauld, L., Chesterman, J. and Judge, K. 2005. The English smoking treatment services: One-year outcomes. *Addiction* 100 (S2): 59–69.

Fletcher, C. and Peto, R. 1977. The natural history of chronic airflow obstruction. *British Medical Journal* 1 (6077): 1645–1648.

Halpin, D., Holmes, S., Calvert, J. and McInerney, D. 2015. Improving inhaler technique. *Nursing Standard* 26 (1): 16–20.

Heslop, K., De Soyza, A., Baker, C., Stenton, C. and Burns, G. 2009. Using individualised cognitive behavioural therapy as a treatment for people with COPD. *Nursing Times* 105 (14): 14–17.

Heslop, K., Newton, J., Baker, C., Carrick-Sen, D., Burns, G.P. and De Soyza, A. 2013. Effectiveness of cognitive behavioural therapy (CBT) interventions for anxiety and depression in patients with chronic obstructive pulmonary disease (COPD) undertaken by respiratory nurses. The COPD CBT CARE Study. *BMC Pulmonary Medicine* 13 (1): 62–68.

Kim, V., Crappo, J., Zhao, H., Jones, P.W., Silverman, E.K., Comellas, A., Make, B.J., Criner, G.J., and the COPDGene Investigators. 2015. Comparison between an alternative and the classic definition of chronic bronchitis in COPDGene. *Annals of the American Thoracic Society* 12 (3): 332–339.

Medical Research Council. 1981. Long term domiciliary oxygen therapy in chronic hypoxic cor pulmonale complicating chronic bronchitis and emphysema. Report of the Medical Research Council Working Party. *Lancet* 317 (8222): 681–686.

NHS. 2011. Hone Oxygen Service: Assessment and Review. Good Practice Guide. Available at http://improvementsystem.nhsiq.nhs.uk/ImprovementSystem/ViewDocument.aspx?path=Lung%2FNational%2FHome%20Oxygen%2Fhome_oxygen_service_assessment_and_review.pdf

National Institute of Health and Care Excellence (NICE). 2010. *COPD Management of Chronic Obstructive Pulmonary Disease in Adults in Primary and Secondary Care. Clinical Guidelines 101.* NICE, London.

O'Driscoll, B.R., Howard, L.S. and Davison, A.G. 2008. British Thoracic Society guideline for emergency oxygen use in adult patients. *Thorax* 63 (Suppl 6): vi1–vi73.

Primary Care Respiratory Society – UK (PCRS-UK). 2010. *Diagnosis and Management of COPD in Primary Care.* Primary Care Respiratory Society-UK, Leeds.

Royal College of Physicians., British Thoracic Society and Intensive Care Society. 2008. *Non-Invasive Ventilation in Chronic Obstructive Pulmonary Disease: Management of Acute Type 2 Respiratory Failure*. Royal College of Physicians, London.

Tashkin, D.P., Celli, B., Senn, S., Burkhart, D., Kesten, S., Menjoge, S., Decramer, M. for the UPLIFT Study Investigators 2008. A 4-Year trial of tiotropium in chronic obstructive pulmonary disease. *New England Journal of Medicine* 359 (Suppl 15): 1543–1554.

West, R., McNeill, A. and Raw, M. 2000. Smoking cessation guidelines for health professionals: An update. *Thorax* 55 (12): 987–999.

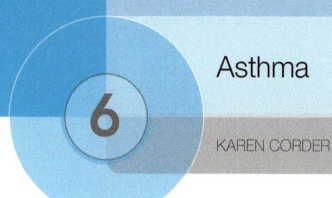

Asthma

6

KAREN CORDER

LEARNING OBJECTIVES

Upon completion of this chapter the reader should be able to:

- Provide a definition of asthma and discriminate between the different classifications
- Describe the clinical investigations performed that support a diagnosis of asthma
- Identify genetic susceptibility and environmental factors that may trigger or worsen symptoms
- Discuss the management of asthma
- Understand and follow the stepwise approach to treatment

INTRODUCTION

Asthma is a non-communicable long-term condition affecting the lungs. Inhaled substances and particles can irritate the airways or trigger an allergic reaction, which results in inflammation. The resulting inflammation causes the airways in the lungs to become narrowed, leading to symptoms of breathlessness, chest tightness, cough and wheeze (Asthma UK, 2014). According to the World Health Organisation (WHO) some 235 million people suffer from asthma globally, yet they believe it remains under-diagnosed and under-treated (WHO, 2013). The National Institute for Health and Care Excellence (NICE, 2013) state that asthma is the most common long-term condition in the UK, with 5.4 million people currently receiving treatment, of which 1.1 million

are children. The causes of asthma are not well understood and with the exception of some cases of occupational asthma, a cure is not usually possible. Therefore, the management goal for people with asthma is symptom control to allow them to lead a normal active life (NICE, 2013).

An annual audit undertaken by the British Thoracic Society regarding adult hospital admissions for acute asthma concluded that readmission rates for asthma were relatively unchanged from previous audits, and remained disappointingly high (Lindsay and Heaney, 2013). Their data show that 7.5% of patients were readmitted to hospital within a month of discharge and a further 8.2% had been discharged in the previous 1–3 months, whereas 64.5% had either not had a previous admission or none within the last 12 months. A similar audit carried out in relation to paediatric asthma (Paton, 2013) noted that over 70% of children admitted to hospital were less than 5 years of age, reporting that the evidence base for acute asthma management in this group of young children is weak. Both reports indicate that based on published evidence, significant improvements can be made by educating patients in the correct use of their inhaled devices and ensuring that a written action plan for further exacerbations is supplied.

This chapter aims to provide an overview of asthma and will include a definition and classification of asthma with reference to relevant anatomy and physiology regarding the respiratory system. Clinical investigation and diagnosis of asthma will be discussed. Genetic and environmental factors that may trigger or worsen symptoms will be identified along with the consideration of co-factors. Finally, a case study will be used to consider the management and stepwise approach to treatment for asthma.

DEFINITION AND CLASSIFICATION

Hargreave and Nair (2009) state that defining asthma is controversial as there is no single genetic or environmental cause. They offer a simple definition of 'abnormality of airway function'. According to the Global Initiative for Asthma (GINA, 2015), central to all definitions are the symptoms (more than one of wheeze, breathlessness, chest tightness and cough) and variable airflow obstruction. Furthermore, they note that more recent descriptions of asthma have included hyper responsiveness and airway inflammation. There is no gold standard definition that makes evidence-based recommendations for asthma diagnosis impossible. Difficulty in defining asthma leads to difficulty in diagnosing asthma. Hargreave and Nair (2009) recommend caution when making such a diagnosis, suggesting that asthma may not be a disease entity but perhaps an abnormality of one component such as airflow limitation or airway hyper-responsiveness.

Bourke and Burns (2011) advocate that asthma is not a fixed consistent disease, suggesting it has added complications owing to its heterogeneous and dynamic nature. They offer the example that asthmatic patients with well-controlled disease are often asymptomatic and possess normal lung function between attacks. However, they report

that further investigations of those asymptomatic patients would reveal evidence of airway inflammation and increased responsiveness.

According to the latest report 'Global Strategy for Asthma Management and Prevention' from GINA (2014), based on consideration of characteristics that are typical of asthma, and therefore to distinguish it from other respiratory diseases the following definition was reached by consensus:

Asthma is a heterogeneous disease, usually characterised by chronic airway inflammation. It is defined by the history of respiratory symptoms such as wheeze, shortness of breath, chest tightness and cough that vary over time and intensity, together with variable expiratory airflow limitation (GINA, 2014, p. 2).

Although asthma diagnosis in children and adults shares many features, there are important differences. Diagnosing asthma relies upon the recognition of a characteristic pattern of symptoms and the absence of an alternative explanation for them. The key to accurate diagnosis lies in taking a careful clinical history as the differential diagnosis, history of wheeze and ability to perform as well as the diagnostic value of investigations can all be influenced by age (British Thoracic Society/Scottish Intercollegiate Guidelines Network [BTS/SIGN], 2013).

Clinical features that increase the probability of an individual having asthma include the presence of more than one of the following symptoms: wheeze, cough, difficulty breathing, chest tightness. This is particularly likely if these symptoms:

- Occur frequently and are recurrent
- Are worse at night or early morning
- Occur in response to, or are worse after exercise
- Occur in response to, or are worse after other triggers such as contact with pets, exposure to cold or damp air, or emotions or laughter
- There is a history of atopic disorder
- There is a family history of atopic disorder or asthma
- There is widespread wheeze heard on auscultation
- There has previously been an improvement in symptoms or lung function in response to treatment (BTS/SIGN, 2013)

Clinical features that lower the probability of asthma include:

- Symptoms with colds only, with no interval symptoms
- Isolated cough in the absence of wheeze or difficulty breathing
- History of moist cough
- Prominent dizziness, light-headedness, peripheral tingling
- Repeatedly normal physical examination of chest when symptomatic
- Normal peak expiratory flow (PEF) or spirometry when symptomatic
- No response to a trial of asthma therapy
- Clinical features pointing to alternative diagnosis (BTS/SIGN, 2013)

The National Review for Asthma Deaths (Royal College of Physicians [RCP], 2014) states that the underlying pathological process that results in features of asthma varies between individuals.

Therefore, it is likely that their asthma triggers and response to treatment will be variable. Uncontrolled episodes and attacks can be life threatening and at times fatal. An average of three people die every day from asthma, and around 90% of those are considered to be preventable. Based on these facts, RCP (2014) advocate that each patient has their asthma triggers identified and their treatments tailored to meet their individual needs (see Table 6.1).

PATHOPHYSIOLOGY

The pathophysiology of asthma is complex and involves airway inflammation, intermittent airflow obstruction, bronchial hyper responsiveness and ultimately airway remodelling in response to persistent inflammation. According to Bourke and Burns (2011) asthma symptoms are triggered when a series of factors work together to produce increasing airway inflammation, airway responsiveness and finally bronchoconstriction. They promote the theory of a two-phase response, which includes an 'early asthmatic reaction' to an inhaled allergen, within a maximum of 20 minutes, followed by a second phase around 6–12 hours later referred to as a 'late asthmatic reaction'.

Inflammation in the airways is caused by dilation in the small blood vessels in the mucosa. This dilation causes the small pores in the walls of the blood vessels to become larger. According to Hasan-Arshad and Suresh-Babu (2008), water cells and proteins are released from the blood vessels into the mucosa. These blood cells then become deactivated, which allows the inflammatory cells (including mast cells, eosinophils, B and T lymphocytes and neutrophils) to release their contents which contain chemicals known as mediators given that they mediate inflammation. The resulting mediators cause production of mucus as they stimulate the glands in the mucsa. The same mediators stimulate the bronchial muscles, which causes constriction and narrowing of the bronchial tubes. As a result of this inflammatory process and subsequent narrowing of the airways, individuals with asthma develop wheezing and breathlessness. Coughing occurs due to the mucosa irritation from the excess mucus. Inflammatory cells which are present in the mucus initiate further airway narrowing as they cause irritation and twitching in the airways. This irritability is referred to as bronchial hyper responsiveness, and it increases the likelihood of a reaction when an irritant such as dust or smoke is introduced. Oni et al. (2010) advocate that non-specific stimuli such as exercise, emotional

Table 6.1 Classifying asthma severity

Components of severity	Age in years	Classification of asthma severity (intermittent vs persistent)			
		Intermittent	Persistent		
			Mild	Moderate	Severe
Symptoms	ALL	≤2 Days/week	>2 Days/week but not daily	Daily	Throughout the day

Source: Adapted from Global Initiative for Asthma. 2014. *Pocket Guide for Asthma Management and Prevention (For Adults and Children over 5 Years): A Pocket Guide for Physicians and Nurses.* Available at: http://ginasthma.org/local/uploads/files/GINA_Pocket_2014_Jun11.pdf.

Note: Classifications of asthma are based on how often symptoms occur and how bad they are.

stress, cold air or pharmacological agents such as histamine or methacholine can also provoke the same reaction.

Rees et al. (2010) suggest that permanent fibrotic damage as a result of irreversible airflow obstruction may occur in poorly controlled asthma. However, they acknowledge that remodelling of the airway wall in response to persistent inflammation can resolve. Bourke and Burns (2011) believe that airway remodelling leading to fibrosis and fixed narrowing of the airway impedes the response to bronchodilator medication.

Please note, in-depth structure of the airways and lungs can be found in Chapter 1, which focusses specifically on respiratory anatomy and physiology.

CLINICAL INVESTIGATIONS AND DIAGNOSIS OF ASTHMA

The BTS/SIGN (2014) state that the key to an accurate asthma diagnosis is to take a careful clinical history; this is because recognition of a characteristic pattern of signs and symptoms in the absence of an alternative explanation is the basis for asthma diagnosis. The NICE (2013) Quality Standard for Asthma outlines the need to diagnose asthma in accordance with the BTS/SIGN guidance. However, they warn that diagnosis is not a one-off event and may need to be reviewed, particularly in younger children. In their draft guidance, NICE (2015) offer simple flow charts for healthcare professionals to use to aid the initial assessment. The diagnostic process for children and adults would include:

- History and clinical examination
- Objective tests if the clinical diagnosis is uncertain
- Response to treatment given in accordance with the BTS/SIGN treatment steps (BTS/SIGN, 2013)

ASTHMA PHENOTYPES

There are recognisable clusters of demographic, clinical and/or pathophysiological characteristics often referred to as 'asthma phenotypes'. GINA (2014) suggests more research is needed to understand phenotype classification in asthma. However, it is reported that some phenotype-guided treatments are available for severe asthmatic patients. Phenotypes:

- *Allergic asthma* – Most easily recognisable as it often commences in childhood and is associated with family history of allergic diseases such as eczema, allergic rhinitis and food and drug allergies.
- *Non-allergic asthma* – This occurs in adults who have no allergy.
- *Late-onset asthma* – Often occurring in adult women, who present with symptoms for the first time in adulthood.
- *Asthma with fixed airflow limitation* – Fixed airflow obstruction develops in some patients with long-standing asthma. This is thought to be as a result of the airway walls remodelling.
- *Asthma with obesity* – Prominent respiratory symptoms can be found in obese asthma patients with little eosinophilic airway inflammation.

GENETIC SUSCEPTIBILITY AND ENVIRONMENTAL FACTORS

There is often a familial history of asthma. Hasan-Arshad and Suresh-Babu (2008) confirm that families often have many members with asthma, spread across generations, which indicates a genetic susceptibility. However, they note that although there is strong evidence of genetic contribution, the hereditary effect is not straightforward. Bourke and Burns (2011) state that evidence shows that a child may not necessarily have asthma even if both parents are asthmatic. They go on to advocate that the development of asthma depends on environmental factors reacting with a genetic predisposition; this they believe is apparent as families share environments as well as genes.

Individuals who demonstrate symptoms of asthma owing to exposure to one or more allergens are said to have 'allergic asthma' or 'atopic asthma' (see information on phenotype above). Atopy is an inherited tendency to produce significant amounts of immunoglobin E (IgE) on minimal exposure to common antigens. IgE refers to antibodies that are produced when an individual experiences exposure to a new allergen. Once produced, these antibodies can react to the same allergen when subsequently exposed. As a result, these individuals are referred to as hyper allergic. Skin prick testing will establish responses to a range of common allergens; however, Rees et al. (2010) state that the results only show an individual's tendency to produce the IgE; confirming atopy. Furthermore, they note that 20% of the population will have positive skin prick test results, yet less than half of those will go on to develop asthma. Elevated total IgE is often seen in those individuals with atopic asthma.

In addition to the genetic effect, environmental factors are of great importance in the aetiology of asthma. Rees et al. (2010) suggest that prior to birth, prenatal stress, cigarette smoke and air pollutants can all have an impact on asthma risk for the unborn child. Asthma studies have been conducted into populations who have migrated from one country to another. One such widely published study reviewed the prevalence of asthma in Tokelauan children aged from birth to 14 years. Bourke and Burns (2011) report that, following a hurricane which devastated the local economy, many Tokelauan children were evacuated to New Zealand. Those who had settled in New Zealand showed a significantly higher prevalence of asthma than those children who remained in Tokelauan. These findings suggest that the increasing prevalence is likely to be attributed to environmental rather than genetic factors. Specific environmental factors cannot be identified; however, it is considered that moving from a rural environment into an urban area increases exposure to allergens such as house dust mites, fungal spores and pollution.

Environmental exposure relates to indoors and outdoors. Bourke and Burns (2011) suggest that overall exposure to air pollutants should be determined by indoor concentrations as they believe that people spend a minimum of 75% of their time indoors. They consider this to be of particular importance to young children as their exposure early in life determines their sensitisation. This theory is supported by Hasan-Arshad and Suresh-Babu (2008) as they remark that our genes do not change significantly over a few decades. Therefore, the increase in asthma and allergic disease must be attributable to environmental exposure. Common indoor and outdoor environmental factors include diet, infection,

allergens and pollution. Rees et al. (2010) report that there is a relationship between asthma and increased salt intake, low selenium or reduced vitamin C and E. However, they observe that no single factor can be held responsible.

As noted above, allergens such as house dust mites found in carpets, or those from pets are common in households. Central heating leads to high humidity and an increase in fungal spores. According to Bourke and Burns (2011), indoor pollution from cigarette smoking, open fires or paraffin stoves (popular again today) has adverse effects on asthma in children in particular as well as other respiratory diseases. Furthermore, studies have shown asthma control to be significantly worse in those who smoke cigarettes compared to those who have never smoked.

Motor vehicle emissions and fuel burning industries contribute to the source of pollution in the outdoor environment. However, Hasan-Arshad and Suresh-Babu (2008), Rees et al. (2010) and Bourke and Burns (2011) all agree that outdoor pollution levels do not correlate with changes in asthma prevalence. However, they state that outdoor air pollution does play a part in triggering exacerbations of pre-existing asthma, although this is not completely understood. This further compounds the notion that asthma is indeed a complex multifactorial condition.

MANAGEMENT OF ASTHMA

For all but the most severely affected patients, the ultimate goal is to prevent symptoms, minimise morbidity from acute episodes, and prevent functional and psychological morbidity to provide a healthy (or near healthy) lifestyle appropriate to the age of the individual. GINA (2014) promotes control-based asthma management. This involves adjusting asthma treatment in accordance with a continuous cycle to assess, adjust treatment and review the response:

Assess
- Diagnosis
- Symptom control and risk factors (including lung function)
- Inhaler technique and adherence
- Patient preference

Adjust treatment
- Asthma medications
- Non-pharmacological strategies
- Treat modifiable risk factors

Review response
- Symptoms
- Exacerbations
- Side-effects
- Patient satisfaction
- Lung function

BTS/SIGN (2014) refer to the aim of asthma management as control of the disease. They go on to define complete control as:

- No daytime symptoms
- No night-time awakening due to asthma
- No need for rescue medication
- No asthma attacks

- No exacerbations
- No limitations on activity including exercise
- Normal lung function (in practical terms forced expiratory volume in 1 second [FEV_1] and/or PEF >80% predicted or best)
- Minimal side effects from medication

BTS/SIGN (2014) advocate using the 'stepwise approach' to management of asthma (see Figures 6.1 to 6.3 below), starting treatment at the most appropriate step depending on initial severity. Control can be maintained by stepping up or down treatment as necessary. They encourage practitioners to check adherence to the current regime, including inhaler technique in an attempt to eliminate trigger factors ahead of initiating new therapies.

According to BTS/SIGN (2014), self-management education incorporating written personalised asthma action plans (PAAPs) improves health outcomes, and

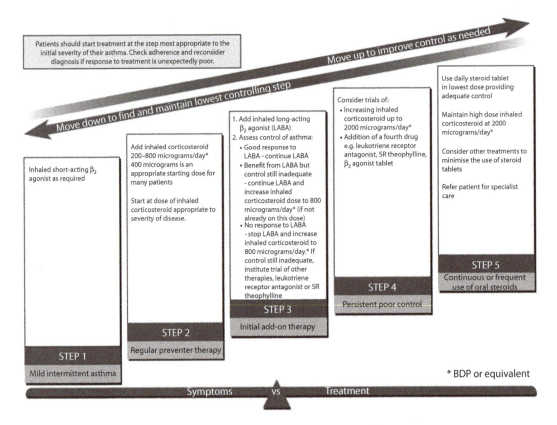

Figure 6.1 Summary of stepwise management in adults. (Adapted from British Thoracic Society/Scottish Intercollegiate Guidelines Network. 2014. *British Guideline on the Management of Asthma: Revised 2014.* Available at: https://www.brit-thoracic.org.uk/document-library/clinical-information/asthma/btssign-asthma-guideline-2014/.)

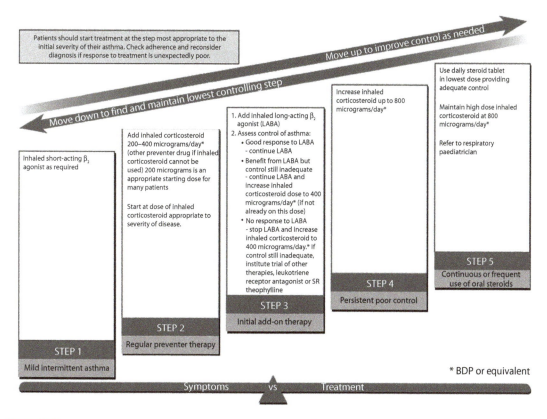

Figure 6.2 Summary of stepwise management in children aged 5–12 years. (Adapted from British Thoracic Society/ Scottish Intercollegiate Guidelines Network. 2014. *British Guideline on the Management of Asthma: Revised 2014.* Available at: https://www.brit-thoracic.org.uk/document-library/clinical-information/asthma/btssign-asthma-guideline-2014/.)

should be offered to all patients on a general practice 'active asthma' register. The benefits of the use of a written action plan alongside educating patients in the correct use of their inhaled devices are echoed in the results from the BTS annual audits looking into hospital admissions for adults and children with asthma (Lindsay and Heane, 2013; Paton, 2013). Self-management action plans are available to download from Asthma UK and should be supplied to all hospital inpatients prior to their discharge by health-care professionals who have expertise in providing asthma education (BTS/SIGN, 2014).

Bourke and Burns (2011) emphasise that, if successful management is to prevail, individuals must understand the nature of their asthma and its treatment. In order to ensure education is consistent they advocate asthma education begins at diagnosis and every subsequent consultation. Offering insight into the multifactorial aetiology and identification

of precipitating factors is deemed a good starting point. Rees et al. (2010) acknowledge the importance of patient education, stating that an explanation of the role of inflammation in the airways is paramount. In addition, medication education is of equal importance. According to GINA (2014), around 80% of patients do not use their inhaler correctly, which leads to poor symptom control and ultimately an exacerbation of their asthma. Patients often get confused about basic aspects such as short-acting β_2 agonists (SABAs) and long-acting β_2 agonists (LABAs) combined with a steroid; advising them of which is a 'reliever' (bronchodilator) and which is the 'preventer' (anti-inflammatory) will support them to use their inhalers appropriately. The practitioner prescribing the medication should also consider the most appropriate device for each individual; taking into account potential difficulties due to physical dexterity such as arthritis.

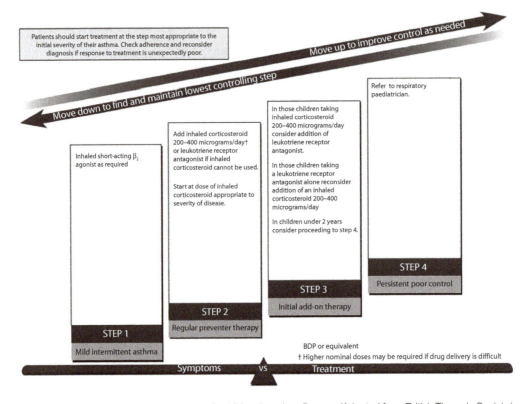

Patients should start treatment at the step most appropriate to the initial severity of their asthma. Check adherence and reconsider diagnosis if response to treatment is unexpectedly poor.

Move up to improve control as needed

Move down to find and maintain lowest controlling step

Refer to respiratory paediatrician.

In those children taking inhaled corticosteroid 200–400 micrograms/day consider addition of leukotriene receptor antagonist.

In those children taking a leukotriene receptor antagonist alone reconsider addition of an inhaled corticosteroid 200–400 micrograms/day

In children under 2 years consider proceeding to step 4.

Add inhaled corticosteroid 200–400 micrograms/day† or leukotriene receptor antagonist if inhaled corticosteroid cannot be used.

Start at dose of inhaled corticosteroid appropriate to severity of disease.

Inhaled short-acting β₂ agonist as required

STEP 4
Persistent poor control

STEP 3
Initial add-on therapy

STEP 2
Regular preventer therapy

STEP 1
Mild intermittent asthma

BDP or equivalent
† Higher nominal doses may be required if drug delivery is difficult

Symptoms   vs   Treatment

Figure 6.3 Summary of stepwise management in children less than 5 years. (Adapted from British Thoracic Society/ Scottish Intercollegiate Guidelines Network. 2014. *British Guideline on the Management of Asthma: Revised 2014.* Available at: https://www.brit-thoracic.org.uk/document-library/clinical-information/asthma/btssign-asthma-guideline-2014/.)

Peak flow meters that measure the peak expiratory flow of the airways can be used effectively with patients as it allows them to see the daily variability of their airway obstruction. Bourke and Burns (2011) believe that asthma patients can self-manage their disease in a similar vein to those who have diabetes and monitor their blood sugar levels in order to adjust their insulin therapy, using the peak flow readings to influence treatment and/or seek further medical advice.

Non-pharmacological management of asthma includes avoidance of precipitating factors. Environmental control is difficult as most households have dust mites in mattresses, carpets and other soft furnishings. Bourke and Burns (2011) state that dust mite levels can be reduced by using mattress covers and washing bedding frequently. Furthermore, humidity, which is responsible for creating an environment conducive to dust mites, can be reduced through improved home ventilation. Conversely, BTS/SIGN (2014) state that physical and chemical methods used to reduce house dust mite levels are not effective and as a result should not be recommended by healthcare practitioners. Avoidance of allergens from cats or dogs is possible, although pet allergens may remain in the home for up to six months after removal of the pet and results are often disappointing. Weight loss should be supported in overweight patients owing to the many health benefits and potential to improve asthma symptoms. Breathing exercise programmes are considered to be useful in reducing symptoms and improving quality of life and should be offered as an adjuvant to pharmacological treatment.

Management of asthma will not be complete unless co-factors are considered, controlled and, if possible, treated. Respiratory infections may aggravate airways due to increased response from inflammatory cells; the resulting mediators will cause airway narrowing and bronchoconstriction. Hasan-Arshad and Suresh-Babu (2008) comment that cigarette smoking is known to increase IgE levels, thus increasing susceptibility to allergens. Passive smoking is also shown to have an adverse effect on asthma as well as other respiratory diseases. BTS/SIGN (2014) state that patients should be advised about the dangers of smoking to themselves and others and provided smoking cessation support. Beta blocking drugs are known to potentially induce bronchoconstriction in patients with asthma; even when administered through the conjunctiva in the form of eye drops. Bourke and Burns (2011) also report worsening asthma symptoms owing to use of non-steroidal anti-inflammatory drugs such as ibuprofen. Once sensitivity is known, these patients should avoid aspirin preparations.

STEPWISE APPROACH TO TREATMENT

According to GINA (2014), a stepwise approach to asthma treatment takes into account the effectiveness of available medications, their safety and their cost. It is advocated that regular preventer treatment, particularly with inhaled corticosteroids (ICS), reduces the frequency and severity of asthma symptoms as well as reduces the risk of flare-ups. ICSs are indicated on step two of the stepwise management in adults, children 5–12 years and children aged less than five years.

CASE STUDY

Julie is a 39-year-old estate agent who has a cough which is worse at night and in the mornings. Although no longer a smoker, she attributes the cough to lung damage caused by cigarette smoking and therefore she has not sought advice from her GP. Overweight and unfit, in an effort to improve her lifestyle and lose weight ahead of her 40th birthday Julie joined a gym. Initially Julie experienced difficulty participating in 30-minute exercise classes, suffering with dyspnoea and chest tightness within ten minutes. At that time Julie considered the symptoms she experienced to be related to her lack of fitness and excess weight. After six weeks Julie noticed that, although she considered her fitness to have improved, she was still experiencing dyspnoea and chest tightness when exercising. Julie is divorced from her husband and she lives in a two-bedroomed house with her 14-year-old daughter. Julie is an ex-smoker and only drinks alcohol socially (around 10 units of wine at the weekend). There are no pets within the home.

Julie attended her GP surgery at their request for a health check. During the consultation Julie discussed with her GP her recent change in lifestyle, new fitness regime and subsequent symptoms upon exertion. Julie has a past medical history of menorrhagia, endometriosis and mild eczema. Julie smoked cigarettes and has a 10 pack year history. Julie has no known allergies. Julie's GP took a detailed clinical history from her and a diagnosis of asthma or chronic obstructive pulmonary disease (COPD) was considered. Upon physical examination, everything was normal and her lung sounds were clear. However, spirometry revealed her baseline results suggested mild airway obstruction:

	Baseline (pre bronchodilator)	% of Predicted
FVC (forced vital capacity)	3.6 L	69
FEV_1	2.9 L	76
FEV_1/FVC	70%	

Spirometry was repeated after 15 minutes post inhaled bronchodilator to ascertain if any improvement and therefore clarify diagnosis of asthma or mild COPD. Her results showed a marked improvement post bronchodilator:

	Post bronchodilator	% of predicted
FVC	4.2 L	77
FEV_1	3.4 L	93
FEV_1/FVC	87%	

The large positive response to the use of a bronchodilator is consistent with a diagnosis of asthma. Julie's spirometry results, considered along with her non-significant physical examination results and her detailed clinical history, led to a diagnosis of asthma.

In accordance with the BTS/SIGN (2014) stepwise management of asthma in adults (see Figure 6.1), Julie was prescribed a short-acting β_2 agonist as required. In addition, Julie was encouraged to use the inhaler approximately 15 minutes prior to her exercise classes for maximum benefit. Julie was given a follow-up appointment to attend the asthma clinic four weeks later in order to assess her response to treatment.

CASE STUDY DISCUSSION

This case study demonstrates that asthma can be diagnosed at any age. Although Julie was relatively young at 39 years, the GP did consider a diagnosis of COPD because of Julie's history of smoking (see Chapter 5). The use of spirometry was essential in forming an accurate diagnosis for Julie. The spirometry showed a marked improvement between pre- and post-bronchodilator therapy (see Chapter 3). According to national guidelines, Julie was started on the treatment most appropriate to the severity of her asthma and was followed up (BTS/SIGN, 2014). It is important that Julie is regularly assessed at her GP asthma clinic, that she understands the nature of her disease and its management, and what to do if she suffers an exacerbation. Her inhaler technique should also be assessed at every follow up.

SUMMARY

Asthma is a non-communicable long-term condition affecting the lungs which is usually characterised by chronic airway inflammation. It is a multifactorial disease that occurs due to a complex interaction of genetic and environmental factors. Airflow obstruction is a clinical characteristic of asthma that can be reversed over short periods of time or with treatment. Most patients can experience a good level of asthma management through the use of inhaled medication. Patient education is vital to ensure understanding of the disease, its severity and the importance of preventative medication. Self-management should be encouraged through the use of personalised asthma action plans (PAAP). Medication adherence and correct use of inhaled devices should be checked at every contact and prior to stepping up treatment.

REFERENCES

Asthma UK. 2014. www.asthma.org.uk.

Bourke, S.J. and Burns, G.P. 2011. *Respiratory Medicine: Lecture Notes* (8th ed.). Wiley-Blackwell, Chichester.

British Thoracic Society/Scottish Intercollegiate Guidelines Network. 2013. *British Guideline on the Management of Asthma: Quick Reference Guide.* [updated online]. Available at: https://www. brit-thoracic.org.uk/document-library/clinical-information/asthma/btssign-asthma-guideline-quick-reference-guide/.

British Thoracic Society/Scottish Intercollegiate Guidelines Network. 2014. *British Guideline on the Management of Asthma: Revised 2014.* Available at: https://www.brit-thoracic.org.

uk/document-library/clinical-information/asthma/btssign-asthma-guideline-2014/.

Global Initiative for Asthma. 2014. *Pocket Guide for Asthma Management and Prevention (For Adults and Children over 5 Years): A Pocket Guide for Physicians and Nurses.* Available at: http://ginasthma.org/local/uploads/files/GINA_Pocket_2014_Jun11.pdf.

Global Initiative for Asthma. 2015. *Pocket guide for Asthma Management and Prevention (For adults and children over 5 years): A Pocket Guide for Physicians and Nurses.* Available at: http://www.ginasthma.org/local/uploads/files/GINA_Pocket_2015_Jun11.pdf.

Hargreave, F.E. and Nair, P. 2009. The definition and diagnosis of asthma. *Clinical and Experimental Allergy* 39 (11): 1652–1658.

Hasan-Arshad, S. and Suresh-Babu, K. 2008. *Asthma: The Facts*. Oxford University Press, Oxford.

Lindsay, J. and Heaney, L. 2013. British Thoracic Society *Adult Asthma Audit*. Available at: https://www.brit-thoracic.org.uk/document-library/audit-and-quality-improvement/audit-reports/bts-adult-asthma-audit-report-2012/.

National Institute for Health and Care Excellence. 2013. *Quality Standard for Asthma: NICE Quality Standard 25*. Available at: guidance.nice.org.uk/qs25.

National Institute for Health and Care Excellence. 2015. *Asthma: Diagnosis and Monitoring of Asthma in Adults, Children and Young People. [Draft Guidance]*. Anticipated publication date: July 2015. Available at: https://www.nice.org.uk/news/article/draft-guideline-to-improve-asthma-diagnosis.

Oni, A.O., Eweka, A.O. and Otuaga, P.O. 2010. The relevance of co-factors in asthma. *International Journal of Biomedical and Health Sciences* 6 (1): 7–12.

Paton, J. 2013. British Thoracic Society *Paediatric Wheeze/Asthma Audit Report*. Available at: https://www.brit-thoracic.org.uk/document-library/audit-and-quality-improvement/audit-reports/bts-paediatric-asthma-audit-report-2012/.

Rees, J., Kanabar, D. and Pattani, S. 2010. *ABC of Asthma*. (6th ed.). Wiley-Blackwell, Chichester.

Royal College of Physicians. 2014. *Why Asthma Still Kills: The National Review of Asthma Deaths (NRAD)*. Available at: https://www.rcplondon.ac.uk/sites/default/files/why-asthma-still-kills-full-report.pdf.

World Health Organisation. 2013. *Asthma: Fact Sheet No. 307*. Available at: http://www.who.int/mediacentre/factsheets/fs307/en/.

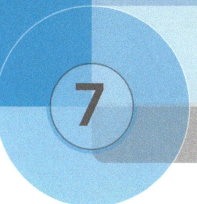

Tuberculosis

7

VANESSA GIBSON AND CHRIS STENTON

LEARNING OBJECTIVES

Upon completion of this chapter the reader should be able to:

- Discuss the cause of tuberculosis
- Provide a definition of tuberculosis and differentiate between the different classifications of tuberculosis
- Identify risk factors for the development of tuberculosis
- Discuss the treatment and prevention of the disease

INTRODUCTION

Tuberculosis (TB) is one of the commonest communicable diseases in the world. The World Health Organisation (WHO) estimated that in 2014 approximately 10 million people developed TB and 1.5 million died from it (WHO, 2015a). Most of those affected live in low-income countries of Africa, Asia and South America. In several sub-Saharan African countries more than 1 in 200 people develop the disease each year. TB is second only to human immunodeficiency virus (HIV) as the world's greatest killer from a single infectious agent (WHO, 2015b).

Almost all cases of TB are contracted via the respiratory route (Public Health England [PHE], 2013). TB can spread to almost any part of the body,

but this chapter will focus on pulmonary TB, which accounts for approximately 60% of cases in the United Kingdom (UK). This chapter will discuss the pathogenesis and classification of the disease. It will also discuss risk factors for contracting TB, current treatment and complications, and prevention strategies. Finally, a case study will be presented.

DEFINITION AND CLASSIFICATION

Tuberculosis is a bacterial infection caused by either *Mycobacterium tuberculosis* (*M. tuberculosis*), *Mycobacterium bovis* (*M. bovis*) or *Mycobacterium africanum* (*M. africanum*) (PHE, 2013). *M. tuberculosis* is the main cause of TB in humans. *M. bovis* infects cattle, badgers and other wild animals, but can also infect humans, particularly those who drink unpasteurised milk from infected cattle. *M. africanum* is very similar to *M. tuberculosis* and is found almost exclusively in West Africa where it causes up to a quarter of TB infections.

Mycobacteria are rod-shaped bacteria that have a layer of the lipid mycolic acid on their cell surface. This gives them a waxy, hydrophobic coating (Madigan et al., 2015) and makes them resistant to drying, acidity, alkalinity and antibiotics. It also gives them some unique properties that help them evade hosts' immune systems (Sakamoto, 2012) and remain alive but dormant for many years. Mycobacteria have an unusual staining pattern when examined microscopically. They resist staining by dyes unless these are combined with phenol, but once stained the dye is difficult to remove with acidified organic solvents. The organism is described as 'acid-fast' (Lawn and Zumla, 2011). Traditionally, a Ziehl-Neelsen (ZN) stain was used to identify mycobacteria, but now other techniques are more generally used.

PATHOPHYSIOLOGY

Individuals with active pulmonary TB are a source of infection and can spread it to others by droplets that are expelled when they cough or sneeze. The particles can remain airborne for several days. Inhaled bacteria enter the lungs of the new host and begin to multiply. The immune system mounts a response, as explained in detail in Chapter 10. Neutrophils and macrophages arrive to try to phagocytose the bacteria. At this point the immune system may:

1. Completely eliminate the bacteria so that the person does not develop any disease and is not infectious.
2. Contain the bacteria but fail to kill them. The leucocytes at the site of infection secrete cytokines that in turn attract other macrophages and lymphocytes. These encircle and enclose the mycobacteria in granulomas, which then develop a peripheral fibrous capsule that seals off the infection. The mycobacteria are not killed off but they cannot spread. They may remain dormant for the whole of the host's lifetime but they may be reactivated if

the immune system is weakened, for example by age, immunosuppression or other illness (Haney and Stenton, 2010; Ahmad, 2011; PHE, 2013; Zumla et al., 2013). This is known as latent TB. The infected individual has no symptoms and cannot spread the disease to others.

3. Fail to mount an adequate response so that the bacteria continue to replicate, leading to the development of symptoms and active TB. The centres of the granulomas undergo necrosis with caseous (cream cheese-like) material derived from lipids and proteins of dead macrophages in their centres. These 'caseating granulomas' are diagnostic of TB. If the TB is eventually eradicated, the granulomas contract to form a scar or calcify. A small TB nodule in the lungs is sometimes known as a Ghon focus (Sakamoto, 2012).

Symptomatic disease develops in only approximately 10% of those who are infected with TB (Ahmad, 2011). The remainder develop latent TB. There are several reasons why some people go on to develop active TB while others do not. These include immune suppression, an initial high bacterial load, infection with particularly virulent bacteria, or genetic susceptibility (Sakamoto, 2012). In most cases the disease progresses within the chest but it may spread to distant organs either by the lymphatics or via the blood. Lymph nodes, kidneys, the meninges and bones are often involved but TB can affect any part of the body (Lawn and Zumla, 2011). Miliary TB is the term for widespread TB with multiple small (millet seed-sized) nodules that can be easily seen on a chest X-ray.

RISK FACTORS AND EPIDEMIOLOGY

Tuberculosis was known in ancient times and features of infection can be found for example in Egyptian mummified human remains. It became common in Europe at the time of the industrial revolution when mass migration into towns and very poor, overcrowded living conditions promoted rapid spread of the disease. It is estimated that in the seventeenth and eighteenth centuries TB was responsible for a quarter of adult deaths in Europe (Griffith and Kerr, 1996). In the UK, TB is now much less common, affecting approximately 12 per 100,000 of the population. The decline of TB occurred mostly because of improvement in housing, nutrition and general health rather than any drug treatment.

TB was at one time thought to be under control in the UK, but rates have increased by approximately 40% from their lowest point in 1987. Initially this was because of the HIV epidemic of the 1980s, but more recently rates have risen because of increased movement of people to and from countries where the disease is more common. The rate of TB in the UK is relatively high and is, for example, over 4 times higher than that in the USA. Approximately 6000–7000 cases are diagnosed each year (Public Health England [PHE], 2014).

HIV is the most important individual risk factor for TB. It increases the risk 20–40 times and accounts for much of the persistence of TB in regions of the world where HIV prevalence is high (Griffith and Kerr, 1996). The WHO (2015a) estimate that of the 10 million people who developed TB in 2014, 12% were HIV positive and 74% of these were from Africa. TB is the leading killer of HIV positive people (WHO, 2015b).

Other important risk factors for TB include diabetes, cigarette smoking, treatment with corticosteroids, and drug or alcohol abuse. Silicosis (see Chapter 9) increases the risk of developing TB up to 80 times. Men are slightly more likely than women to develop TB. It can affect any age group, but is commonest in young adults (PHE, 2015a).

More recently, treatment of rheumatoid arthritis and other inflammatory conditions with anti-tumour necrosis factor (TNF) monoclonal antibodies such as Inflixamab has been recognised to increase the risk of TB (Gomez-Reino et al., 2003). TNF is a cytokine that is important in maintaining the integrity of granulomas. Anti-TNF antibodies disrupt granulomas and allow TB to spread. Guidelines generally recommend screening for TB before starting treatment with these agents (Ormerod et al., 2005).

Migration from countries with a high TB prevalence now makes an important contribution to TB in the UK. While the annual risk of TB in UK-born citizens is four per 100,000, the risk in those born abroad and now living in the UK is approximately 10 times higher at 40 per 100,000. The risk is highest in the first few years after moving to the UK and the disease is probably triggered by stresses of moving, reduced exposure to sunlight and changes in diet. Imprisonment, overcrowding and poor general health increases the risk of TB in refugees and asylum-seekers. Screening of those entering or about to enter the UK from countries where TB is an important public health procedure.

Migration patterns largely explain the marked geographic differences in TB prevalence within the UK. London accounts for the highest proportion of cases in England at 40% followed by the West Midlands at 12%. The north-east and south-west have the lowest incidences. TB in those born abroad is more likely to be non-pulmonary, affecting lymph nodes or other organs.

DIAGNOSIS

ACTIVE TB

Active TB can develop within a few weeks of infection or may occur after many years due to reactivation of latent disease. With pulmonary disease the individual is likely to be infectious and spread the disease via droplet infection (PHE, 2013; Oliphant, 2015). The key to establishing a diagnosis of TB is to consider the possibility. Initial symptoms are often mild and might include a persisting cough, fever and night sweats, poor appetite and weight loss, chest pain or erythema nodosum (WHO, 2014; Oliphant, 2015; Ward et al., 2015). If left untreated, the symptoms will worsen and the TB is likely to prove fatal.

A chest X-ray is usually the first investigation and will almost always be abnormal with pulmonary TB. Mycobacteria tend to favour the apical and posterior segments of the lungs where there is higher oxygen pressure but poor perfusion (Sakamoto, 2012; Oliphant, 2015). Cavities develop as the disease progresses (see Figure 7.1). Non-pulmonary disease may be more difficult to diagnose and a CT scan may be needed to identify for example lymph node TB.

Three sputum samples should be obtained if pulmonary TB is suspected, and stained and cultured for TB. If a large number of mycobacteria are present in the sputum, they can be seen microscopically and

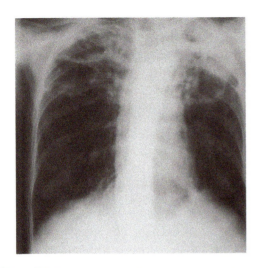

Figure 7.1 Posterior–anterior (PA) chest X-ray of a patient with TB demonstrating typical shadowing in the upper and posterior zones. (Reproduced from Davies, P.D.O., Lalvani, A. and Thillai, M. 2015. *Clinical Tuberculosis: A Practical Handbook*. CRC Press, London. With permission.)

the specimen is said to be 'smear positive'. If there are fewer organisms, they may not be seen and the specimen is 'smear negative', but they can still be grown in culture. Smear-positive patients are more infectious

than smear negative. *M. tuberculosis* is a slowly growing organism that may take up to 6 weeks to culture in the laboratory. When it has been cultured its sensitivity to anti-tuberculous drugs can be tested and that helps guide treatment (see Table 7.1).

The genetic makeup of *M. tuberculosis* is well characterised and modern molecular techniques are increasingly being used to help with diagnosis. Polymerase chain reactions (PCR) can be used to rapidly identify *M. tuberculosis* genes in sputum and other samples. The gene that makes *M. tuberculosis* resistant to treatment with rifampicin is also known and can be identified in sputum and other samples using PCR. The GeneXpert™ test combines testing for both *M. tuberculosis* genes and rifampicin resistance and can provide rapid information about the diagnosis and treatment. This is potentially particularly useful in low-income countries (WHO, 2013).

Attempts should always be made to obtain samples for culture and drug sensitivity testing, but sometimes treatment has to be started while awaiting these results. Extra-pulmonary TB is often only diagnosed from biopsies that show caseating granulomas. Unfortunately, often TB is not suspected when the biopsy is obtained and samples are not sent for culture

Table 7.1 Investigations used in the diagnosis of TB

Investigation	Procedure and rationale
Posterior-anterior chest X-ray	Abnormal findings on chest X-ray may suggest TB but are not diagnostic. Chest X-ray appearance consistent with TB should lead to further investigations.
Sputum samples	Spontaneously produced sputum should be obtained. If this is not possible bronchoscopy and lavage may be used. At least three sputum samples should be obtained (one early morning) for TB microscopy and culture. These should be obtained prior to starting treatment or with 7 days of commencing treatment. A sputum smear should be performed for acid-fast bacilli, but this is only likely to be positive with rates of 5000 organisms per millilitre. Culture may take 2–6 weeks depending on media used.
Sputum samples from children	These should be produced spontaneously, or via induction of sputum expectoration or via gastric washings.
Tuberculin skin test	The Mantoux test is used and purified tuberculin protein is injected intra-dermally. The Mantoux test should be read 48–72 hours after administration. The site of the test should be inspected and palpated for a hard, raised, dense area of swelling (induration). The area should be measured using a ruler and an induration of greater than 5 mm indicates a response by the immune system to either TB infection, infection with environment mycobacteria or previous BCG vaccination.
Blood tests	Single blood tests are now available to test for TB antigens. Two tests are available and known as QuantiFERON-TB Gold and T-SPOT. Results are available in 16–24 hours. These are also known as Interferon-Gamma Release Assays (IGRAs).

(Haney and Stenton, 2010). For a range of investigations used in the diagnosis of TB see Table 7.1.

LATENT TB

The diagnosis of latent TB depends on finding evidence that the immune system has been stimulated by *M. tuberculosis*. The Mantoux test involves injecting mycobacterial protein (tuberculin) intradermally and measuring the diameter of the swelling after 72 hours. A positive test indicates that the immune system has previously been in contact with tuberculin and recognises it as foreign. Bacillus Calmette–Guerin (BCG) immunisation stimulates the immune system to react to tuberculin, and that limits the usefulness of the test in those who have been immunised.

Modern tests for the identification of latent TB rely on stimulating blood lymphocytes in the laboratory by incubating them with proteins from *M. tuberculosis* and measuring the amount of the inflammatory mediator interferon gamma that is released. They are known as interferon gamma release assays or IGRAs. A positive test indicates that the blood contains lymphocytes that have been in contact with mycobacteria. IGRAs have a major advantage over tuberculin skin tests as they use proteins that are found in *M. tuberculosis* but not in other mycobacteria such as BCG. They are not positive in those who have been immunised with BCG and so are more specific for TB. They are often negative in active TB and their main use is in diagnosing latent disease.

TREATMENT

ACTIVE TB

The discovery of antibiotics in the mid twentieth century led to most patients being cured of TB. Previously infected individuals were isolated in sanatoria where rest, fresh air and good nutrition were provided to try to combat the disease. *M. tuberculosis* is highly oxygen dependent for its growth, and a variety of techniques were developed to deprive the lungs of oxygen. These included inducing artificial pneumothoraces, crushing the phrenic nerve to reduce the function of the diaphragm, or breaking the ribs and pushing in the chest wall – a thoracoplasty (Daniel,

2006). Older patients are still occasionally seen with X-ray abnormalities caused by these procedures.

In 1946 streptomycin was discovered and found to be effective against *M. tuberculosis*. This was followed by isoniazid in 1952 and rifampicin in 1970 (Griffith and Kerr, 1996). Modern drug treatment of TB is very effective, with more than 98% of patients being cured provided they take their medication regularly. Multiple antibiotics are required as *M. tuberculosis* readily develops resistance to single antibiotics, and a long period of treatment is needed to be sure that all dormant or slowly growing bacteria are killed. The standard regimen recommended by the National Institute of Health and Care Excellence (NICE) (2016) involves 6 months of isoniazid and rifampicin supplemented in the first 2 months with pyrazinamide and ethambutol. These drugs are usually given as fixed-dose combination tablets as that reduces the risk that the patient will take one tablet but not the others and so develop drug resistance.

Hepatotoxicity is the most important side effect of TB treatment and liver function needs to be monitored carefully (Joint Formulary Committee [JFC], 2015). Patients should be given advice that the drugs, particularly rifampicin, will interact with other medications, especially oral contraceptives and corticosteroids. They should be advised that bodily secretions, particularly urine, might turn a red/orange colour. Isoniazid depletes vitamin B6 and can cause a peripheral neuropathy, particularly in those who are susceptible because of diabetes or alcohol abuse. Other common side effects of TB treatment include optic neuritis with ethambutol, gastrointestinal disturbances, rashes, joint pains, hypersensitivity reactions and blood abnormalities.

Patients diagnosed with TB will need a number or pre-treatment screening investigations. Pre-treatment checks should include:

- Full blood count
- Urea and electrolyte
- Liver function tests
- Visual acuity and colour vision
- HIV, Hepatitis B and C testing (NICE 2016)

The treatment of TB is long and complex. Patients often do not speak English, could be homeless, substance abusers or mentally ill and potentially difficult to engage with (Haney and Stenton, 2010). Monitoring for compliance with medication and side effects requires treatment by an expert multidisciplinary team. Partial treatment of TB leads to the development of drug-resistant disease and that adds hugely to the complexity, cost and risks of treatment.

Patients should be allocated a key worker, usually a nurse specialist, to oversee treatment. Consideration should be given to factors that might improve adherence. These include joint decision making about the setting and frequency of treatment, home visits, advice on social security benefits, housing and social services support, use of interpreters and health education advice. Directly observed therapy (DOT) involves a skilled worker watching the patient taking their medication and is an important approach to ensuring compliance. All patients should have their risk of non-compliance assessed and DOT considered if it is likely to be poor (NICE, 2016). DOT can be given using a thrice-weekly regimen (NICE, 2016), but it is not possible to manage TB giving the medication less often than that. TB medication is exempt from NHS prescription charges in the UK when prescribed by specialist TB centres (Haney and Stenton, 2010).

Every effort should be made to enable those with TB to adhere to treatment. In exceptional circumstances when patients refuse treatment they can be detained under the Health and Social Care Act 2008 in order to protect the public. They cannot be forced to take treatment.

Patients with TB should not be treated in hospital unless they are acutely unwell. If hospital admission is necessary, they should be given a single room and separated from any immunocompromised patients. Each hour of close contact with a TB patient carries approximately a 1 in 10,000 chance of developing the disease. There is no need for healthcare professionals to wear masks or gowns unless multi-drug-resistant TB (MDR-TB) is suspected, or aerosol generating procedures such as bronchoscopy, chest physiotherapy or using nebulised saline to generate sputum samples are being performed. Aerosol-generating procedures should be performed in appropriately engineered and ventilated rooms. Infectivity decreases rapidly with treatment and after 2 weeks patients are non-infectious and no longer need to be separated from others. If a patient with TB has to leave their room, they should wear a surgical mask until they have completed 2 weeks of treatment (NICE, 2016).

Patients often need reassurance and psychological support. Other supportive measures such as analgesia, hydration, nutrition, rest and activity need to be addressed. Any visitors to a child with TB in hospital should be screened for TB and kept separate from other patients until they are excluded as a source of infection.

If the patient does have MDR-TB, then healthcare professionals and visitors should wear FFP3 masks during contact with patients. The patient should be isolated in a negative pressure room under the care of a consultant experienced in complex MDR-TB cases. Before a patient with MDR-TB is discharged from hospital the case should be discussed with the infection control team, the microbiologist, the local TB service and the consultant in communicable diseases control. Secure arrangements for the supervision and administration of drugs should be agreed with patients and carers (NICE, 2016).

LATENT TB

Those with latent TB have far fewer infecting mycobacteria than patients with active TB. Their treatment still needs to be prolonged to be sure that slowly growing organisms are killed but the risk of developing drug resistance is much less and so fewer drugs can be used. A variety of treatment regimens are used. Isoniazid alone can be given for up to 6 months. In the UK a combination of rifampicin and isoniazid for 3 months is most commonly used (NICE, 2016). NICE (2016) gives detailed advice about treating neonates and children for latent TB.

The treatment of latent TB only reduces the risk of developing active TB by about two-thirds. There is no test for its effectiveness and IGRA tests often remain positive after treatment for latent TB. It is important to consider the possibility of active TB in someone with the appropriate symptoms even if they have undergone previous treatment for latent disease.

The risks of side effects of treating latent TB are similar to the risks of treating active disease and careful monitoring is still required. The risk of hepatitis increases with age and so guidelines often recommend offering treatment only to those aged less than 65 years, although with regular checking of liver function the treatment can be given to older individuals (see Table 7.2).

DRUG-RESISTANT TB

Micro-organisms including mycobacteria have developed resistance to antibiotics over the decades since antibiotics were first discovered. Drug-resistant TB can be classified as primary or secondary. Primary resistance occurs in patients who have been infected by someone with drug-resistant disease, usually from travel to or living in a part of the world where drug-resistant TB is common. High-risk countries include India, China and the Russian Federation. Acquired or secondary drug resistance in TB occurs in patients who have been incompletely treated for TB and the treatment has failed usually because of poor compliance (Haney and Stenton, 2010; Oliphant, 2015).

About 7% of TB in the UK is resistant to isoniazid. This is relatively easily managed with a more prolonged course of treatment. Resistance to rifampicin is much more serious and is often accompanied by resistance to other anti-tuberculous antibiotics. Multiple-drug-resistant (MDR) TB is TB that does not respond to at least rifampicin and isoniazid, which are the most powerful, first line anti-TB drugs (WHO, 2015b). About 1% of TB in the UK is MDR. The WHO (2015a) estimate that globally 3.3% of new cases and 20% of previously treated cases have MDR-TB.

Early identification of MDR-TB is very important as the treatment is very different from that for drug-sensitive disease. A range of 'second-line' drugs is used, and treatment may need to be continued for at least 20 months (WHO, 2011). The treatment is complex and side effects are common and so MDR-TB must be managed in one of a small number of specialist centres. Features that point to MDR-TB

Table 7.2 Treatment of latent TB in the UK

Consider treatment for latent tuberculosis (NICE, 2016)
Entrants from countries with high TB prevalence
Household contacts under 65 years old. Older people have an increasing risk of hepatoxicity
Immunocompromised patients — including HIV
Prisoners; substance abusers
Healthcare workers
Children who are Mantoux or IGRA positive
Diabetes, chronic renal disease, silicosis

include a history of prior TB treatment, contact with a known case of MDR-TB, residence in an area with a high incidence of MDR-TB or HIV infection (NICE, 2016). However, PCR testing for the gene for rifampicin resistance which indicates MDR-TB should be used in all positive sputum or culture samples.

Recently, extensively drug-resistant disease (XDR-TB) has been described. This form of MDR-TB is resistant to some or all of the second-line anti-TB drugs and presents even greater treatment and public health challenges (WHO, 2015b). XDR-TB had been reported in 105 countries by 2015 and it is estimated that 9.7% of people with MDR-TB have XDR-TB.

IMMUNISATION

Bacillus Calmette–Guerin (BCG) immunisation was first used in humans in 1921 and was an important step in the control of TB. BCG is a form of *M. bovis* that has been modified in culture to reduce its virulence. When injected into the skin it causes localised inflammation and ulceration that heals over a few days. That stimulates the immune system and offers protection against developing TB. The protection is not complete and has varied between 0% and 80% in different studies, probably related to variations in exposure to non-tuberculous environmental mycobacteria. BCG is most effective in early life, particularly in reducing the risk of TB meningitis in children.

The BCG school vaccination programme was introduced in the UK in 1953 and targeted children aged 14. The programme was stopped in 2005 because of uncertainty about its cost-effectiveness given the falling rates of TB. Currently TB immunisation in the UK is a risk-based programme (PHE, 2013) and is recommended for some previously non-immunised tuberculin skin test negative groups:

- Infants 0–12 months living in areas with a high incidence of TB (40/100,000 or above)
- Infants and children under 15 years with a parent or grandparent born in a country with a high incidence of TB
- Children under 16 years who are contacts of cases of respiratory TB with a parent or grandparent born in a country with a high incidence of TB

- Children under 16 years who were born, or who have lived for a prolonged period in a country with a high incidence of TB
- Adults under 35 years working in high-risk occupations including healthcare and laboratory staff, veterinary and abattoir staff, prison staff and staff working in care homes and hostels for the homeless (PHE, 2013)

PUBLIC HEALTH ISSUES

TB would not exist if it did not spread from one person to another by the inhalation of infected droplets or particles. Stopping the spread of infection by early identification and treatment of infectious patients, those who have recently been infected but have not yet developed disease, and those with latent TB is an important public health measure.

CONTACTS

Tuberculosis is a 'notifiable disease' and any doctor who has diagnosed a case must report it to a proper officer of the local authority, usually the public health consultant, within 3 days. This requirement for notification of infectious diseases has been a vital health protection measure since the late nineteenth century. Similar schemes are found in many countries. Early reporting allows the prompt identification of contacts of those with TB, and treatment before they themselves become infectious. It also allows for the collection of data for epidemiological surveillance and the identification of patterns of spread. This can help monitor the effectiveness of treatment and inform the planning of healthcare services (PHE, 2010). In the UK this is now facilitated by PCR genetic fingerprinting of most cultures of *M. tuberculosis*. When samples from two patients have identical genetic fingerprints it is very likely that one has infected the other.

The person with TB is known as the index case. Others who have had close contact with the index case should be identified and systematically investigated for TB. Close household contacts are those who live with the index case and share meals, etc. Typically, approximately one in 10 close household contacts will have been infected by the index case and if left untreated 1 in 100 will develop active disease.

Others will be left with latent disease that may reactivate later in life. Sometimes work colleagues, intimate friends or frequent visitors to the home have the same amount of exposure as household contacts and need to be screened. Casual contacts include the vast majority of work colleagues and do not need to be screened except occasionally when the index case is very infectious (NICE, 2016).

The main aim of contact screening is to identify anyone who might have been infected by the index case using an IGRA and treat them before they themselves develop active disease. If there is any suspicion that the individual might have active TB, then a chest X-ray should be obtained.

Many individuals who feel perfectly well are reluctant to take prolonged courses of treatment, and compliance rates are often very low. Those who decline treatment for latent TB should have a chest X-ray at 3 and 12 months. All contacts should be advised of the risks and given 'inform and advise' information about the symptoms to watch out for should they develop TB.

ENTRANTS

In the UK at present approximately half of all TB develops in those who were born abroad. New entrants to the country from areas where there is a high prevalence of TB are at high risk and require screening for TB.

Since 2014 anyone living in a country with an incidence of TB of more than 40 per 100,000 who intends to stay in the UK for more than 6 months has been required to obtain a chest X-ray before they obtain a visa. In 2014, a total of 233,000 people were screened in this way, and 224 cases of TB were identified.

A new UK latent tuberculosis infection (LTBI) screening programme aims to screen all migrants who entered the UK in the last five years from a country of high incidence using IGRAs (PHE, 2015b) and offer treatment to those with positive tests. Screening for latent TB should be incorporated into larger health screening programmes including testing for HIV and hepatitis and ensuring adequate immunisation.

OTHER GROUPS

In the past, mobile chest X-ray programmes screened large numbers of the population. This is no longer cost effective but occasionally screening of high-risk groups such as the homeless, drug and alcohol abusers or prisoners might be necessary.

The WHO has set a target of a 95% reduction in deaths and a 90% decline in TB incidence by 2035, bringing the incidence in low-income countries down to that of more economically developed countries (WHO, 2015c). In England, Public Health England has recently stated its aim of reducing the incidence of TB year on year and eliminating it as a public health problem. Continued effort, improved resources and vigilance will be necessary to achieve that.

CASE STUDY

Mr O'Reilly is a 74-year-old gentleman who had been complaining of fatigue, weight loss, night sweats and a persistent cough for the last 5 weeks. He is a widower but is frequently visited by his adult children and grandchildren. His daughter finally persuaded Mr O'Reilly to go to his GP because she was concerned about his persistent cough and weight loss and privately thought that her father might have lung cancer. The GP sent Mr O'Reilly for a chest X-ray which revealed cavitation in the right upper lobe and he was immediately recalled to the surgery. Mr O'Reilly was asked to provide sputum samples, which later cultured positive for TB. A sputum smear was positive for acid fast bacilli. The GP followed the relevant procedures for notification and referral to a specialist physician and Mr O'Reilly was commenced on a four drug regimen (NICE, 2016).

Baseline blood tests were taken and Mr O'Reilly was monitored throughout his treatment. He complained of gastric disturbance and numbness in his hands and feet but was able to complete his six-month course of antibiotics and was cleared of TB.

Mr O'Reilly lived alone but was active in his local community, he had an allotment and socialised regularly with friends as well as receiving frequent visits from his family.

CASE STUDY DISCUSSION

Mr O'Reilly had fairly typical symptoms for TB (Oliphant, 2015; Ward et al., 2015). However, as TB is relatively uncommon in UK-born citizens it never occurred to him that he could have TB (PHE, 2015a). He was not in a high-risk group and it was never discovered how he caught TB, the most likely cause being reactivation of latent TB. Mr O'Reilly's symptoms of weight loss and a persistent cough were concerning to his daughter, but she also never suspected TB and was concerned that her father may have lung cancer as he was an ex-smoker.

Cavitation in the upper lobe is a common finding on chest X-ray as the *M. tuberculosis* favours the upper lobe (Sakamoto, 2012; Oliphant, 2015). The finding of the chest X-ray immediately prompted the GP into action, but he also had not suspected TB because Mr O'Reilly lived in a fairly affluent area in a low-incidence region of the UK.

At 74 Mr O'Reilly was in danger of suffering severe side effects from his treatment and he was monitored with regular blood tests as hepatoxicity was a particular concern. Mr O'Reilly's peripheral neuropathy was probably a side effect of the isoniazid but this was monitored and did not need to be stopped (Haney and Stenton, 2010).

Mr O'Reilly was assessed for risk of non-adherence but was deemed low risk and did not require directly observed therapy. Despite Mr O'Reilly having no household contacts, contact tracing was needed. Mr O'Reilly was sputum-smear positive and therefore frequent visitors to his home who were his children and grandchildren were assessed. Casual contacts which included his friends from the allotment were not assessed but 'inform and advise' information was given out (NICE, 2016). Mr O'Reilly's children were all over 40 years old and had been vaccinated under the old BCG schools' vaccination scheme. However, they were offered treatment for latent TB under the new NICE guidelines (NICE, 2016). Mr O'Reilly did have an 18-month old granddaughter. Because she was not in a high-risk category, she had never had a BCG vaccination as a baby (PHE, 2013) and was therefore started on isoniazid and given a Mantoux test, which was negative. In accordance with NICE (2016) guidelines the Mantoux test was repeated after six weeks together with an interferon gamma test, which were both negative. At that point the isoniazid was stopped and the grandchild was vaccinated (NICE, 2016).

SUMMARY

TB is second only to HIV as the greatest killer worldwide from a single infectious agent. Mycobacteria that cause tuberculosis possess properties that make them resilient and difficult to eradicate. TB can remain latent, but alive, in a host for the entirety of their life but can be reactivated for example by immunosuppression. Typical symptoms of TB are a chronic cough, night sweats, anorexia and weight loss. TB is a notifiable disease. Treatment is complex and patients should be treated by physicians with expertise supported by a multidisciplinary team. Several potentially toxic drugs are needed for long periods of time, with the minimum duration being 6 months. Patients need close monitoring during treatment as poor compliance leads to drug-resistant disease. MRD-TB and XDR-TB are concerning developments as these strains are resistant to multiple antibiotics, making treatment very complex and prolonged. BCG immunisation has been available for almost a century but its effectiveness is variable. These combined factors make TB very difficult to eradicate.

REFERENCES

Ahmad, S. 2011. Pathogenesis, immunology, and diagnosis of latent *Mycobacterium tuberculosis* infection. *Clinical and Developmental Immunology*. 2011: 17. Article ID 814943, doi:10.1155/2011/814943.

Daniel, T.M. 2006. The history of tuberculosis. *Respiratory Medicine* 100 (11): 1862–1870.

Davies, P.D.O., Lalvani, A. and Thillai, M. 2015. *Clinical Tuberculosis: A Practical Handbook.* CRC Press, London.

Gomez-Reino, J.J., Carmona, L., Valverde, V.R., Mola, E.M. and Montero, M.D. 2003. Treatment of rheumatoid arthritis with tumor necrosis factor inhibitors may predispose to significant increase in tuberculosis risk. *Arthritis and Rheumatism* 48 (8): 2122–2127.

Griffith, D.E. and Kerr, C.M. 1996. Tuberculosis: Disease of the past, disease of the present. *Journal of PeriAnaesthesia Nursing* 11 (4): 240–245.

Haney, S. and Stenton, S.C. 2010. Tuberculosis and the older patient. *Reviews in Clinical Gerontology* 20 (2): 81–91.

Joint Formulary Committee (JFC). 2015. *British National Formulary* (68th ed.). British Medical Association and Royal Pharmaceutical Society of Great Britain, London.

Lawn, S.D. and Zumla, A.I. 2011. Tuberculosis. *Lancet* 378 (9785): 57–72.

Madigan, M.T., Martinko, J.M., Bender, K.S., Buckley, D.H. and Stahl, D.A. 2015. *Brock Biology of Micro-Organisms* (14th ed.). Person, Boston.

National Institute of Health and Care Excellence (NICE). 2016. *Tuberculosis. Clinical Diagnosis and Management of Tuberculosis, and Measures for Its Prevention and Control.* Clinical Guideline NG33. NICE, London.

Oliphant, C.M. 2015. Tuberculosis. *The Journal for Nurse Practitioners* 11 (1): 87–94.

Ormerod, L.P., Milburn H.J., Gillespie, S., Ledingham, J. and Rampton, D. 2005. BTS recommendations for assessing risk for managing *Mycobacterium tuberculosis* infection and disease in patients due to start anti-TNF-α treatment. *Thorax* 60 (10): 800–805.

Public Health England (PHE). 2010. *The Health Protection (Notification) Regulations 2010.* Public Health England, London.

Public Health England (PHE). 2013. Tuberculosis. In: *The Green Book in Immunisation against Infectious Diseases*, Salisbury, D., Ramsay, M. and Noakes, K. (eds.). Public Health England, London, Chapter 32, pp. 391–409.

Public Health England (PHE). 2014. *Tuberculosis in the UK 2014 Report.* Public Health England, London.

Public Health England (PHE). 2015a. *Tuberculosis in England 2015 Report (Presenting Data to the End of 2014).* Public Health England, London.

Public Health England (PHE). 2015b. *Annual TB Update 2015.* Public Health England, London.

Sakamoto, K. 2012. The pathology of *Mycobacterium tuberculosis* infection. *Veterinary Pathology* 49 (3): 432–439.

Ward, J.P.T., Ward, J. and Leach, R.M. 2015. *The Respiratory System at a Glance.* John Wiley and Sons Ltd, Chichester.

World Health Organisation (WHO). 2011. *Guidelines for the Programmatic Management of Drug-Resistant Tuberculosis*. WHO, Geneva.

World Health Organisation (WHO). 2013. *Automated Real-Time Nucleic Acid Amplification Technology for Rapid and Simultaneous Detection of Tuberculosis and Rifampicin Resistance: Xpert MTB/RIF Assay for the Diagnosis of Pulmonary and Extrapulmonary TB in Adults and Children. Policy Update.* WHO, Geneva.

World Health Organisation (WHO). 2014. *Global Tuberculosis Report 2014.* WHO, Geneva.

World Health Organisation (WHO). 2015a. *Global Tuberculosis Report 2015.* WHO, Geneva.

World Health Organisation (WHO). 2015b. *Tuberculosis. Fact Sheet 104.* WHO, Geneva.

World Health Organisation (WHO). 2015c. *The End TB Strategy.* WHO, Geneva.

Zumla, A., Raviglione, M., Hafner, R. and von Reyn, F. 2013. Tuberculosis. *The New England Journal of Medicine* 368 (8): 745–755.

Pleural Conditions

8

DAVID WATERS

LEARNING OBJECTIVES

Upon completion of this chapter the reader should be able to:

- Understand the underlying pathophysiology associated with pleural disease
- Describe the common signs, symptoms and diagnostic tests associated with pleural disease
- Explain the key treatment interventions and care considerations for patients with diseases of the pleura

INTRODUCTION

Pleural disease refers to a wide spectrum of disorders and disease processes that affect the lung pleura; these include conditions such as pneumothorax, pleural effusion, pleural infection or inflammation and pleural malignancy. Pleural disease presents a significant health challenge globally, with over 3000 people per million each year being affected (Du Rand and Maskell, 2010). Consequently, pleural disease contributes to a considerable workload and resource burden for healthcare professionals caring for this patient group. Owing to the diverse nature of pleural disease, healthcare professionals may encounter this patient group in a variety of clinical settings, for example in emergency departments, respiratory centres, within critical care facilities and also within the community setting.

This chapter aims to explore the more common pleural diseases, with specific reference to pneumothorax, pleural effusion and pleural infection. These conditions will each be defined, their pathophysiology explored and key treatment interventions discussed. Particular focus will be directed towards the role of the multidisciplinary team in delivering care to this patient group. In addition, this chapter will end with a pleural disease case study, which aims to illustrate key patient considerations and associated interventions.

PNEUMOTHORAX

DEFINITION

The term 'pneumothorax' refers to an abnormal accumulation of air between the visceral and parietal layers of the lung pleura (MacDuff et al., 2010). In normal respiratory physiology, the difference between the sub-atmospheric (negative) pressure in the pleural cavity and the atmospheric (positive) pressure in the respiratory tract ensures continual lung inflation (Marieb and Hoehn, 2010). In the context of a pneumothorax, atmospheric (positive) pressure air fills some of the pleural space, resulting in elastic recoil of the lung away from the chest wall. The possible lung collapse subsequently results in a reduced functional residential capacity (FRC) and potential respiratory compromise (West, 2013). The existence of pre-existing respiratory disease and the degree of lung collapse will influence the severity of symptoms observed.

TYPES OF PNEUMOTHORAX

A pneumothorax can occur as a spontaneous event, secondary to a traumatic event or due to an iatrogenic injury. There are distinct categories of pneumothorax, these include:

- Primary spontaneous pneumothorax
- Secondary spontaneous pneumothorax
- Traumatic or iatrogenic pneumothorax
- Tension pneumothorax

PRIMARY SPONTANEOUS PNEUMOTHORAX

A pneumothorax that occurs in an otherwise healthy person, with no underlying respiratory disease, is described as a primary spontaneous pneumothorax (PSP). PSP is the commonest type of pneumothorax, with a global prevalence of 8/100,000 per year (Ward et al., 2010). Concerning the aetiology of PSP, a possible contributory factor is abnormal lung anatomy. It has been noted that a large proportion of patients presenting with PSP have either subpleural blebs or bullae (MacDuff et al., 2010); these are small cystic spaces of around 1 to 2 cm in diameter within the visceral pleura. Smoking has also been identified as a possible causative factor in the development of PSP, with otherwise healthy smokers having an increased risk of developing a PSP, compared to healthy non-smokers (MacDuff et al., 2010). Height is also considered a risk factor for development of PSP, with those presenting with a PSP often being taller than control groups (Sadikot et al., 1997). PSP frequently reoccurs, with 54% of patients representing with a PSP within 4 years (Lippert et al., 1991). Clinical observations

commonly associated with PSP include chest pain and dyspnoea; however, these may be minimal or even absent in some cases. Additional clinical characteristics might include reduced lung expansion, hyper-resonance on percussion and reduced breath sounds on auscultation on the affected side (MacDuff et al., 2010). Imaging of the thorax is a vital component to assist in the diagnosis of any type of pneumothorax. This will commonly be facilitated through a standard erect posterior–anterior (PA) chest X-ray taken during inspiration; however, the use of computerised tomography (CT) scanning can be useful in the diagnosis of more challenging cases (MacDuff et al., 2010).

Concerning the treatment options for patients with PSP, those who are asymptomatic or who have minimal dyspnoea can be monitored conservatively, which might include close observation as an inpatient, or discharge home and subsequent review in an outpatient capacity (MacDuff et al., 2010). For larger sized PSPs and when the patient exhibits moderate dyspnoea, oxygen therapy and needle aspiration is recommended (MacDuff et al., 2010) (see Figure 8.1). Oxygen administration will primarily correct any hypoxia associated with the PSP. However, its use is associated with a fourfold increase in pneumothorax resolution time (MacDuff et al., 2010); this is thought to cause a reduction in the partial pressure of nitrogen, allowing oxygen to be more readily absorbed. To facilitate needle aspiration, a 14–16-gauge intravenous cannula is inserted into the pleural cavity at the intersection of the mid-clavicular line and the second intercostal space. This is then attached to a three-way-tap, followed by a large syringe. Using the syringe, air is then aspirated. Needle aspiration has been noted to be as effective as large-bore (gauge >20 F) chest drains in treatment of pneumothoraces (Noppen et al., 2002; Zehtabchi and Rios, 2008) and has also been associated with a reduced length of hospital stay (Ayed et al., 2006; Zehtabchi and Rios, 2008). In addition, patients have reported less pain associated with the needle aspiration method, as opposed to chest drain insertion (Harvey and Prescott, 1994; Zehtabchi and Rios, 2008). Needle aspiration has been observed to be successful in around 60% of patients (MacDuff et al., 2010); insertion of a small-bore chest drain is recommended for those patients where needle aspiration has failed.

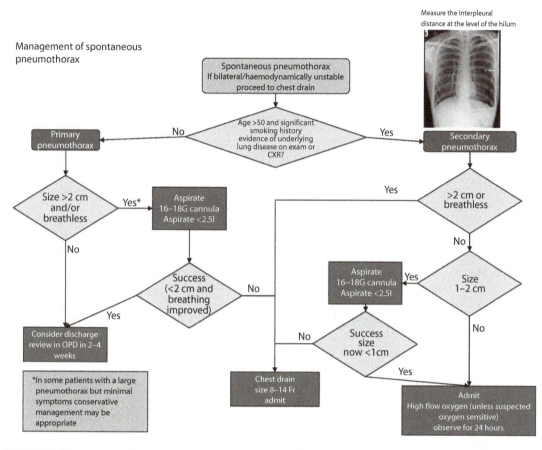

Figure 8.1 Management of spontaneous pneumothorax. (From MacDuff, A., Arnold, A. and Harvey, J. 2010. *Thorax*, 65 (Suppl 2), ii21. With permission.)

SECONDARY SPONTANEOUS PNEUMOTHORAX

In contrast to PSP, secondary spontaneous pneumothorax (SSP) is attributed to an existing respiratory disease process, for example chronic obstructive pulmonary disease (COPD), tuberculosis or cystic fibrosis. Owing to their underlying respiratory disease, patients with SSP have less pulmonary reserve, often resulting in a more life-threatening presentation (in comparison to PSP) and a more urgent requirement for drainage (Yarmus and Feller-Kopman, 2012). The clinical symptoms noted within SSP will echo those observed in cases of PSP (i.e. chest pain and dyspnoea), but will frequently be more severe, with patients often experiencing profound breathlessness (MacDuff et al., 2010).

Treatment for SSP is similar to that recommended for PSP, with oxygen and needle aspiration being recommended for patients with minimal symptoms and/or a smaller pneumothorax (MacDuff et al., 2010). For patients that are symptomatic with dyspnoea and/or have a larger pneumothorax, the insertion of a small-bore chest drain (with a gauge <14 F) is recommended as first-time intervention, rather than needle aspiration (MacDuff et al., 2010) (see Figure 8.1).

TRAUMATIC/IATROGENIC PNEUMOTHORAX

Traumatic or iatrogenic pneumothoraces can be associated with traumatic injuries, such as blunt trauma sustained from a road traffic accident, penetrating trauma from a knife wound or as a consequence of medically initiated invasive procedures, such as sub-clavian vessel puncture during central line insertion, intercostal nerve blocks or transthoracic lung biopsy. A further cause of iatrogenic pneumothoraces could be mechanical ventilation, potentially associated with ventilation of non-compliant lungs with abnormally large tidal volumes. These types of pneumothorax are sometimes referred to as non-spontaneous and their incidence has been suggested to be higher than that of PSP and SSP (MacDuff et al., 2010).

Concerning treatment, the majority of iatrogenic pneumothoraces resolve independently and require no intervention. In cases of larger iatrogenic pneumothoraces or when the patient becomes symptomatic, needle aspiration is indicated and this has been noted to be successful in the majority of cases (Delius et al., 1989; Loiselle et al., 2013), the remainder requiring chest drain insertion.

TENSION PNEUMOTHORAX

A tension pneumothorax in contrast, is any large pneumothorax that is associated with significant haemodynamic and pulmonary compromise. This occurs when air accumulates within the pleural cavity during inspiration and is unable to escape during exhalation, usually due to the presence of a pleural defect, which might act as a 'flap valve'. The increasing pressure within the pleural cavity causes the major anatomical structures within the mediastinum to be displaced to the opposite hemithorax, causing compression of functioning lung tissue and inhibition of venous return, leading to symptoms of severe shock (West, 2013). Owing to the rapid progression and severe symptoms associated with a tension pneumothorax, its presentation is considered a medical emergency and warrants urgent intervention. Specific symptoms of a tension pneumothorax include: significant respiratory deterioration, demonstrated by tachypnoea, dyspnoea and hypoxaemia, absent breath sounds on auscultation on the affected side and signs of haemodynamic compromise, i.e. tachycardia and hypotension, potentially leading to cardiac arrest (Coombs et al., 2013). A tension pneumothorax often occurs in the following clinical situations: patients receiving non-invasive ventilation (NIV), those who are mechanically ventilated within critical care settings, following

traumatic injury, following an episode of cardiopulmonary resuscitation, patients with chronic lung disease (such as COPD or asthma) or due to chest drain complications (blocked, clamped or displaced chest drain tubing) (MacDuff et al., 2010).

As a tension pneumothorax can be a life-threatening situation, it warrants urgent and immediate management. Recommended treatment is high concentration oxygen and urgent needle decompression (MacDuff et al., 2010) using a 12-gauge intravenous cannula inserted through the anterior surface of the chest on the affected hemithorax, at the point of the second intercostal space in the mid-clavicular line (MacDuff et al., 2010; Resuscitation Council United Kingdom, 2011). A standard intercostal drain should then be inserted to facilitate pleural expansion and to prevent reoccurrence of the tension pneumothorax.

CHEST DRAINS

When needle aspiration is not recommended or unsuccessful, the use of an intercostal chest drain is advocated for the treatment of a pneumothorax (see Figure 8.1). The following section aims to explore some key care considerations related to chest drains.

A chest drain is a tube that is inserted through the chest wall into the pleural cavity, to facilitate drainage of air or fluid, allowing for lung re-expansion (Coombs et al., 2013). Once it exits the patient's chest wall, the chest drain tube is connected to an underwater seal drain system. This water-filled container acts as a one-way valve, allowing any liquid or air to be removed from the patient's pleura, while preventing any backflow of liquid or air (see Figure 8.2). To expedite liquid or air removal and lung re-expansion, the underwater seal system may be attached to a dedicated thoracic suction unit connected to a wall suction supply (delivering 10–20 cm H_2O of suction); however, there is no clear evidence to support this practice, although its use is common practice for non-resolving pneumothoraces (Havelock et al., 2010).

While the chest drain is *in situ*, the patient should be closely monitored; this will alert the healthcare team to any potential issues that may arise as a consequence of the chest drain itself, or the underlying pathology that prompted its insertion (Coombs et al., 2013). In addition to physiological observations,

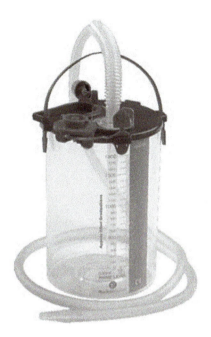

Figure 8.2 Diagram of an intercostal drain (a R54500 Rocket Blue drain from Rocketmedical). Image kindly reproduced with permission from Rocketmedical.

regular attention should be directed to the drain itself: the volume, appearance and characteristics of the drainage should be acknowledged and documented, as this may highlight any complications or could be a guide towards further interventions or possible drain removal (Coombs et al., 2013). If the chest drain is patent and in the correct position, any fluid within the system should be noted to 'swing'; this is observed as a very slight rise and fall of fluid level. In self-ventilating patients, their inspiratory breath will cause the fluid level to move towards them; the opposite is noted with those on mechanical ventilation (Coombs et al., 2013). A chest drain system that is not 'swinging' could be suggestive of a blocked or kinked tube and should be communicated to the relevant member of the healthcare team. In situations where a chest drain is required to facilitate lung re-expansion, i.e. for a pneumothorax, the presence of 'bubbling' within the system may be noted. Bubbles or 'bubbling' within the chest drain canister is indicative of air being displaced from the pleural cavity and in the context of a pneumothorax, can suggest lung re-expansion. When the pneumothorax has been fully drained, 'bubbling' within the drain

system should cease. However, a drain that is not 'bubbling' may also indicate tube blockage or kinking and warrants further investigation or communication among the healthcare team. The presence of a 'swing' or 'bubbling' should also be documented in the patient's medical notes, in addition to the volume and characteristics of the drainage. Patients may experience pain and discomfort as a consequence of chest drain insertion; because of this the requirement analgesic medications should be routinely assessed by the healthcare team.

PLEURAL EFFUSION

DEFINITION AND CLASSIFICATION

Pleural effusions are associated with increased pleural fluid formation and/or impaired pleural fluid reabsorption by the lymphatic system (Marieb and Hoehn, 2010). The pleural space usually contains around 20 mls of viscous fluid; its function is to lubricate the internal surfaces of the pleura and to prevent any friction between the pleural layers as the lungs move during respiration (Cohen, 2014). The pleural fluid within the pleural cavity is in a state of constant change, with it being continually secreted and absorbed to maintain a sufficient volume and composition (Cohen, 2014). As a consequence of different disease processes, the normal mechanisms for regulating the amount of pleural fluid can be disrupted, leading to accumulation of excess pleural fluid and eventual development of pleural effusions.

Pleural effusions have traditionally been classified as either transudative or exudative. A transudative pleural effusion results from *systemic* factors that influence pleural fluid movement. This is associated with changes to hydrostatic or oncotic pressures, causing excessive secretion or reduced reabsorption of pleural fluid (Light, 2005; Cohen, 2014). Clinical causes for transudative pleural effusions include: congested heart failure affecting the left, right or both sides of the heart, cirrhosis of the liver, pericardial inflammation and nephrotic syndrome (Light, 2005; Hooper et al., 2010). Typically, a transudative effusion will be watery and straw coloured or clear in appearance; it will also have a low protein content (<3 g/dL) (Cohen, 2014). This type of effusion is also usually free flowing, rather than loculated, making drainage easier to achieve if required.

In contrast, an exudative pleural effusion is associated with changes from local factors that contribute to pleural fluid movement, such as increased permeability and fluid shift into the pleural cavity associated with inflammation or an obstructed lymphatic drainage system perhaps due to a malignancy (Light, 2005; Cohen, 2014). Specific clinical causes for exudative pleural effusions include: malignancy (which could be primary or secondary in nature), infarcted pulmonary tissue associated with a pulmonary embolus, infection (such as tuberculosis or parapneumonic), as a consequence of an inflammatory process (i.e. pancreatitis or lupus) or an obstruction (perhaps to a lymphatic vessel) (Hooper et al., 2010). The appearance of an exudative pleural fluid sample can vary; it can be clear or straw coloured, stained with blood or could resemble frank pus (Light, 2005). Commonly it will have a high protein content (>3 g/dL). Exudative pleural effusions, in contrast to free-flowing transudative effusions, are often loculated or compartmentalised. These individual pockets of effusion can be difficult to drain percutaneously, so surgical thoracotomy and decortication procedure is often utilised instead (Cohen, 2014).

DIAGNOSIS

To assist the healthcare team in making a diagnosis of pleural effusion, various tests and investigations are recommended; these include a comprehensive patient assessment, radiology and pleural fluid analysis (see Figure 8.3 for additional detail). The provisional diagnosis of pleural effusion can often be made by a healthcare professional following a thorough physical examination and by taking the patient's medical history. During the physical examination and through the history-taking process, specific observations that could be suggestive of a pleural effusion include: symptoms of dyspnoea, cough or sharp non-radiating chest pain (McGrath and Anderson, 2011). Additional findings might also include: a dull percussion note over the affected area and reduced or absent breath sounds over the effusion (Cohen, 2014). The patient's medical history may also guide the healthcare professional as to whether the effusion is a transudate or an exudate,

i.e. in the presence of heart failure symptoms, the pleural effusion is likely to be transudative, or in cases of known malignancy more likely exudative (Hooper et al., 2010). During the patient assessment, attention should be directed towards their drug history, as several commonly prescribed medications are associated with development of pleural effusions, these include: Methotrexate, Amiodarone, Phenytoin, Nitrofurantoin and a number of beta-blockers (Hooper et al., 2010).

A PA chest X-ray is vital to establish the diagnosis of pleural effusion. Radiographic findings will vary depending on the size of the effusion. Smaller pleural effusions may produce blunting of the costophrenic angle (where the diaphragm meets the chest wall laterally), or the small meniscus sign could be present (when fluid fills the cavity between the lung and the chest wall, indicated by a white opaque crescent) (Cohen, 2014). See Figure 8.4 for a typical chest X-ray depicting a pleural effusion. With larger pleural effusions, a complete whiteout of the affected hemithorax may be observed, possible obscuring of the hemidiaphragm may occur and in more severe cases mediastinal shift may be noted (Cohen, 2014). An erect PA chest X-ray (taken with the patient standing up) is preferable to a supine PA chest X-ray (where the patient may be lying flat), as better assessment of air and fluid levels can be made in the erect position. In critical care settings, an erect PA chest X-ray might not be possible, as the patient's condition may not facilitate them standing. Instead, a supine PA chest X-ray would be used, and consequently any free pleural fluid would lay posteriorly within the chest cavity while the patient is laid in the supine position. A pleural effusion on a supine PA chest X-ray would be seen as an area of increased hemithorax opacity, with preserved vascular shadows (Hooper et al., 2010).

Ultrasound also offers an additional diagnostic tool, which can be especially useful in quantifying the size of an effusion. Furthermore, the use of ultrasound is recommended to aid safe positioning for needle aspiration of pleural fluid (Hooper et al., 2010).

Needle aspiration is utilised to establish the aetiology of a pleural effusion, which in turn can inform the ongoing management of the condition. The procedure should be guided by ultrasound; this ensures safe positioning, has been shown to increase

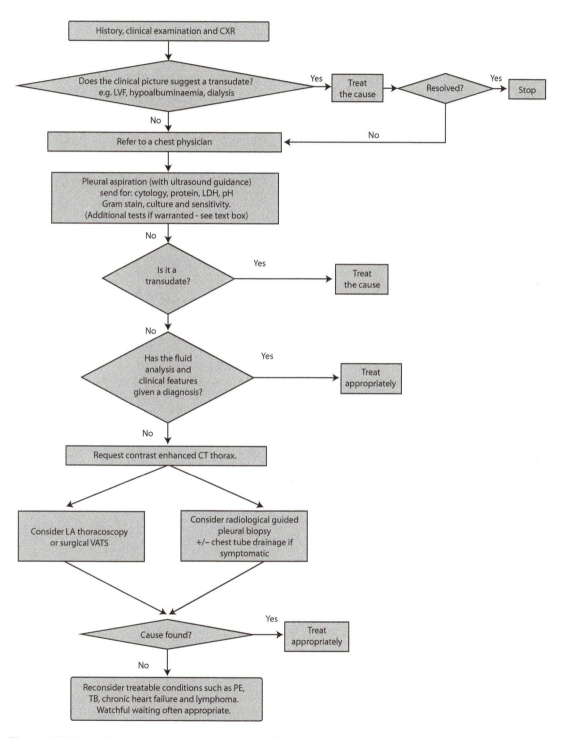

Figure 8.3 Diagnostic investigations for pleural effusion. (From Hooper, C., Lee, Y.C.G. and Maskell, N. 2010. *Thorax*, 65 (Suppl 2): ii5. With permission.)

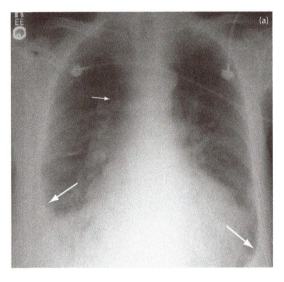
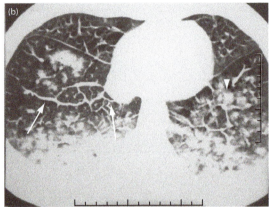

Figure 8.4 (a) Typical chest X-ray of a pleural effusion. (b) Typical CT scan of a pleural effusion depicting a dorsal collection. (From Light, R.W. and Lee, Y.C.G. (eds.). 2016. *Textbook of Pleural Diseases* (3rd ed.). CRC Press, London. With permission.)

aspiration success and reduces the need for repeated attempts (Diacon et al., 2003). A lateral puncture site is recommended, rather than posterior or medial positions, as fewer intercostal vessels are located within the lateral chest wall (Hooper et al., 2010). Prior to aspiration, the chest wall should be instilled with a local anaesthetic agent to reduce any pain or discomfort for the patient. To facilitate aspiration, a green needle (21 gauge) can be attached to a 50 mL Luer Lock syringe and 50–60 mls of pleural fluid should be removed (Hooper et al., 2010). Samples of aspirated fluid should then be sent for biochemical, microbiological and cytological assessment.

MANAGEMENT

The exact management of a pleural effusion is guided by the patient's symptoms and the effusions aetiology. For transudative pleural effusions, the treatment focus is very much orientated towards addressing the cause, i.e. if the pleural effusion is associated with biventricular heart failure, the management will involve optimisation of heart failure medications and diuretic therapy.

Exudative pleural effusions, which are often associated with systemic issues such as a malignancy, may require more invasive interventions such as

thoracoscopy, surgical video-assisted thoracoscopic surgery (VATS) (see Chapter 14) or insertion of a chest drain (Hooper et al., 2010).

PLEURAL INFECTION

DEFINITION

Pleural infections are a common respiratory disorder, with a significant annual incidence globally, with around 80,000 cases each year in the United Kingdom and the United States combined (Davies et al., 2010). The incidence of pleural infection is noted to be increasing, with highest prevalence among children and the elderly (Finley et al., 2008). Risk factors associated with the development of pleural infections mirror those of pneumonia, i.e. lifestyle factors such as smoking, alcohol abuse, low body weight, poor dental hygiene, in addition to co-morbidities, such as respiratory and cardiac disease (Torres et al., 2013). Pleural infections can also have an iatrogenic cause, for example occurring following pleural procedures, upper gastrointestinal or thoracic surgery (Davies et al., 2010). A high proportion of pleural infections are associated with an episode of pneumonia; up to 57% of cases of pneumonia result in the development of parapneumonic pleural effusions (Sahn, 2007), which usually manifest as a short, self-limiting pleural infection that resolves promptly with appropriate antibiotic therapy. However, in some situations, the pleural effusion may be more severe, multi-loculated and associated with signs of systemic sepsis. This more severe form of pleural infection presentation is likely to be associated with significant respiratory compromise and warrants urgent treatment (Davies et al., 2010). The term 'empyema' refers to the presence of frank pus within the pleural cavity and also may be noted in more severe cases of pleural infection.

Bacterial pathogens associated with pleural infections can be categorised as either community acquired or hospital acquired. Gram-positive aerobic pathogens are more commonly associated with community-acquired pleural infections, which often are due to *Streptococcus aureus* or *Streptoccus milleri*. In contrast, hospital-acquired pleural infections are usually Gram-negative anaerobic pathogens, such as Methicillin-resistant *Staphylococcus aureus* (MRSA).

DIAGNOSIS

A comprehensive patient assessment and medical history is vital to establish a diagnosis of pleural infection. Symptoms associated with pleural infection include: pyrexia, malaise, chest pain of a pleuritic nature (sharp chest pain noted during respiration), dyspnoea and a cough (Sahn, 2007). In patients who have had a history of recent pneumonic illness, with continued symptoms of infection (such as tachypnea, pyrexia and a raised C reactive protein), there should be a high degree of suspicion towards a diagnosis of pleural infection.

Radiological investigations can be useful in confirming findings noted through the patient physical assessment process. On a chest X-ray, the presence of a pleural effusion, in addition to pulmonary infiltrates, is highly suggestive of a parapneumonic pleural effusion (Davies et al., 2010). Ultrasonography is also commonly used alongside chest X-rays, to assist with diagnosis. Computerised tomography (CT) and magnetic resonance imaging (MRI) are also useful for more complex cases; however, their routine use is not recommended for straightforward pleural infection presentations.

Examination of pleural fluid, obtained through needle aspiration, can also provide valuable data to assist with the diagnosis of pleural infections. The visual characteristics of a pleural fluid should be noted, i.e. the presence of frank pus is highly suggestive of an empyema. Samples should be obtained for biochemical analysis, with tests to include protein level, pH and glucose. An infected pleural fluid sample will have a raised protein level, an acidotic pH and a raised glucose (Davies et al., 2010). In addition, a sample should be sent for microbiological culture; however, it has been noted that around 40% of pleural aspirate samples fail to grow any pathogens (Maskell et al., 2006). The taking of blood cultures is also recommended as a diagnostic tool, as this can also help identify the specific pathogen causing the pleural infection.

MANAGEMENT

Pleural infection is associated with significant mortality, so prompt treatment by specialists within a respiratory unit is recommended (Davies et al., 2010). See Figure 8.5 for a more detailed exploration of the management of pleural infection. Appropriate antibiotic therapy should be prescribed to all patients once pleural infection has been diagnosed; this should be guided by culture and sensitivity results from pleural aspirate and blood culture samples. However, in situations where samples have not cultured pathogen growth, empirical antibiotics should be prescribed that are appropriate for the likely causative organisms (Davies et al., 2010). Early engagement with respiratory physicians and microbiologists is advocated in cases of pleural infection, to ensure safe and appropriate use of antibiotic therapy.

Insertion of a chest drain is urgently required, if frank pus, purulent or cloudy pleural fluid is observed during a diagnostic needle aspiration (Davies et al., 2010). Chest drainage is also indicated when pathogens are identified through Gram stain and/or culture in cases of non-purulent pleural fluid aspirates; this is suggestive of a simple pleural effusion into a more complex parapneumonic effusion warranting intervention (Davies et al., 2010). Other patient groups for whom chest drainage is recommended include patients who have an acidotic pleural fluid sample (pH <7.2) and also those who have been commenced

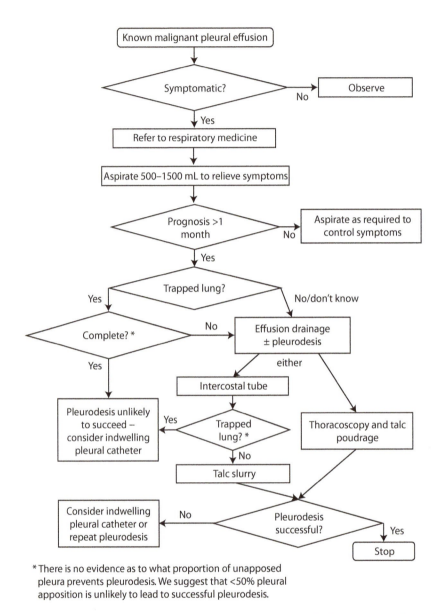

Figure 8.5 Management of pleural infection. (Based on Davies, H.E., Davies, R.J.O. and Davies, C.W.H. 2010. *Thorax*. 65 (Suppl 2): ii42.)

on antibiotic therapy but are showing poor clinical improvement (Davies et al., 2010). In the context of pleural infection drainage, a smaller bore chest drain catheter is advocated (10–14 F); however, these often require regular flushing to promote catheter patency (Davies et al., 2010). Small bore chest drain catheters are associated with less trauma on insertion and increased patient comfort.

Possible surgical intervention is recommended for patients that have ongoing sepsis, associated with their pleural infection, despite antibiotic therapy and chest drainage. Early referral to thoracic surgeons is advocated in cases for pleural infection related sepsis which fails to resolve after 5–7 days of conventional therapy (Davies et al., 2010). Specific surgical procedures for the treatment of severe pleural infections may include VATS, which is more commonly employed, or a thoracotomy and decortication. For additional content thoracic surgical procedures, see Chapter 14.

CONCLUSION

This chapter has explored three common pleural diseases (namely pneumothorax, pleural effusion and pleural infection). Pleural disease has a high prevalence within the UK; it is also associated with significant mortality and morbidity. Members of the healthcare team must possess the relevant skills and knowledge to participate in the care of this complex patient group. A comprehensive patient assessment and the use of radiological investigations are vital tools that will assist the clinical team in the diagnosis of such diseases. Interventions such as oxygen therapy, needle aspiration and the use of chest drains feature heavily in the management of this patient group.

CASE STUDY

James Wilson is a 25-year-old gentleman who self-presented at his local Emergency Department (ED) following a 2-day history of dyspnoea and chest discomfort, which has progressively worsened. He has no past medical history of note. He smokes heavily, around 20 cigarettes a day. He is tall, of normal weight and is otherwise healthy.

On arrival, he is triaged and moved immediately into the urgent assessment area. His initial observations and findings from his patient assessment are:

Airway: He is able to talk normally and has no abnormal airway sounds.
Breathing: Respiration rate of 32 bpm, SpO_2 of 88%, no cyanosis noted and minimal use of accessory muscles. He has notable dyspnoea. On chest auscultation he has reduced breath sounds on the right middle and upper hemithorax, no added sounds were noted. On percussion the right chest was noted to be hyper-resonant in the middle and upper zones.
Circulation: Heart rate of 98 bpm, blood pressure of 135/79 mmHg and capillary refill time of 2 seconds. James reports a sharp stabbing chest pain that is worse upon taking deep breaths.
Disability: James is fully alert; his Glasgow Coma Score is 15/15.
Exposure: Apyrexial. No issues of concern noted during a 'top-to-toe' assessment.

James is reviewed by the ED physician, who suspects a diagnosis of Primary Spontaneous Pneumothorax (PSP) affecting the right hemithorax. Blood samples are requested, a 12 lead electrocardiograph recorded and an urgent chest X-ray were taken. Oxygen therapy (15 L via non-rebreath mask) and intravenous analgesia were also given.

The chest X-ray confirmed the provisional diagnosis of a right-sided PSP and following consultation with a senior colleague and following consultation with a senior colleague the ED physician undertakes an urgent needle aspiration. During the procedure a volume of air is aspirated, which significantly eases James' dyspnoea and improves his SpO_2. A repeat chest X-ray indicates complete resolution and after a period of monitoring James is discharged home with outpatient follow-up.

CASE STUDY DISCUSSION

James has many risk factors for the development of a PSP; namely his age, gender, his height and his heavy smoking habit. Awareness of these risk factors will assist the healthcare professional in making a provisional diagnosis when presented with such patients with symptoms of a PSP. James had a 2-day history of mild dyspnoea and chest discomfort with a delayed engagement with medical services; often the symptoms of PSP are minor and sometimes completely absent, this can result in patients presenting to primary or secondary care facilities several days after the onset of symptoms (MacDuff et al., 2010). Conservative management is recommended for patients who are asymptomatic or who have small PSPs (MacDuff et al., 2010); James, however, exhibited signs of compromise, with a worsening dyspnoea and a low SpO_2, indicating the need for more immediate invasive treatment.

Worsening dyspnoea in the context of a PSP can sometimes be suggestive of a tension pneumothorax, so urgent medical intervention is required in these situations. In response to his low SpO$_2$ (88%) and his respiratory distress, James was administered high flow oxygen; this intervention will not only correct his hypoxic state, but has also been shown to quicken pneumothorax resolution (MacDuff et al., 2010). The physician undertook a needle aspiration to treat this confirmed PSP. Needle aspiration is preferable over the use of large bore chest drains for the treatment of PSP, and is associated with reduced lengths of hospital stay and improved patient comfort (Ayed et al., 2006). Following needle aspiration, James made a prompt recovery and was discharged home for outpatient review.

REFERENCES

Ayed, A.K., Chandrasekaran, C. and Sukumar, M. 2006. Aspiration versus tube drainage in primary spontaneous pneumothorax: A randomised study. *European Respiratory Journal* 27 (3): 477–482.

Cohen, Z. 2014. Chest imaging. In: Heuer, A.J. and Scanlan, C.L. (eds.). *Wilkins' Clinical Assessment in Respiratory Care* (7th ed.). Elsevier, Maryland Heights.

Coombs, M., Dyos, J., Waters, D. and Nesbitt, I. 2013. Assessment, monitoring and interventions for the respiratory system. In: Mallett, J., Albarran, J.W. and Richardson, A. (eds.). *Critical Care Manual of Clinical Procedures and Competencies*. Wiley Blackwell, Oxford, 64–171.

Davies, H.E., Davies, R.J.O. and Davies, C.W.H. 2010. Management of pleural infection in adults: British Thoracic Society pleural disease guideline 2010. *Thorax* 65 (Suppl 2): ii41–ii53.

Delius, R.E., Obeid, F.N., Horst, H.M., Sorensen, V.J., Fath, J.J. and Bivins, B.A. 1989. Catheter aspiration for simple pneumothorax. Experience with 114 patients. *Archives of Surgery* 124 (7): 833–836.

Diacon, A.H., Brutsche, M.H. and Soler, M. 2003. Accuracy of pleural puncture sites. A prospective comparison of clinical examination with ultrasound. *Chest* 123 (2): 436–441.

Du Rand, I. and Maskell, N. 2010. Introduction and methods: British Thoracic Society pleural disease guideline 2010. *Thorax* 65 (Suppl 2): ii1–ii3.

Finley, C., Clifton, J., Fitzgerald, J.M. and Yee, J. 2008. Empyema: An increasing concerning in Canada. *Candian Respiratory Journal* 15 (2): 85–89.

Harvey, J. and Prescott, R.J. 1994. Simple aspiration versus intercostal tube drainage for spontaneous pneumothorax in patients with normal lungs. *British Medical Journal* 309 (6965): 1338–1339.

Havelock, T., Teoh, R., Laws, D. and Gleeson, F. 2010. Pleural procedures and thoracic ultrasound: British Thoracic Society pleural disease guideline 2010. *Thorax* 65 (Suppl 2): ii61–ii71.

Hooper, C., Lee, Y.C.G. and Maskell, N. 2010. Investigation of a unilateral pleural effusion in adults: British Thoracic Society pleural disease guideline 2010. *Thorax* 65 (Suppl 2): ii4–ii17.

Light, R.W. 2005. Diseases of the pleura, mediastinum, chest wall and diaphragm. In: George, R.B., Light, R.W., Matthay, M.A. and Matthay, R.A. (eds.). *Chest Medicine. Essentials of Pulmonary and Critical Care Medicine* (5th ed.). Lippincott Williams and Wilkins, Philadelphia, 415–447.

Light, R.W. and Lee, Y.C.G. (eds.). 2016. *Textbook of Pleural Diseases* (3rd ed.). CRC Press, London.

Lippert, H.L., Lund, O., Blegvad, S. and Larsen, H.V. 1991. Independent risk factors for cumulative recurrence rate after first spontaneous pneumothorax. *European Respiratory Journal* 4: 324–331.

Loiselle, A., Parish, J.M., Wilkens, J.A. and Jaroszewski, D.E. 2013. Managing iatrogenic pneumothorax and chest tubes. *Journal of Hospital Medicine* 8 (7): 402–408.

MacDuff, A., Arnold, A. and Harvey, J. 2010. Management of spontaneous pneumothorax: British Thoracic Society pleural disease guideline 2010. *Thorax* 65 (Suppl 2): ii18–ii31.

Marieb, E.N. and Hoehn, K. 2010. *Human Anatomy & Physiology* (8th ed.). Pearson Benjamin Cummings, San Francisco.

Maskell, N.E., Batt, S., Hedley, E.L., Davies, C.W., Gillespie, S.H. and Davies, R.J. 2006. The bacteriology of pleural infection by genetic and standard methods and its mortality significance. *American Journal of Respiratory Critical Care* 174 (7): 817–823.

McGrath, E. and Anderson, P.B. 2011. Diagnosis of pleural effusion: A systematic approach. *American Journal of Critical Care* 20 (2): 119–128.

Noppen, M., Alexander, P., Driesen, P., Slabbynck, H. and Verstraeten, A. 2002. Manual aspiration versus chest tube drainage in first episodes of primary spontaneous pneumothorax. *American Journal of Respiratory Critical Care Medicine* 165 (9): 1240–1244.

Resuscitation Council United Kingdom (RCUK). 2011. *Advanced Life Support* (6th ed.). Resuscitation Council, London.

Sadikot, R.T., Greene, T., Meadows, K. and Arnold, A.G. 1997. Recurrence of primary pneumothorax. *Thorax* 52: 805–809.

Sahn, S.A. 2007. Diagnosis and management of parapneumonic effusions and empyema. *Clinical Infectious Diseases* 45 (11): 1480–1486.

Torres, A., Peetermans, W.E., Viegi, G. and Blasi, F. 2013. Risk factors for community-acquired pneumonia in adults in Europe: A literature review. *Thorax* 68 (11): 1057–1065.

Ward, J.P.T., Ward, J., Wiener, C.M. and Leach, R.M. 2010. *The Respiratory System at a Glance* (3rd ed.). Blackwell Science Ltd, Oxford.

West, J.B. 2013. *Pulmonary Pathophysiology: The Essentials* (8th ed.). Lippincott Williams and Wilkins, Baltimore.

Yarmus, L. and Feller-Kopman, D. 2012. Pneumothorax in the critically Ill patient. *Chest* 141 (4): 1098–1105.

Zehtabchi, S. and Rios, C.L. 2008. Management of emergency department patients with primary spontaneous pneumothorax: Needle aspiration or tube thoracostomy? *Annals of Emergency Medicine* 51 (1): 91–100.

Occupational lung disease

9

CHRIS STENTON

LEARNING OBJECTIVES

Upon completion of this chapter the reader should be able to:

- Recognise the contribution of occupational exposures to lung disease
- Understand the importance of obtaining a careful occupational history
- Recognise the key features of occupational asthma and its investigation
- Recognise the key features of lung disease caused by coal, silica and asbestos

INTRODUCTION

The lungs are the body's main interface with the environment. Every minute around 5 litres of air is breathed in and out, and interfaces with an alveolar surface the size of a tennis court. It is therefore not surprising that most lung disease is caused by inhaled environmental agents. Cigarette smoke is the commonest cause of lung disease but people often encounter their most challenging environments at work. Occupational exposures contribute substantially to the common lung diseases such as asthma, chronic obstructive pulmonary disease (COPD) and cancer, and they cause a number of unique problems such as pneumoconiosis.

There is still a considerable legacy in the United Kingdom (UK) and other industrialised countries from past exposures to coal and asbestos that are now largely controlled, but hundreds of new chemicals are introduced into industry each year. New occupational lung diseases continue to appear and established conditions reappear in new guises.

This chapter discusses first occupational asthma as it is the commonest work-related lung disease and management decisions early in its course can have profound implications for the individual's health and future employment. Asbestos is discussed next as it is still the commonest cause of occupational lung disease in the UK, usually presenting many years after exposure has occurred. Coal and silica are discussed as they remain important in the differential diagnosis of conditions such as tuberculosis and lung cancer, and silicosis in particular still occurs in new and unusual circumstances. Occupational COPD and lung cancer appear the same as their non-occupational counterparts and so the contribution of work often goes unrecognised. A range of other occupational diseases will be discussed and a case of occupational asthma illustrated. The emphasis throughout this chapter is on diagnosis as the clinical management of most occupational diseases is similar to that of their non-occupational forms and is dealt with elsewhere.

The key to identifying occupational lung disease lies in a detailed occupational history. Many occupational diseases develop years after the exposure occurred, but all too often patients are simply described as 'retired', and a clue to their illness is missed. When asked, they may describe only their most recent job or the one they consider the most prestigious and they may well need prompting to remember other relevant exposures. In someone with asbestos-related disease it may have been a few months' work in a shipyard or on a building site at the start of their career that is relevant but has been completely forgotten. Equally, it may not be the individual's own work that was the cause of the problem. Often those handling a toxic material wear proper protective clothing but others working alongside or undertaking repair or maintenance are exposed. Some detective work may be necessary. Cases of occupational asthma have occurred when the fumes extracted from a factory were drawn into the ventilation system of a neighbouring office and caused disease in the workers there (Carroll et al., 1976). The language of work can be complex and difficult to understand. Job descriptions such as 'engineer', 'fitter' or 'mechanic' can give very little information about what someone does. However, most people enjoy talking about their work and taking an occupational history can be a useful way of establishing rapport with an anxious or reticent patient.

OCCUPATIONAL ASTHMA

Occupational asthma is the most important of the occupational lung diseases. It is common, it is not easy to diagnose and proper management at an early stage can make a huge difference to the outcome. The term refers to asthma that is caused by exposure to some chemical, dust or fume at work (Tarlo and Lemiere, 2014). Typically, the individual is well, changes jobs or starts to work with a new material, and after a latent interval of a few months begins to develop breathlessness and wheezing. These symptoms worsen to the point where the individual has to leave work. The asthma typically improves but may not disappear completely. It is estimated from epidemiological studies that around 1 in 6 cases of asthma in adults is caused by work (Nicholson et al., 2010), although at present far fewer than that are diagnosed (McNamee et al., 2008).

There are around 500 agents that are recognised to cause occupational asthma (see Table 9.1). They fall into two categories: large molecular allergens and reactive chemicals. Large molecular weight allergens such as flour in bakeries, fish protein in food processers or animal proteins in laboratory animal handlers stimulate the production of IgE antibodies and these underpin the asthmatic reactions.

Table 9.1 Causes of occupational asthma

High molecular weight agents	
Agent	**Occupation/industry**
Flour/grain	Bakers/cooks
Animal protein	Laboratory animal workers
Latex	Rubber glove users
Enzymes	Detergent manufacturer
Fish/seafood	Food processors
Solder flux (colophony)	Solderers
Wood dust	Joiners
Low molecular weight agents	
Agent	**Occupation/industry**
Isocyanates	Polyurethane production, paint spraying
Epoxy resins	Resins, paints
Cyanoacrylates	Superglue users
Persulphates	Hairdressers
Glutaraldehyde	Sterilising solutions
Stainless steel fume	Welders
Cooling oils	Engineering workshop
Cleaning agents	Cleaners
Pharmaceuticals	Drug manufacturers

The mechanism is akin to that involving house dust mite, pollen and domestic pets in non-occupational asthma. The other group of agents causing occupational asthma are reactive chemicals such as isocyanates used in some paints or in polyurethane foam production, glues such as cyanoacrylate superglue, or detergents. Generally, it is not possible to demonstrate the IgE antibodies on skin prick or blood testing with these agents. These chemicals are believed to cause asthma by reacting with proteins in the airway, altering their structure, rendering them 'foreign' to the immune system and triggering a response (Vandenplas, 2011).

Because occupational asthma is caused by allergy, there is a latent period after the onset of exposure when the worker is asymptomatic but the allergy is developing. Typically, this lasts several months or years. Occasionally asthma can be triggered by a sudden massive exposure to an irritant gas or fume such as concentrated chlorine (Shakeri et al., 2008). This acute irritant asthma, sometimes known as the reactive airway dysfunction syndrome, develops through a completely different non-allergic mechanism.

Patients with occupational asthma experience work-related symptoms. Breathlessness can develop immediately on exposure or can be delayed for several hours, and often symptoms are worst toward the end of a shift or even after work. As each exposure makes the asthma slightly worse, symptoms tend to worsen as the week goes on and improve over weekends or on holidays. Often there is also work-related rhinitis and conjunctivitis which can precede the asthma. Work-related symptoms are not always clear-cut for a variety of reasons. Some individuals are poor perceivers of bronchoconstriction and are not aware of the problem. Some will not report symptoms for fear of losing their job (Cullinan et al., 2003). Others become very anxious about their exposures and develop symptoms of hyperventilation, or have symptoms caused by irritant dusts or fumes. Because of the importance of occupational asthma to the individual it is essential to consider the diagnosis in any adult who develops asthma or whose asthma substantially worsens during their working life (Nicholson et al., 2010). It is essential also to try to confirm the diagnosis objectively.

Serial measurements of peak flow can demonstrate work-related changes in lung function and should be made in anyone suspected of having occupational asthma. The OASYS programme (Huggins et al., 2005) is freely available (www.occupationalasthma.com) and can assist with displaying and interpreting peak flow measurements (see Figure 9.1). The presence of specific IgE antibodies

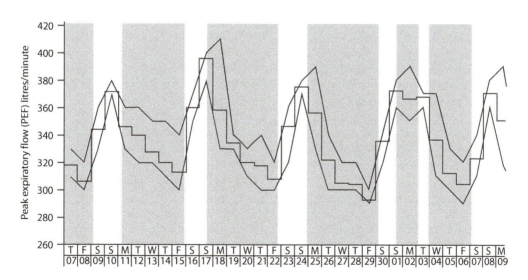

Figure 9.1 Serial peak expiratory flow measurements in occupational asthma. Serial peak expiratory flow measurements plotted using OASYS-2 (www.occupationalasthma.com). Daily maximum, minimum and average values are shown. Work days are shaded. A progressive decline over each period of several days at work can be seen with improvements at weekends.

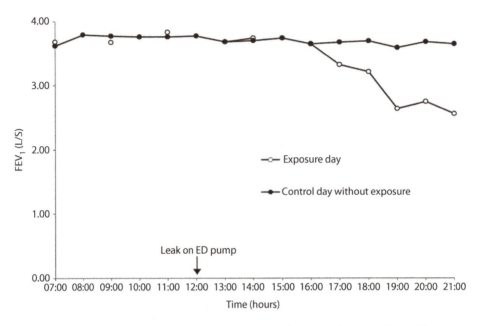

Figure 9.2 Late asthmatic reaction following exposure at work. A workplace challenge test in a subject exposed to ethylene diamine (ED). Day 1 (open circles) was spent in an office and day 2 (solid circles) on a chemical plant where there was a brief exposure around 12.00. A late asthmatic reaction began about 4 hours later and persisted for the rest of the day.

can be identified from skin prick tests or blood radio-allergosorbent tests (RASTs) and are particularly useful with high molecular weight allergens although antibodies can be found in many individuals who are exposed to a particular agent but do not have asthma (Tarlo et al., 2008). Airway responsiveness measurements can quantify the severity of asthma and can be used to demonstrate improvements away from work, for example on holidays (Tarlo et al., 2008). Often some form of more detailed workplace challenge test or laboratory challenge tests is required to demonstrate that a particular agent is responsible for the symptoms (see Figure 9.2). This is a highly specialised area and referral to a respiratory physician is generally required.

Occupational asthma tends to worsen with continued exposures. If it is diagnosed early then it can disappear when the individual stops being exposed, but after about 2 years of symptomatic exposure the asthma tends to continue indefinitely even if the individual leaves work or stops being exposed (Chan-Yeung and Malo, 1995). Two years is a relatively short time: it often takes many months for the developing symptoms to be recognised as those of asthma

rather than repeated colds, for example, and patients are often tried on several inhalers before an occupational cause is suspected. Currently the average time between the start of symptoms and a diagnosis of occupational asthma is around 4 years (Fishwick et al., 2007). Treating the asthma may mask the work-related symptoms and make the occupational cause more difficult to establish and remedy. If occupational asthma is suspected, it is better to clarify the diagnosis at an early stage rather than prescribe increasing amounts of treatment.

The impact of a diagnosis of occupational asthma can be devastating. Most affected workers suffer financially either because they can no longer work or they can no longer do the job for which they have been trained (Ayres et al., 2011). A skilled baker or welder may become a labourer or become unemployed. A good employer will redeploy an affected worker away from exposures, but often workers face the dilemma of risking their health by continuing with their job or facing the emotional and financial consequences of giving up their work. The worst possible outcome is when someone with occupational asthma continues to work, suffers worsened asthma and then is no longer fit to do any work. Sometimes it is possible for the individual to continue in their job with reduced exposures, but because the asthma is caused by hypersensitivity to something at work even very small levels of exposure are sufficient to perpetuate and worsen the asthma. By analogy, people who are not allergic to pollen can tolerate high exposures, but it does not require a lot of pollen in the air to affect those who are sensitised. It can be the same with occupational exposures.

Once the diagnosis is established and exposures are controlled, occupational asthma is treated in the same way as non-occupational disease (see Chapter 6). The asthma may get better or disappear completely. It is likely to worsen again if the worker comes into contact with the causative agent once again.

Non-occupational asthma is common and affects about 5%–10% of the population (Anderson et al., 2007). Many workers are exposed to extreme temperatures, dust or fumes at work and if they have asthma, even it is not caused by work, their symptoms may be worse at work. This is termed work-exacerbated asthma. It is estimated to affect around 20% of asthmatics and may be sufficiently severe for them not to be able to carry out their work (Lemiere et al., 2012). It can be difficult to distinguish from occupational asthma, asthma caused by work, although it should not be associated with a latent interval of asymptomatic exposures and is unlikely to progressively worsen with repeated exposures.

ASBESTOS

Asbestos is a mineral that unlike most other minerals occurs naturally in the form of fibres rather than crystals (American Thoracic Society [ATS], 2004). The fibres can be woven to form cloth, fluffed to make insulation material or added to cement to make it less brittle. Asbestos was widely used in the insulation of buildings and ships and for a variety of other purposes through much of the twentieth century. The fibres are easy to inhale into the lung but then get trapped and are difficult to remove. White (crysotile) asbestos does disappear from the lung and is less harmful than brown (amosite) or blue (crocidilite) asbestos. Although asbestos use came under control from the 1970s and its import was banned in the UK in 2000, because of its persistence in the lung the peak of asbestos-related deaths in the UK will not occur until around 2020 (see Figure 9.3). Altogether around 150,000 deaths are anticipated as a consequence of asbestos exposure in the UK. As of 2015 there are more people in the UK who are destined to die of asbestos-related malignancy than have already died, and asbestos will continue to cause death on a large scale for several decades (Darnton et al., 2012).

Asbestos pleural plaques are fibrotic and usually calcified areas on the parietal pleura, the pleural layer lining the inside of the ribs. They can occur following very low-level exposures to asbestos. They do not

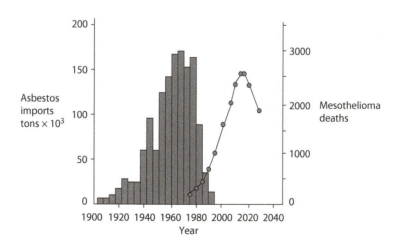

Figure 9.3 UK asbestos imports and mesothelioma deaths. UK asbestos imports from 1900 (histogram), and actual and predicted mesothelioma deaths. (Adapted from Peto, J. et al. 1995. *Lancet* 345 (8949): 535–539.)

cause the parietal and visceral pleura to adhere and generally they do not cause symptoms or affect lung function. They are easily spotted on a chest X-ray and indicate that the individual has worked with asbestos. They can cause a lot of anxiety and their significance often needs to be carefully explained.

Pleural effusions and diffuse pleural thickening can also be caused by asbestos exposures. Typically, an individual develops a pleural effusion many years after working with asbestos. That resolves leaving pleural fibrosis that causes the visceral and parietal pleura to adhere, interferes with lung movements and leads to breathlessness. Often the process starts on one side, after a few months the same happens on the other side, and then the fibrosis remains essentially stable thereafter. The trigger for the disease is not known (Jeebun and Stenton, 2012).

Malignant mesotheliomas are tumours of the pleura that are closely associated with asbestos exposure. They can occur following very low-level exposures, for example in wives who washed the overalls of men who worked with asbestos, and 30 or more years after exposure. They present with pleural effusions, often with chest pain, and with features of malignancy such as fatigue, anorexia and weight loss. They are poorly responsive to treatment and the average life expectancy is around 12 months from the onset of symptoms (Stenton and Peel, 2013).

Asbestosis is a form of diffuse lung fibrosis. It is a disease of those with heavy asbestos exposures and is now relatively uncommon. It presents with slowly progressive breathlessness, fine basal crackles on examination of the chest and basal interstitial fibrosis on the chest radiograph. The features are the same as those of idiopathic pulmonary fibrosis except that asbestosis tends to be slowly progressive over many years or decades, whereas idiopathic pulmonary fibrosis often progresses rapidly. There is no effective treatment (Roggli et al., 2010).

Asbestos also increases the risk of lung cancer. The risk is multiplicative with that of smoking so that a smoker may have a 20-times increased risk and someone with asbestosis a 5-times increased risk. Someone who smokes and has asbestos then has a 100-times increased risk (Selikoff, 1979). There are no features that allow the cause of the cancer to be determined and in many cases the contribution of asbestos exposures goes unrecognised.

PNEUMOCONIOSIS

The term pneumoconiosis is used to describe lung disease associated with diffuse chest radiograph abnormalities and caused by exposures to mineral dusts. Asbestosis is a form of pneumoconiosis. Coal workers' pneumoconiosis and silicosis are the other important types of fibrotic pneumoconiosis. Some metals such as iron from welding and barium from mining are very radio-dense and can cause striking abnormalities on the radiograph without causing symptoms or abnormalities of lung function.

Coal workers' pneumoconiosis became common in the 1950s when mechanisation in coal mines led to greatly increased dust exposures (Pestonk et al., 2013). In its milder forms it is characterised by multiple small nodules on the chest radiograph (simple pneumoconiosis) that have little effect on lung function (Brichet et al. 2002). Its main significance in current miners is that it is associated with a risk of more severe pneumoconiosis and so exposures should be reduced. In ex-miners its main significance is that it can be confused with other diseases that cause diffuse lung nodules, particularly tuberculosis and sarcoidosis. As the disease progresses the nodules coalesce to form larger masses of progressive massive fibrosis. These occur predominantly in the upper zones and can be several centimetres across. They can be confused with lung cancer and tuberculosis. A careful occupational history is important and could save the patient an unnecessary lung biopsy.

Silicosis is caused by exposure to crystalline silica or quartz (Leung et al., 2012). One of its commonest sources is sand. Sand on the beach is harmless because the particles are too large to get into the lungs – only particles of less than 10 μm in diameter get beyond the upper airways. If the same particles are broken down by blasting them against a surface as in sandblasting or heating them to high temperatures, they become highly toxic. Historically, silicosis was commonest in miners, foundry workers who used sand to form moulds for molten metal and pottery workers. It still occurs sporadically in quarry workers, stonemasons and others. Concrete can contain a lot of silica and construction workers are exposed when they cut, polish or drill into it. A recent outbreak was described in workers making composite worktops for kitchens (Kramer et al., 2012). In another outbreak, several teenagers who were sandblasting jeans to artificially age them suffered fatal silicosis (Akgun et al., 2006).

The radiological picture of silicosis is very similar to that of coal worker's pneumoconiosis. Sometimes the unusual feature of 'eggshell' calcification around the edges of mediastinal lymph nodes can be seen. The disease is easily mistaken for sarcoidosis for example, but the clue to the diagnosis lies in a careful occupational history. Very heavy silica exposures can cause a different picture of acute silicosis which appears more like pulmonary oedema and can be rapidly fatal. Silica exposures are associated with a marked increase in the risk of tuberculosis and also cause lung cancer (Scarselli et al., 2011).

CHRONIC OBSTRUCTIVE PULMONARY DISEASE AND LUNG CANCER

Occupational asthma, pneumoconiosis and asbestos-related disease can be identified by their clinical features. Occupational COPD and cancer, however, are identical to the non-occupational forms of the diseases. They can be shown to be more common in some groups of workers but in any individual it is generally impossible to determine whether their disease was caused by work rather than by smoking.

It can be very difficult to demonstrate that a disease is more common than it should be in a particular workplace (Pearce et al., 2007). People in work tend to be healthier than the rest of the population – the healthy worker effect – and so for example lung function measurements tend to be better than predicted. A study that showed that lung function measurements in a group of workers were on average 100% of predicted could miss an effect of work. Those who are most susceptible to an adverse effect of work tend to leave, so only the healthy remain – the survivor effect. A study of cancer in workers in a factory might find no one affected but others could have already left or be dead. Occupational effects can be confounded by

smoking for example. Teenagers who smoke are more likely to look for jobs such as welding that expose them to fumes and so an adverse effect could be due either to the smoking or the welding fumes (Beach et al., 1996). As a rule, few records are kept of workers' exposures.

Studies from the 1960s showed that coal miners developed COPD that was related to their dust exposure (Stenton, 2002) and was unrelated to any pneumoconiosis on their chest radiographs. The average effect of heavy dust exposure was similar to that of smoking. As with smoking most workers are little affected, but a minority develop severe disease. Later studies showed that a variety of dusts and fumes had the same effect, and overall it is felt that about 15% of COPD is caused by occupational exposures (Balmes et al., 2003). Some individuals have COPD only because of their work and many have disease that has been worsened by their occupational exposures. In the past the term 'nuisance dust' was often used to describe exposures that were felt not to be harmful, but that term is no longer appropriate and it is likely that almost any occupational exposure to a vapour, gas, dust or fume has some harmful effect.

There are a number of chemicals and exposures that are known to increase the risk of lung cancer. Asbestos, coal tar from coking plants, ionising radiation and chromium are well-recognised risks. Animal studies do not predict well the effects in humans and because of the problems with occupational epidemiology discussed above there is a range of exposures, such as to welding fume, for which it is uncertain whether or not there is a risk (Field and Withers, 2012).

HYPERSENSITIVITY PNEUMONITIS (EXTRINSIC ALLERGIC BRONCHIOLOALVEOLITIS)

Hypersensitivity pneumonitis is an immunologically mediated lung disease that often has an occupational cause. Bird-fancier's lung caused by the 'bloom' that coats feathers, and farmer's lung caused by micro-organisms that contaminate mouldy hay are traditional causes (Lacasse et al., 2012). A more important newer form of the disease is caused by contaminated cooling fluids used to cool drills and cutting blades in industry (Robertson et al., 2007). The fluid is recirculated and can become contaminated in sumps. When it is resprayed onto a rapidly rotating drill it becomes aerosolised and can be inhaled. There is an acute form of hypersensitivity pneumonitis that presents as a flu-like illness with fever, breathlessness and joint aches several hours after the exposure. The chest radiograph shows a diffuse abnormality. It is relatively easy to recognise as the symptoms are associated with the exposure and a CT scan can confirm the diagnosis. The chronic form of the disease presents with progressive breathlessness and fibrosis on the chest radiograph with a less clear relationship with exposures and can be difficult to diagnose. It is like budgerigar fancier's lung, which can be notoriously difficult to diagnose unless the question about birds at home is asked. Corticosteroids can help but the mainstay of the treatment is a reduction or avoidance of the exposure.

NEW OCCUPATIONAL LUNG DISEASES: POPCORN AND FLOCK WORKERS LUNG

In 2002 a 42-year-old lady developed breathlessness over the course of about 9 months with a dramatic fall in lung function. Investigations including a CT scan and lung biopsy revealed bronchiolitis with inflammation and narrowing of the small airways. Because of the severity of her disease she was assessed for a possible lung transplant. It was then noticed that there were three others from her workplace on the same transplant list. The butter flavouring diacetyl used to flavour microwavable popcorn was identified as the cause of their lung disease (Kreiss et al., 2002). Since then, numerous other cases of popcorn worker's lung have been reported. Workers making flock coverings for car seats and the like can develop diffuse lung fibrosis caused by inhaling small polyethylene fibres (Eschenbacher et al., 1999). These conditions illustrate that new occupational diseases are continually arising with the introduction of new industrial processes and chemicals. The clinician needs to be constantly alert to that possibility and the importance of a careful occupational history.

OTHER OCCUPATIONAL LUNG DISEASES

Occupational exposures cause a wide range of lung diseases. Infection with TB is a recognised risk in healthcare workers. *Legionella pneumophila* can live in warm water systems such as cooling towers; if these are not properly maintained, this can lead to outbreaks of legionnaires disease. Acute inhalation injuries occur with a variety of gases and chemicals. Soluble gases and fumes such as chlorine tend to dissolve in the airways and cause irritation or asthma. Insoluble gases such as nitrogen dioxide penetrate to the alveoli and cause pulmonary oedema. Exposure to a variety of substances can cause alveolitic-like symptoms with fever, aching joints and breathlessness often developing several hours after exposures. Metal fume fever is caused by zinc fumes generated by welding galvanised metal. Polymer fume fever is caused by heated polytetrafluoroethylene (Teflon©), for example when tape used to seal joints adheres to plumber's cigarettes and gets inhaled (Greenberg and Vearrier, 2015). Byssinosis is caused by contaminants of cotton and other fibre. Alveolitic symptoms that get better with repeated exposure are typical, giving rise to Monday morning fever (Fishwick and Pickering, 1992).

CONTROL AND PREVENTION OF OCCUPATIONAL LUNG DISEASE

Occupational lung disease is generally preventable by proper control of exposures. Widespread exposure to mineral dusts is now less common in developed countries so that coal workers' pneumoconiosis, silicosis and asbestosis are relatively rare. However, these exposures have been replaced in industry by a variety of reactive chemicals that cause a different range of diseases such as asthma and alveolitis. Much occupational disease has been 'exported' in recent decades to less economically developed countries where exposures are less carefully controlled.

In Europe, employers are under obligations set out in the Control of Substances Hazardous to Health (COSHH) regulations to inform and protect workers exposed to a potentially harmful process or material (HMSO, 2012). A risk assessment needs to be undertaken and there is a hierarchy of steps that should be taken to reduce risks. If a chemical or process does not need to be used, then it should not be: In the past, rubber gloves were coated in powder that became contaminated by rubber proteins in storage and was breathed in when the gloves were put on, giving rise to asthma (LaMontagne et al., 2006). If a material can be replaced with something less hazardous, then it should be: rubber gloves have generally been replaced by nitrile gloves. If a process can be enclosed, then it should be: endoscopes in hospitals are now sterilised in enclosed machines rather than in open baths. If it cannot be enclosed, then any fumes should be extracted at source: welding and soldering require fume extraction equipment. Sometimes a less hazardous form can be used: liquids and pellets give rise to less dust than powders. Only if none of these steps can control exposures should facemasks be used as they are often not worn properly or not worn all the time and are of limited effectiveness.

Early detection of disease is important and so lung function surveillance programmes are mandatory in some workplaces such as bakeries where there are exposures to flour or paint shops where there are exposures to isocyanate paints. To be of value a surveillance programme requires a disease that has an asymptomatic early stage, a test that is sensitive and specific for the disease and which causes no harm, and an effective intervention. There is currently debate about the value of CT scans to detect early lung cancer, for example in asbestos workers who are at high risk (Ollier et al., 2014). For some conditions such as malignant mesothelioma there is no good means of detecting the disease early or no good means of treating it if it is detected early and so screening is inappropriate.

MANAGEMENT OF AND COMPENSATION FOR OCCUPATIONAL LUNG DISEASE

Most occupational diseases are treated in exactly the same way as their non-occupational counterparts with the additional step of reducing or eliminating exposure. Early treatment may mask the effect of work and generally it is better to explore and establish the correct diagnosis before escalating treatment.

Most countries have schemes for compensating individuals with occupational lung disease. In the UK, Industrial Injuries Disablement Benefit is a no-fault scheme that compensates individuals who are suffering one of a number of prescribed diseases, for more information visit https://www.gov.uk/industrial-injuries-disablement-benefit/further-information. Disability is assessed on a scale from 0%–100% and a weekly pension is paid depending on the level of disability. The benefit is not means-tested but individuals may lose other means-tested benefits if they are awarded Industrial Injury Benefit. There are separate schemes for members of the armed forces, coal miners, and some individuals with mesothelioma who are unable to obtain compensation in other ways.

In the UK and most other countries individuals can take a civil action against an employer who has caused them harm. In that case it is necessary to show not only that the disease was caused by the work but that the employer was negligent in allowing the exposures. If the individual is successful then a lump sum is awarded that can take into account not just the level of disability but loss of earnings, care needs and any risk of premature death.

Prevention is more important than compensating occupational disease. Healthcare professionals have a key role in being aware of the risks associated with occupational exposures and making proper enquiries about work when they come into contact with someone with almost any respiratory disease.

CASE STUDY

Sue Potter is a 19-year-old lady who had worked as an apprentice baker for 2 years. Her job involved mixing flour, yeast and other ingredients in large bowls, and some dust was given off when she did this. Sue had no previous history of asthma or hay fever and she was in generally good health. Sue began to notice a runny nose and chest tightness starting about half an hour into her work shifts and lasting for an hour or more after she went home. She started wakening at nights coughing. Her symptoms only occurred on days when she was at work, and at weekends she was entirely well. Sue was given a salbutamol inhaler that helped initially but her symptoms gradually worsened.

Lung function tests showed mild airflow obstruction, tests for specific IgE antibodies to alpha amylase, an enzyme used in bread production, were positive and serial measurements of peak expiratory flow showed a work-related pattern similar to that of Figure 9.1. Occupational asthma and rhinitis were diagnosed and Sue was redeployed to the confectionary area where she did not have to handle flour. Sue was not able to complete her apprenticeship, has taken a considerable drop in earnings and she still has mild ongoing asthma requiring low inhaled corticosteroids and 1–2 puffs of salbutamol per day.

CASE STUDY DISCUSSION

Unfortunately, occupational asthma is a common occupational lung disease and Sue's allergy to flour dust is also fairly common (Fishwick et al., 2008). Occupational asthma is also the most common form of adult-onset asthma for which a cause can be found. Sue was also typically well until starting work in the bakery and had a latent period of working in the bakery for 2 years before developing symptoms. Sue's symptoms followed a pattern of being triggered while at work but absent when she was off duty. Fishwick et al. (2008) recommend a detailed medical history as the type/cause of Sue's symptoms need to be distinguished from other diseases, especially non-work-related asthma and work-exacerbated asthma because a diagnosis of occupational asthma may have serious financial consequences for the sufferer (Ayres et al., 2011). While Sue received appropriate treatment for asthma (see Chapter 6) unfortunately she could no longer work as a baker, which is often the case. In one sense Sue was fortunate because her employer redeployed her to an area where she was not exposed to flour, but she did receive a reduction in earnings. Fishwick et al. (2008) report that deployment may not be utilised and workers often continue to suffer in silence due to of fear of contract termination, or until their symptoms render them unable to work. The prognosis for occupational asthma is better if the individual is removed from the exposure as soon as possible.

SUMMARY

Occupational lung disease is common. Exposures at work cause a number of specific lung conditions such as pneumoconiosis but they also cause all the common lung diseases such as asthma, COPD and lung cancer. Often the occupational contribution goes unrecognised, and a careful occupational history is important. Occupational asthma is a prime example. Only about one fifth of cases are identified, yet early diagnosis and modification of exposures can have a profound effect on the outcome of the disease. Anyone with new-onset asthma or asthma that has got a lost worse should be questioned about whether their symptoms are related to their work and investigated further if occupational asthma is a possibility. Similarly, pneumoconiosis can mimic other conditions such as idiopathic pulmonary fibrosis, tuberculosis and sarcoidosis. As new chemicals and processes are constantly being introduced new occupational disease are likely to continue to occur and the clinician needs to maintain a high level of vigilance.

REFERENCES

American Thoracic Society. 2004. Diagnosis and initial management of nonmalignant diseases related to asbestos. *American Journal of Respiratory and Critical Care Medicine* 170 (6): 691–715.

Anderson, H.R., Gupta, R., Strachan, D.P. and Limb, E.S. 2007. 50 years of asthma: UK trends from 1955 to 2004. *Thorax* 62 (1): 85–90.

Akgun, M., Mirici, A., Ucar, E.Y., Kantarci, M., Araz, O. and Gorguner, M. 2006. Silicosis in Turkish denim sandblasters. *Occupational Medicine* 56 (8): 554–558.

Ayres, J.G., Boyd, R., Cowie, H. and Hurley, F.J. 2011. Costs of occupational asthma in the UK. *Thorax* 66 (2): 128–133.

Balmes, J., Becklake, M., Blanc, P., Henneberger, P., Kreiss, K., Mapp, C., Milton, D., Schwartz,

D., Toren, K. and Viegi, G. 2003. American Thoracic Society Statement: Occupational contribution to the burden of airway disease. *American Journal of Respiratory Critical Care Medicine* 167 (5): 787–797.

Beach, J.R., Dennis, J.H., Avery, A.J., Bromly, C.L., Ward, R.J., Walters, E.H., Stenton, S.C. and Hendrick, D.J. 1996. An epidemiologic investigation of asthma in welders. *American Journal of Respiratory and Critical Care Medicine* 154 (5): 1394–400.

Brichet, A., Desurmont, S. and Wallaert, B. 2002. Coal workers pneumoconiosis. In: Hendrick, D., Burge, P., Beckett, W. and Churg, A. (eds.). *Occupational Disorders of the Lung.* WB Saunders, Philadelphia.

Carroll, K.B., Secombe, C.J. and Pepys, J. 1976. Asthma due to non-occupational exposure to toluene (tolylene) di-isocyanate. *Clinical Allergy* 6 (2): 99–104.

Chan-Yeung, M. and Malo, J.L. 1995. Occupational asthma. *New England Journal of Medicine* 333 (2): 107–112.

Cullinan, P., Tarlo, S. and Nemery, B. 2003. The prevention of occupational asthma. *European Respiratory Journal* 22 (5): 853–860.

Darnton, A., Hodgson, J., Benson, P. and Coggon, D. 2012. Mortality from asbestosis and mesothelioma in Britain by birth cohort. *Occupational Medicine* 62 (7): 549–552.

Eschenbacher, W.L., Kreiss, K., Lougheed, M.D., Pransky, G.S., Day, B. and Castellan, R.M. 1999. Nylon flock-associated interstitial lung disease. *American Journal of Respiratory and Critical Care Medicine* 159 (6): 2003–2008.

Field, R.W. and Withers, B.L. 2012. Occupational and environmental causes of lung cancer. *Clinics in Chest Medicine* 33 (4): 681–703.

Fishwick, D., Barber, C.M., Bradshaw, L.M., Harris-Roberts, J., Francis, M., Naylor, S., Ayres, J. et al. 2008. British Thoracic Society standards of care subcommittee guidelines on occupational asthma. *Thorax* 63 (3): 240–250.

Fishwick, D., Bradshaw, L., Davies, J., Henson, M., Stenton, C., Burge, S., Niven, R. et al. 2007. Are we failing workers with symptoms suggestive of occupational asthma? *Primary Care Respiratory Journal* 16 (5): 304–310.

Fishwick, D. and Pickering, C.A. 1992. Byssinosis – A form of occupational asthma? *Thorax* 47 (6): 401–403.

Greenberg, M.I. and Vearrier, D. 2015. Metal fume fever and polymer fume fever. *Clinical Toxicology (Phila)* 53 (4): 195–203.

Her Majesty's Stationary Office (HMSO). 2012. *Working with Substances Hazardous to Health: A Brief Guide to COSHH.* HMSO, London.

Huggins, V., Anees, W., Pantin, C. and Burge, S. 2005. Improving the quality of peak flow measurements for the diagnosis of occupational asthma. *Occupational Medicine* 55 (5): 385–388.

Jeebun, V. and Stenton, S.C. 2012. The presentation and natural history of asbestos-induced diffuse pleural thickening. *Occupational Medicine* 62 (4): 266–268.

Kramer, M.R., Blanc, P.D., Fireman, E., Amital, A., Guber, A., Rhahman, N.A. and Shitrit, D. 2012. Artificial stone silicosis: Disease resurgence among artificial stone workers. *Chest* 142 (2): 419–424.

Kreiss, K., Gomaa, A., Kullman, G., Fedan, K., Simoes, E.J. and Enright, P.L. 2002. Clinical bronchiolitis obliterans in workers at a microwave-popcorn plant. *New England Journal of Medicine* 347 (5): 330–338.

Lacasse, Y., Girard, M. and Cormier, Y. 2012. Recent advances in hypersensitivity pneumonitis. *Chest* 142 (1): 208–217.

LaMontagne, A.D., Radi, S., Elder, D.S., Abramson, M.J. and Sim, M. 2006. Primary prevention of latex related sensitisation and occupational asthma: A systematic review. *Occupational Environmental Medicine* 63 (5): 359–364.

Lemiere, C., Bégin, D., Camus, M., Forget, A., Boulet, L-P. and Gérin, M. 2012. Occupational risk factors associated with work-exacerbated asthma in Quebec. *Occupational Environmental Medicine* 69 (12): 901–907.

Leung, C.C., Yu, I.T.S. and Chen, W. 2012. Silicosis. *Lancet* 379 (9830): 2008–2018.

McNamee, R., Carder, M., Chen, Y. and Agius, R. 2008. Measurement of trends in incidence of work-related skin and respiratory diseases, UK 1996–2005. *Occupational Environmental Medicine* 65 (12): 808–814.

Nicholson, P.J., Cullinan, P., Burge, P.S. and Boyle, C. 2010. *Occupational Asthma: Prevention, Identification & Management: Systematic Review & Recommendations.* British Occupational Health Research Foundation, London.

Ollier, M., Chamoux, A., Naughton, G., Pereira, B. and Dutheil, F. 2014. Chest CT scan screening for lung cancer in asbestos occupational exposure: A systematic review and meta-analysis. *Chest* 145 (6): 1339–1346.

Pearce, N., Checkoway, H. and Kriebel, D. 2007. Bias in occupational epidemiology studies. *Occupational Environmental Medicine* 64 (8): 562–568.

Peto, J., Hodgson, J.T., Matthews, F.E. and Jones, J.R. 1995. Continuing increase in mesothelioma mortality in Britain. *Lancet* 345 (8949): 535–539.

Petsonk, E.L., Rose C. and Cohen R. 2013. Coal mine dust lung disease new lessons from an old exposure. *American Journal of Respiratory and Critical Care Medicine* 187 (11): 1178–1185.

Robertson, W., Robertson, A.S., Burge, C.S.G., Moore, V.C., Jaakkola, M.S., Dawkins, P.A., Burd, M. et al. 2007. Clinical investigation of an outbreak of alveolitis and asthma in a car engine manufacturing plant. *Thorax* 62 (11): 981–990.

Roggli, V.L., Gibbs, A.R., Attanoos, R., Churg, A., Popper, H., Cagle, P., Corrin, B. et al. 2010. Pathology of asbestosis- An update of the diagnostic criteria: Report of the Asbestosis Committee of the college of American pathologists and pulmonary pathology society. *Archives Pathology and Laboratory Medicine* 134 (3): 462–480.

Selikoff, I.J. 1979. Mortality experience of insulation workers in the United States and Canada, 1943–1976. *Annals New York Acadamcy of Sciences* 330 (1): 91–116.

Scarselli, A., Binazzi, A., Forastiere, F., Cavariani, F. and Marinaccio, A. 2011. Industry and job-specific mortality after occupational exposure to silica dust. *Occupational Medicine* 61: 422–429.

Shakeri, M.S., Dick, F.D. and Ayres, J.G. 2008. Which agents cause reactive airways dysfunction syndrome (RADS)? A systematic review. *Occupational Medicine* 58 (3): 205–211.

Stenton, S.C. 2002. Asthma. In: Hendrick, D., Burge, P., Beckett, W. and Churg, A. (eds.) *Occupational Disorders of the Lung.* WB Saunders, Philadelphia.

Stenton, S.C. and Peel, T. 2013. Pleural effusions and mesothelioma. In: Bourke, S.J. and Peel, T.E. (eds.). *Integrated Palliative Care of Respiratory disease.* Springer, London.

Tarlo, S.M., Balmes, J., Balkissoon, R., Beach, J., Beckett, W., Bernstein, D., Blanc, P.D. et al. 2008. Diagnosis and management of work-related asthma: American College of Chest Physicians consensus statement. *Chest* 134(Suppl 3): S1–S41.

Tarlo, S.M. and Lemiere, C. 2014. Occupational asthma. *New England Journal of Medicine* 370 (7): 640–649.

Vandenplas, O. 2011. Occupational asthma: Etiologies and risk factors. *Allergy Asthma Immunology Research* 3 (3): 157–167.

Pneumonia

10

VANESSA GIBSON

LEARNING OBJECTIVES

Upon completion of this chapter the reader should be able to:

- Describe the defence mechanisms of the respiratory system that protect against invasion by micro-organisms
- Provide a definition of pneumonia and discriminate between the different classifications of pneumonia
- Identify risk factors for the development of community-acquired and hospital-acquired pneumonia
- Discuss the management of community-acquired and hospital-acquired pneumonia
- Identify significant complications of pneumonia
- Discuss the importance of severity assessment tools

INTRODUCTION

Despite developments in antibiotic therapy over the last few decades, pneumonia remains a significant cause of death in the United Kingdom (UK) and for those who do recover the process may take many months (Moussaoui et al., 2006). One study undertaken in general practice suggested that people with a diagnosis of pneumonia have a significantly increased mortality in the short term, with cases 46 times more likely to die in the first 30 days after diagnosis, but some increase in mortality persists during longer-term follow-up (Myles et al., 2009). The British Thoracic Society (BTS) audit, which reviewed

hospital admissions for community-acquired pneumonia (CAP), found that out of 5652 admissions the average age was 72 years and that during the last 4 years in which the audit took place in-patient mortality rates at 30 days had reduced (Lim and Rodrigo, 2013). Pneumonia can affect any age group and the World Health Organisation (WHO) (2013) suggests that pneumonia is the biggest killer of children worldwide. Pneumonia can be acquired in the community, in the acute hospital setting or in long-term care facilities. While there are some well-documented risk factors such as smoking or co-morbidities such as asthma, pneumonia can affect anyone. In addition, some groups of patients, such as the elderly, will not have what would be considered character-istic signs and symptoms. There may be an absence of fever and symptoms might be much subtler. It is therefore necessary that healthcare professionals have a detailed understanding of pneumonia.

This chapter aims to provide an overview of pneumonia and will include: a definition and classification of pneumonia, reference to relevant anatomy and physiology regarding the defence of the respiratory system, CAP and its management, severe complications of pneumonia with specific reference to invasive pneumococcal disease and severity assessment tools. Hospital-acquired pneumonia (HAP) will be discussed briefly with reference to ventilator-acquired pneumonia (VAP) as there is some overlap between the two conditions. Finally, a case study will be presented that illustrates the challenges associated with the diagnosis of CAP in the elderly.

DEFINITION AND CLASSIFICATION

A very simple definition of pneumonia is an infection of the lung tissue (Campbell, 2003). Hansall and Padley (1999) define pneumonia as an inflammation and infection of the terminal bronchioles and alveoli resulting in consolidation. A more comprehensive definition has been developed by Lim et al. (2009) who define pneumonia diagnosed in the community as symptoms of an acute lower respiratory tract illness (cough and at least one other symptom), new focal chest signs on examination, at least one systemic feature such as fever and no other explanation for the illness. A definition of the diagnosis of pneumonia for patients admitted to hospital, however, included signs and symptoms consistent with an acute lower respiratory tract infection associated with new radiographic shadowing for which there is no other explanation and the illness is the primary reason for hospital admission. However, there are a number of different approaches to the classification of pneumonia which include:

- Where the pneumonia was contracted, i.e. in the community or in hospital (see later)
- In relation to the part of the lung affected, i.e. lobar where one or more lobes are consolidated

or bronchial pneumonia where the infection is more widespread and appears as patchy consolidation around the terminal bronchioles
- In relation to the causative organism, i.e. bacterial, viral or fungal

However, there are other types of pneumonia which are often labelled atypical pneumonia and include Legionnaire's disease; mycoplasma pneumonia; *Chlamydia psittaci*; *Coxiella burnetti*; in addition, there is aspiration pneumonia (Mendleson's Syndrome), HAP/VAP and more recently healthcare-associated pneumonia (Davies and Moores, 2010; Cascini et al., 2013).

PATHOPHYSIOLOGY

The delicate walls of the alveoli need to be protected from damage. Davies and Moores (2010) suggest that the respiratory system has evolved to offer protection to the very fine, vascular and moist surface of the alveoli. The upper and conducting airways play a major role in protecting the respiratory surface by filtering out particles and vapours from the air. The anatomy and physiology of the respiratory system is more fully described in Chapter 1. However, the relevant defence mechanisms of the respiratory system will be discussed here as pneumonia occurs when these defences are breached and micro-organisms penetrate deep into the lungs.

The size and shape of inhaled particles will determine how far they penetrate into the lungs and the site of penetration will determine how they are dealt with. The mechanisms for dealing with particles that infiltrate the lungs include impaction, sedimentation, the mucociliary escalator, diffusion and the reticular-endothelium system of fixed macrophages. An aerosol is a cloud of particles or droplets that remain stable when suspended in air for some time. However, not all particles or droplets are the same size and large ones will fall faster than small ones. Ninety-five percent of particles that are >5 μm are trapped by the mucus of the nose and pharynx. This is described by Davies and Moores (2010) as impaction and is the result of turbulence in the nose which throws them out of the airstream. The particles are then wafted by the cilia to the pharynx and are coughed out or swallowed. Slightly smaller particles (1–5 μm) manage to penetrate further into the airways and are removed by sedimentation, which is the settling of particles under gravity. This usually takes place in the small airways due to their narrow diameter. The particles then travel up the mucociliary escalator to the pharynx and are coughed out or swallowed. Smaller particles (<0.1 μm) finally bump into the walls of the small airways by a process known as Brownian motion whereby they are deposited on the walls of the alveoli by the diffusion of gases (Davies and Moores, 2010).

Macrophages in the alveoli, also known as dust cells, are part of the reticulo-endothelial system, which is a system of tissue or fixed macrophages that play an important role in defence against micro-organisms (Tortora and Derrickson, 2012). Any particles, including micro-organisms, that manage to reach the terminal bronchioles or alveoli are engulfed by the macrophages, which either carry them up to the mucociliary escalator or into the blood or lymph. If the dust load is particularly large, the macrophages deposit the particles around the bronchioles and these can often be seen on postmortem examination as halos or dark rings (Davies and Moores, 2010). The macrophages release a number of chemicals known as cytokines, which are designed to kill any micro-organisms that have made it down into the air surfaces. However, this cytokine activity also damages the delicate alveoli and accounts for some of the symptoms displayed by the patient with pneumonia, e.g. productive cough, fever, pain. However, just because micro-organisms have penetrated deep down into the lungs does not mean an individual will develop pneumonia. The development of pneumonia will depend on the pathogen, the size of the inoculum and a number of host factors such as smoking, age and co-morbidities (Driver, 2012a) (see below for a discussion about risk factors).

The classic characteristics of inflammation are redness (vasodilation), swelling (vessel permeability), pain and heat (fever) (Tortora and Derrickson, 2012). When these are applied to the delicate tissue of the alveoli they can be disastrous. Free radicals and proteases released by the macrophages would normally be neutralised to prevent them damaging the lungs (Davies and Moores, 2010). However, owing to the quantities released in pneumonia, these have a chemostatic effect (chemical distress signal) that attracts neutrophils to the alveoli from the vascular compartment (Monton and Torres, 1998). Cytokine activity leads to the classic characteristics described above and includes tumour necrosis factor, proteases, interleukins etc. (Moldoveanu et al., 2009). These cytokines result in permeability of the vessels and a fibrin-rich exudate fills the alveoli rendering them airless (Driver, 2012b) (see Figure 10.1). This leads to consolidation. Each lobe of the lungs is divided into bronchopulmonary segments, which may play an important role in compartmentalising infections such as pneumonia (Campbell, 2003). Despite this compartmentalisation, micro-organisms can spread from alveolus to alveolus and can therefore affect a whole lobe or indeed a whole lung. In the consolidated areas of lung, gas flow is deficient, whereas perfusion remains normal, causing a ventilation/perfusion (V/Q) mismatch where blood flows through the alveoli but does not pick up oxygen (or give up carbon dioxide) and this results in hypoxaemia and sometimes hypercapnia (Boldt and Kiresuk, 2001). The physiological mechanisms described above result in a patient who is hypoxic and often in respiratory distress, is in pain, has a fever and a productive cough.

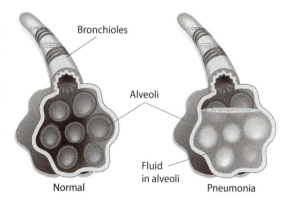

Figure 10.1 Normal and infected alveoli. (From Shutterstock Image ID: 214353118. With permission.)

COMMUNITY-ACQUIRED PNEUMONIA

CAP is a pneumonia that is contracted outside of a hospital or long-term care setting (Schultz, 2003). Public Health England (PHE) (2013) suggest that CAP is a major cause of morbidity and mortality in the UK with an incidence of 5–11 adults per 1000 population, it is also a major cause of admission to hospital. Moussaoui et al. (2006) suggest that most patients with mild to moderate pneumonia will make a full recovery within six months and if symptoms persist beyond 28 days this is likely to be attributable to age and co-morbidity. However, whereas in industrialised countries mortality for pneumonia is more common in the elderly, a study by Myles et al. (2009) suggests that pneumonia appears to be an independent predictor of mortality irrespective of age, sex or coexisting co-morbidity. Therefore, identifying the causative organism and utilising a valid and reliable risk stratification tool are essential. Other risk factors include co-morbidity such as asthma, cystic fibrosis, chronic obstructive pulmonary disease (COPD), bronchiectasis, extremes of age such as the very young or very old, immunocompromised individuals, heart disease, diabetes, malnutrition, altered mental status, smoking, alcohol or substance misuse and overcrowded living conditions or homelessness (Dunn, 2005; Brown, 2012). Micro-organisms that cause CAP can be bacterial, viral or fungal (Brown, 2012). However, a study by Gutierrez et al. (2005) reviewed the prevalence and consequences of mixed aetiology pneumonia. Patients with mixed aetiology were more likely to have co-morbidities and a more severe form of the disease.

Streptococcus pneumoniae (*S. pneumoniae*) is accredited with being the most common bacteria to cause pneumonia outside of hospitals (Davies and Moores, 2010; Brown, 2012). *S. pneumoniae* is a bacterium which has a mucus-like 'coat' that enables it to evade the immune system (Murphy, 2008). Van der Poll (2011) describes this pathogen as truly remarkable in its ability to bind to respiratory surfaces, avoid host immune clearance, compete with other micro-organisms present in the respiratory tract, resist antibiotic therapy and invade the host. Ben-David and Rubinstein (2002) suggest that it is a major pathogen in adults and is responsible for not only causing pneumonia but also otitis media, sinusitis, meningitis and septicaemia. Individuals can have asymptomatic colonisation of the nasopharynx and it is transmitted via droplets or contact with infected pulmonary secretions. There are estimated to be over 90 serotypes and a new serotype will persist for weeks in adults and months in children usually without any harmful effects (van der Poll, 2011). Other bacteria that commonly cause pneumonia are haemophilus influenza, which is common in patients with pre-existing lung disease, and *staphylococcus aureus*, which is common in children and intravenous drug users (Davies and Moores, 2010).

Influenza is also an important cause of CAP; it is a highly infectious virus that affects the respiratory system and has been the cause of many large epidemics (Driver, 2012c). Three types of influenza virus have been identified:

- Type A, which is associated with animals, especially wild aquatic birds, and results in very severe disease.
- Type B, which only affects humans and is associated with less severe disease.
- Type C, which can be asymptomatic or cause only mild disease.

Generally, there will be one type of influenza prevailing in humans at any one time and this allows for the development of immunity within the population. However, in order to survive, the virus mutates and changes its surface antigens. This cycle of change is thought to occur every 2–3 years (Murphy, 2008). Influenza is usually seasonal, occurring in the UK between October and May. Symptoms appear suddenly and include sore throat; headache; weakness and fatigue; muscle ache; feeling unwell; loss of appetite; insomnia; and a dry, unproductive cough. Pneumonia is a severe complication of influenza that can be fatal (National Institute of Health and Care Excellence [NICE], 2013).

MANAGEMENT OF COMMUNITY-ACQUIRED PNEUMONIA IN ADULTS

The BTS Guidelines for the Management on Community Acquired Pneumonia in Adults (Lim et al., 2009) have recently been updated by NICE

(2014) and provide useful recommendations for investigation and management of patients, but it must be remembered that patients will require other supportive measures. Where this support cannot be performed by the patient or given by relatives or 'hospital at home' teams, then admission to hospital should be considered especially in the elderly. Assessing severity accurately is vital and a number of severity assessment tools will be discussed later in the chapter.

Lim et al. (2009) recommend that a chest X-ray is not necessary for patients who remain in community care unless there is doubt about diagnosis or suspicion of underlying lung pathology such as lung cancer or progress is not satisfactory. Similarly, general and microbiology investigations are not necessary, but if pulse oximeters are available oxygen saturation (SpO_2) would be a useful non-invasive check on the patient. Patients should be followed up to assess progress after 48 hours or sooner if clinically indicated. NICE (2014) recommend the use of C-reactive protein testing to guide antibiotic prescription where the diagnosis of pneumonia is not certain. For patients with a C-reactive protein of less than 20 mg/L antibiotics are not recommended. C-reactive protein is produced by the immune system and is associated with inflammation (Du Clos and Mold, 2004).

With regard to antibiotic therapy, the first anti-pneumococcal sulphonamide was introduced in 1939 (Podolsky, 2005). As discussed earlier *S. pneumoniae* remains the most likely causative micro-organism (Gutierrez and Masia, 2008). O'Driscoll et al. (2008) therefore recommend amoxicillin 500 mgs three times daily for 7 days or doxyclycline or clarithromycin for those patients with sensitivities to penicillin. Penicillins act to prevent transpeptidation (stabilisation of bacterial cell walls). Penicillins bind on to sites on the bacterial cell wall and activate autolysin, which destroys the cell wall. The cell wall becomes porous and alters the osmotic pressure within the bacterium and causes the cell to break down (Banning, 2005). NICE (2014) have recently updated this advice to a 5-day course of a single antibiotic, which should be extended if there is no improvement in the patient after 3 days.

For moderate to severe CAP, antibiotics should be continued for 7–10 days and the possibility of dual antibiotic therapy should be considered. This would consist of amoxicillin and a macrolide. Glucocorticosteroids should not be routinely prescribed for patients with CAP unless they have a co-morbidity for which glucocorticosteroids would be indicated (NICE, 2014).

Other supportive measures and advice need to be given to the patient. Patients should be advised to rest, drink plenty of fluid and take simple analgesia such as paracetamol for pain and to stop smoking (Lim et al., 2009). NICE (2014) advise patients to seek further medical assistance if there is no improvement within 3 days of commencing antibiotics.

Lim et al. (2009) suggest that all patients admitted to hospital should have a chest X-ray performed in time for antibiotics to be given within 4 hours of admission should a diagnosis of CAP be confirmed, and this is supported by NICE (2014). Patients should also have their oxygen saturation measured, bloods taken for urea and electrolytes, full blood count, C reactive protein and liver function tests. For patients with moderate-to-high-severity CAP, sputum and blood cultures should be performed. For patients with high-severity CAP, Gram staining may provide an immediate indicator of the pathogen. For patients with severe CAP, other tests are recommended including investigations for legionella. (For a full version of the BTS guidelines please visit https://www.brit-thoracic.org.uk/ and for the NICE guidelines please visit https://www.nice.org.uk/guidance/cg191.)

Moussaoui et al. (2006) suggest that for the majority of patients, respiratory symptoms will resolve within 14 days. However, there are some very serious complications associated with pneumonia which include pleural effusion, empyema, acute respiratory distress syndrome (ARDS) and sepsis (see Chapter 8). Lim et al. (2009) recommend that for patients who fail to improve as expected a thorough clinical history and examination should be undertaken by an experienced clinician, and further tests are warranted such as repeat chest X-ray, white blood cell count (WCC), C-reactive protein and sputum specimens for culture and sensitivity.

S. pneumoniae can colonise the naso-pharynx of individuals who remain asymptomatic, and damage to the nasal or pharyngeal mucosa can result in localised infections such as otitis media or sinusitis. However, for some individuals *S. pneumoniae* becomes invasive or systemic. Van der Poll (2011) suggests the polysaccharide capsule of *S. pneumoniae* can be altered depending on its immediate environment. *S. pneumoniae* with thinner capsules are better at colonising mucosal surfaces, whereas those with thicker capsules promote invasion. A particular virulence factor of *S. pneumoniae* is pneumolysin, which is a soluble toxin that causes lyses of the host cell, and a specific protein known as pneumococcal serine-rich repeat protein (PsrP) on the surface of the bacterium is essential in the invasion across the alveolar membrane in bacteraemic pneumonia.

Sepsis is a severe complication of pneumonia and PHE (2014) report approximately 5000 cases of invasive pneumococcal disease annually. Driver (2012a) identifies a number of risk factors associated with invasive pneumococcal disease including asplenia, alcoholism, drug-induced immunosuppression, human immunodeficiency virus (HIV), chronic liver or kidney disease, diabetes, sickle cell disease, thalassaemia major and children with cochlear implants. Once the bacteria enter the bloodstream, the immune response is stimulated. Sepsis is a systemic response by the host to infection. The infection can be confirmed or suspected. Sepsis can develop into severe sepsis when the host develops organ dysfunction and into septic shock when there is hypotension which is not reversed by fluid resuscitation (Dellinger et al., 2013). One prevailing theory is that sepsis is a result of an uncontrolled hyper-inflammatory response by the host to an infection. However, the response by the host is likely to be much more complex and involve both inflammation and immune suppression (van der Poll and Opal, 2008). A dynamic interaction exists between the host and invading pathogens. The virulence of the pathogen and bacterial load may determine the outcome for the patient (van der Poll and Opal, 2008).

The classic inflammatory response involves fever, redness or flushing, swelling and pain. These symptoms are all produced by cytokine activity released by the host's neutrophils. Neutrophils are the most prominent of all the leucocytes. This physiological response, often referred to as the systemic inflammatory response syndrome (SIRS), is the basis for

Table 10.1 Early recognition of sepsis

Two or more of the following symptoms Pyrexia > 38c or hypothermia < 36c HR > 90 bpm RR > 20 bpm WCC > 12 or <4 g/L Acutely altered mental state Hyperglycaemia in the absence of diabetes (>6.6 mmol/L)	Slurred speech Extremely painful muscles Passing no urine (in a day) 'I feel like I might die' Skin mottled or discoloured
(Robson and Daniels 2008)	The Sepsis Trust UK (2013)

the early detection and treatment of sepsis advocated by Robson and Daniels (2008) and The Sepsis Trust UK (2013) (see Table 10.1).

Early treatment is vital in the case of invasive pneumococcal disease, as with other forms of sepsis. It has been suggested that nurses' and doctors' knowledge of sepsis on the general ward is poor (Poeze et al., 2004; Fernandez et al., 2005; Robson et al., 2007). Ward nurses need to know about the 'Sepsis Six' and how to instigate implementation of these (Robson and Daniels, 2008) (see Table 10.2).

NICE (2014) recommend antibiotics with 4 hours of admission for CAP. Lim and Rodrigo (2013) report approximately 60% of patients receive antibiotics within the first 4 hours and in accordance with local CAP antibiotic guidelines. However, for sepsis the recommendation is that patients receive antibiotics within the first hour. A study by Kumar et al. (2006), which reviewed over 2000 patients,

Table 10.2 Early treatment of sepsis – the 'Sepsis Six'

1. Give 100% oxygen
2. Take blood cultures
3. Give IV antibiotics
4. Start IV fluid resuscitation
5. Measure haemoglobin and lactate
6. Insert urinary catheter and monitor hourly urine output

Source: Adapted from Robson, W.P. and Daniels, R. 2008. *British Journal of Nursing*, 17 (1): 16–21.

found that if antibiotic therapy was commenced within the first hour of documented hypotension it was associated with increased survival and that for every hour delay in antibiotic therapy mortality increased by 7.6%.

Respiratory failure is often a feature of sepsis and should be managed by administering high-flow oxygen to maintain a saturation of between 94% and 98% (O'Driscoll et al., 2008; Robson and Daniels, 2008; Suh and Hart, 2012; Ward, 2013). Patients with *S. pneumoniae* may already have respiratory impairment/failure, which will be compounded by the development of sepsis. Low saturations may persist despite high-flow oxygen therapy. Circulatory failure is caused by vasodilation and capillary leak as a result of the immune response which manifests as hypotension and should be treated promptly with a bolus of crystalloid IV fluid. Delays in implementing aggressive fluid therapy have been associated with worse outcomes (Rivers et al., 2001). A number of blood tests need to be performed to help diagnose and direct the management of patients. While initial antibiotics should be given within the first hour, antimicrobial therapy should be reviewed daily by the senior medical team and expert microbiologists (Dellinger et al., 2013). Lactate is a measure of global perfusion (normal value 1 mmol/L) and increasing lactate levels signify tissue hypoperfusion and the onset of life-threatening metabolic acidosis. An increased blood lactate has been shown to predict haemodynamic instability and is associated with mortality (Nguyen et al., 2004; Mato et al., 2010). Haemoglobin and haematocrit should also be measured. Urine output is an indicator of perfusion to the kidney and can be a clue to blood flow in general (Robson and Daniels, 2008). Therefore, if the patient does not have a urinary catheter *in situ* already, one should be inserted promptly and hourly urine output should be measured. Adequate urine output should be 0.5–1 mL/kg and should be responsive to fluid therapy. Poor urine output and anuria are a sign of acute kidney injury, which unfortunately is a common complication of sepsis (Penack et al., 2010). Healthcare practitioners need to know how to escalate treatment in these situations, either via their critical care outreach teams (CCOT) or senior medical review.

SEVERITY ASSESSMENT

To prevent morbidity and mortality from pneumonia, it is vital that patients are assessed accurately regarding the severity of their infection. The clinical judgement of the practitioner making the assessment is important, but this can be aided by a simple but validated assessment tool. Early evidence suggests that in using clinical judgement physicians both underestimate and overestimate the severity of CAP, which leads to inappropriate treatment (Tang and Macfarlane, 1993; Neill et al., 1996). In the UK, Lim et al. (2009) and NICE (2014) promote the use of both the CRB65 and the CURB65 tool. The CRB65 tool should be used in the community to assess whether the patient should be treated at home or referred to the hospital. The patient will score a point each for **C**onfusion, **R**aised respiratory rate, low **B**lood pressure and being aged **65** or over (Levy et al., 2010). Patients with a score of 0 are at low risk of death whilst those with a score of 2 or more are at high risk of death and require urgent hospital admission (Lim et al., 2009; NICE, 2014) When deciding on home treatment the practitioner must also take into account the stability of the patient, co-morbidities and social circumstances.

If patients are referred to hospital, the CURB65 tool assesses **C**onfusion, **U**rea, **R**aised respiratory rate, low **B**lood pressure and being aged **65** or over. In this instance patients with a score of 0–1 may be suitable for home treatment but, as above, stability of the patient, co-morbidities and social circumstances must be considered. Patients with a score of 3 or above should be reviewed by a senior physician and may require admission to a critical care unit for specific interventions such as mechanical ventilation (Lim et al., 2009; NICE, 2014).

When using any assessment tool, it is important to consider its accuracy to predict a specific outcome, its applicability to the healthcare setting in which it is being used and its simplicity of use in everyday practice. In addition to the tools mentioned above, there is also the pneumonia severity index (PSI). However, this tool has 20 different demographic, co-morbid and clinical variables to assess and is therefore deemed more complex for use in everyday practice (Singanayagam et al., 2009). This is an important consideration as a small survey of junior doctors reported that only 4% could state all the prognostic indicators of the CURB65 tool (Barlow et al., 2007). In a systematic review and meta-analysis by Chalmers et al. (2010), there were no significant differences in overall test performance between the PSI, CURB65 or CRB65 tools for predicting mortality from CAP.

As discussed earlier in this chapter, sepsis is a severe complication of pneumonia and there are specific tools such as the SIRS criteria and various early warning scores (EWS) that assess the severity of the patient's condition. These generic tools are increasingly being advocated for the identification of high-risk patients. In response to this, Barlow et al. (2007) undertook a comparative study between the CURB65 and generic tools and found that the CRB65 and CURB65 tools were better at predicting mortality from CAP than the generic tools. Therefore, in the initial assessment of CAP, the CRB65 and CURB65 remain useful adjuncts to the thorough clinical assessment of patients, especially for junior staff.

HOSPITAL-ACQUIRED PNEUMONIA

HAP gets it title when the illness becomes apparent more than 48 hours after admission to hospital (Dunn, 2005). HAP is one of the most commonly acquired nosocomial infections; it increases length of hospital stay and mortality (Masterton et al., 2008). HAP can be subdivided into early onset, which occurs within 4–5 days of admission and tends to be caused by antibiotic-susceptible, community-type pathogens, and late onset, which occurs after 5 days and is more likely to be caused by antibiotic-resistant pathogens (Masterton et al., 2008). However, Gastmeier et al. (2009) suggest that this distinction is no longer applicable as the pathogens are similar in both groups of patients. VAP is a form of HAP that occurs in patients who are mechanically ventilated (Dunn, 2005). These patients are susceptible because they are already critically ill, but the presence of an endotracheal tube increases susceptibility as it bypasses the normal respiratory defences described earlier in this chapter. Specific issues related to VAP will not be covered in this chapter as it is an extensive

subject in its own right and is covered in specific critical care textbooks, as well as advice being given by NICE (2008) and Rello et al. (2013).

Risk factors for the development of HAP are similar to those described above for CAP, but other major risk factors include colonisation of oropharynx or stomach, which results from the accumulation of dental plaque. Colonisation of the stomach is common in patients taking antacids or H2 antagonists or who are on enteral feed. Other risk factors include conditions favouring reflux such as initial or repeated intubation, insertion of nasogastric (NG) tube, supine position, neurological impairment and surgical procedures (Dodek et al., 2004). Indeed, the contribution of a contaminated oropharynx and therefore the importance of appropriate mouth care has become paramount in the prevention of HAP and VAP (Raghavendran et al., 2007). Quinn et al. (2014) recommend comprehensive oral care and oral care protocols that include all patients (not just those on ventilators). As well as hand hygiene and universal infection control measures, patient position is another very important factor in the prevention of HAP, in particular aspiration pneumonia. Masterton et al. (2008) recommend the head of the bed be elevated between 30° and 45°.

Treatment of HAP is similar to that of CAP and Masterton et al. (2008) recommend, wherever possible, that antimicrobial monotherapy is used for bacterial HAP. The choice of empirical antibiotic therapy should take into consideration the nature and susceptibility patterns of pathogens that are present on individual units/departments. Liapikou et al. (2014) recommend that continuous evaluation of antimicrobial therapy is vital to optimise treatment and reduce mortality associated with HAP. For a comprehensive review of the literature and guidelines on the management of HAP see Masterton et al. (2008) 'Guidelines for the management of hospital-acquired pneumonia in the UK'.

PREVENTION OF PNEUMONIA

Pneumococcal disease represents a significant risk to public health and there is a global action plan for the prevention and control of pneumonia (Greenwood 2008). In the UK, PHE (2013) recommend that all adults over the age of 65 are vaccinated, all children as part of routine childhood immunisations and children and adults in clinical risk groups, which would include people with asplenia, COPD, asthma etc. The influenza virus has the ability to change its genetic makeup, thereby making it possible to re-infect a previous host (Driver, 2012c). This means that the safest way of protecting the population is via vaccination. Currently PHE (2015) recommend vaccination for everyone over the age of 65, or for anyone who falls into an at-risk group, such as those who have chronic heart or renal disease, diabetes, pregnancy etc. Vaccination should also be offered to people who live in long-stay residential care homes, carers of those at significant risk, healthcare workers and social care workers involved in the care of those at risk. PHE (2015) also give specific guidance for vaccination of children. For full details see The Flu Plan 2015/2016, or the latest version.

CASE STUDY

Florey Greenacre is an 86-year-old lady who presented at the Emergency Department accompanied by paramedics after suffering a fall. On the morning of admission, the patient knocked on her neighbour's door disorientated, with a black eye and blood-stained face. The lady's daughter was called. On arrival the daughter found her mother as described above. The sitting room had blood staining to the carpet and the armchair and the bedroom had blood staining to the pillow and sheets. Florey was a very poor historian, and was unable to give any detail of why there was blood staining in the sitting room and the bedroom. It was unknown whether she blacked out or tripped. It was surmised that she fell in her sitting room and at some point later she managed to get herself into bed. It was unknown how long she spent on the sitting room floor or whether or not she lost consciousness.

Extensive bruising around the left eye was noted with a blood-stained nose and mild confusion. The lady had a very painful left shoulder. Crackles were noted on auscultation of the left lower lobe. Both ankles had pitting oedema. The lady was also dehydrated, undernourished and showing symptoms of tachycardia. Observations were RR 18, Pulse 100, Temp 36.9°C, BP 110/70. A chest, facial and left shoulder X-ray, ECG and routine bloods were obtained. Oxygen saturation was 96% on room air. Urinalysis was negative. All other results were normal, with the exception of the chest X-ray, which revealed consolidation of the left upper lobe (see Figure 10.2). While an in-patient, Florey had a CT scan of her head to ascertain the cause of the fall. The CT revealed nothing abnormal.

Florey had a past medical history of hysterectomy aged 53, hypertension, mild congestive cardiac failure and hiatus hernia. Florey had also had influenza and pneumonia as a young adult.

Florey lives alone in a sheltered housing bungalow, is independent and self-caring. She has been widowed twice and has four adult children who visit regularly. Florey does not smoke, but did until her late forties, and drinks alcohol in small amounts very occasionally. Florey is taking medications that include Omeprazole 10 mg once daily, Aspirin 75 mg once daily, Amlodipine 10 mg once daily, Bendroflumethiazide 2.5 mg once daily and Simvastatin 20 mg once daily. Florey is allergic to penicillin.

Owing to her fall and confusion, Florey was eventually admitted to a respiratory ward because of the changes on her chest X-ray. The consultant respiratory physician diagnosed community-acquired pneumonia. Florey made an uneventful recovery and was discharged home with temporary carers.

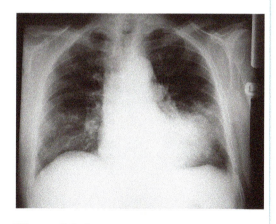

Figure 10.2 Chest X-ray showing consolidation of the upper (lingular segment) lobe consolidation. (From Shutterstock Image ID: 256277077. With permission.)

CASE STUDY DISCUSSION

Perry (2012) suggests that, whereas treatment of pneumonia is the same in the elderly, the presentation of the disease is not, and the case study above acutely demonstrates how difficult it is to diagnose pneumonia in the elderly on clinical signs alone. The weekend before her fall the lady had spent time away with her daughters to celebrate her 86th birthday; she had been well with no respiratory symptoms. On admission, her observations were all within normal limits, with the exception of a fast heart rate; she was not breathless, she had no pleuritic chest pain, no cough and no fever. This is consistent with the suggestion by Perry (2012) that elderly patients will have very subtle symptoms. Driver (2012b) suggests that disorientation which leads to falls is an indicator of pneumonia, and in the case of Florey it was not known if the pneumonia had led to the fall or if the fall, and lying on the floor, had led to the pneumonia. A CT scan of the head had ruled out any obvious cause for the fall. The bungalow was carpeted throughout and the central heating was on, it was also not known how long Florey had lain on the floor. Therefore, if the fall had caused the pneumonia, the warm, comfortable environment had probably mitigated against the development of severe pneumonia overnight. Florey scored 2 on the CURB65 score, one point each for confusion and being over 65. Although hospital staff reported her as being confused, her daughters reported that Florey was no more confused than usual and that what the staff were witnessing was her usual mental state, which had been present for many years. Florey did have several risk factors for the development of pneumonia: she was elderly and frail; malnourished; underweight with muscle wasting; had mild confusion; limited physical activity and was an ex-smoker (Perry, 2012). Florey had a number of co-morbidities cited as risk factors for the development of pneumonia including mild heart failure and a hiatus hernia treated with proton pump inhibitors (PPIs) (Gutierrez and Masia, 2008; Driver, 2014). Gutierrez and Masia (2008) suggest that PPIs have been associated with an increased risk of pneumonia due to their action of increasing gastric pH. The case study demonstrates how investigations of particularly chest X-rays are necessary in the elderly. Despite the high mortality associated with pneumonia in the elderly, Florey made a full recovery with empirical antibiotics, adequate nutrition, hydration and mobilisation.

SUMMARY

Despite advances in health care in the twentieth and twenty-first centuries, CAP remains a communicable disease with a considerable risk of mortality and morbidity. Although pneumonia can be seasonal, it represents a threat at any time of year and to all age groups. Some groups of people are particularly at risk: the WHO (2013) estimates that pneumonia is the biggest killer of children worldwide. Although most people who develop pneumonia will make an uneventful recovery at home, some will develop severe respiratory or systemic disease. Severity assessment tools such as the CRB65 and CURB65 are available and their use is advocated. As well as these tools, thorough patient assessment and clinical judgement are vital in determining the most appropriate environment for treatment. Patient stability, co-morbidities and social circumstances must also be taken into account when deciding on home or hospital treatment. As the case study in this chapter demonstrates, symptoms can be subtle in the elderly who particularly require extra vigilance by healthcare professionals. In the UK, vaccination is available for pneumonia and influenza for certain groups of people. Pneumonia is a vast subject and this chapter has only covered certain aspects. The reader may wish to review other aspects of pneumonia such as atypical pneumonias, necrotising pneumonia (Panton-Valentine Leukocidin) or indeed HAP or VAP in more detail.

REFERENCES

Banning, M. 2005. Community acquired pneumonia: Common causes, treatment and resistance. *Nurse Prescribing* 3 (5): 195–200.

Barlow, G., Nathwani, D. and Davey, P. 2007. The CURB65 pneumonia severity score outperforms generic sepsis and early warning scores in predicting mortality in community-acquired pneumonia. *Thorax* 62: 253–259.

Ben-David, D. and Rubinstein, E. 2002. Appropriate use of antibiotics for respiratory infections: Review of recent statements and position papers. *Current Opinion in Infectious Diseases* 15 (2): 151–156.

Boldt, M.D. and Kiresuk, T. 2001. Community-acquired pneumonia in adults. *The Nurse Practitioner* 26 (11): 14–23.

Brown, J.S. 2012. Community-acquired pneumonia. *Clinical Medicine* 12 (6): 538–543.

Campbell, J.E. 2003. *Campbell's Physiology Notes for Nurses.* Whurr Publishers, London.

Cascini, S., Agabiti, N., Incalzi, R.A., Pinnarelli, L., Mayer, F., Arcà, M., Fusco, D. and Davoli, M. 2013. Pneumonia burden in elderly patients: A classification algorithm using administrative data. *BMC Infectious Diseases* 13: 559 http://www.biomedcentral.com/1471-2334/13/559

Chalmers, J.D., Singanayagam, A.,Akram, A., Mandal, P., Short, P.M., Choudhury, G., Wood, V. and Hill, A.T. 2010. Severity assessment tools for predicting mortality in hospitalised patients with community-acquired pneumonia. Systematic review and meta-analysis. *Thorax* 65: 878–883.

Davies, A. and Moores, C. 2010. *The Respiratory System* (2nd ed.). *Basic Science and Clinical Conditions.* Churchill Livingstone, Edinburgh.

Dellinger, R.P., Levy, M.N., Rhodes, A., Annane, D., Gerlach, H., Opal, S.M., Sevransky, J.E. et al. 2013. Surviving sepsis campaign: International guidelines for management of severe sepsis and septic shock: 2012. *Critical Care Medicine* 41 (2): 580–637.

Dodek, P., Keenan, S., Cook, D., Heyland, D., Jacka, M., Hand, L., Muscedere, J. et al. 2004. Evidence-based clinical practice guideline for the prevention of ventilator associated pneumonia. *Annals of Internal Medicine* 141 (4): 305–114.

Driver, C. 2012a. Pneumonia Part 2: Signs, symptoms and vaccinations. *British Journal of Nursing* 21 (4): 245–249.

Driver, C. 2012b. Pneumonia Part 1: Pathology presentation and prevention. *British Journal of Nursing* 21 (2): 103–106.

Driver, C. 2012c. Pneumonia Part 3: Management and prevention of influenza virus. *British Journal of Nursing* 21 (6): 362–366.

Driver, C. 2014. Understanding pneumonia: Anatomy and physiology. *Nursing and Residential Care* 16 (3): 136–141.

Du Clos, T.W. and Mold, C. 2004. C-reactive protein an activator of innate immunity and a modulator of adaptive immunity. *Immunological Research* 30 (3): 261–277.

Dunn, L. 2005. Pneumonia: Classification, diagnosis and nursing management. *Nursing Standard* 19 (42): 50–54.

Fernandez, R., Boque, M. and Galera, A. 2005. Sepsis: A study of physicians' knowledge about the surviving sepsis campaign. *Critical Care Medicine* 33 (suppl): A160.

Gastmeier, P., Dorit, S., Geffers, C., Ruden, H.,Vonberg, R-P. and Welte, T. 2009. Early and late onset pneumonia: Is it still a useful classification. *Antimicrobial Agents and Chemotherapy* 53 (7): 2714–2718.

Greenwood, B. 2008. A global action plan for the prevention and control of pneumonia (editorial). *Bulletin of the World Health Organisation* 86 (5): 322.

Gutierrez, F. and Masia, M. 2008. Improving outcomes in elderly patients with community-acquired pneumonia. *Drugs and Ageing* 25 (7): 585–610.

Gutierrez, F., Masia, M., Rodriguez, C., Soldan, B., Padilla, S., Hernandez, I., Royo, G. and Martin-Hidaglo, A. 2005. Community-acquired pneumonia of mixed etiology: Prevalence, clinical characteristics and outcome. *European Journal of Clinical Microbiology and Infectious Diseases* 24 (6): 377–383.

Hansall, D. and Padley, S. 1999. Imaging chapter 116. In: Albert, R., Spiro, S. and Jetts, J. (eds.). *Comprehensive Respiratory Medicine.* Harcourt Brace and Company, California.

Kumar, A., Roberts, D., Wood, K., Light, B., Parrillo, J., Sharma, S., Suppes, R. et al. 2006. Duration of hypotension before initiation of effective antimicrobial therapy in the critical determinant of survival in human septic shock. *Critical Care Medicine* 34 (6): 1589–1596.

Levy, M.L., Le Jeune, I., Woodhead, M.A., Macfarlane, J.T. and Lim, W.S. (2010) Primary care summary of British Thoracic Society Guidelines for the management of community acquired pneumonia in adults: 2009 Update. *Primary Care Respiratory Journal* 19 (1): 21–27.

Liapikou, A., Rosales-Mayor, E. and Torres, A. 2014. Pharmacotherapy for hospital-acquired pneumonia. *Expert Opinion Pharmacotherapy* 15 (6): 775–786.

Lim, W.S., Baudouin, S.V., George, R.C., Hill, A.T., Jamieson, C., Le Jeune, I., Macfarlane, J.T. et al. 2009. British Thoracic Society Guidelines for the management of community acquired pneumonia in adults: Update 2009. *Thorax* 64 (suppl III): iii1–iii55.

Lim, W.S. and Rodrigo, C. 2013. *British Thoracic Society Adult Community Acquired Pneumonia Audit 2012–1013.* Available at: https://www.brit-thoracic.org.uk/document-library/audit-and-quality-improvement/audit-reports/bts-adult-community-acquired-pneumonia-audit-report-201213/

Masterton, R.G., Galloway, A., French, G., Street, M., Armstrong, J., Brown, E., Cleverly, J. et al. 2008. Guidelines for the management of hospital-acquired pneumonia in the UK. Report of the working party on hospital acquired pneumonia of the British Society of Antimicrobial Chemotherapy. *Journal of Antimicrobial Chemotherapy* 62: 5–34.

Mato, A.R., Luger, S.M., Heitjan, D.F., Mikkelsen, M.E., Olson, E., Ujjani, C., Jacobs, S. et al. 2010. Elevation in serum lactate at the time of febrile neutropenia in haemodynamically stable patients with haematological malignancies is associated with the development of septic shock within 48 hours. *Cancer, Biology and Therapy* 9: 585–589.

Moldoveanu, B., Otmishi, P., Jani, P., Walker, J., Sarmiento, X., Guardiola, J., Saad, M. and Yu, J. 2009. Inflammatory mechanisms in the lung. *Journal of Inflammatory Research* 2: 1–11.

Monton, C. and Torres, A. 1998. Lung inflammatory response in pneumonia. *Monaldi Archives of Chest Disorders.* 53 (1): 56–63.

Moussaoui, R., Opmeer, B.C., de Borgie, C.A.J.M., Nieuwkerk, P., Bossnyt, P.M.M., Speedman, P. and Prins, J.M. 2006. Long-term symptom recovery and health-related quality of life in patients with mild to moderate-severe community-acquired pneumonia. *Chest* 130 (4): 1165–1172.

Murphy, K. 2008. *Janeway's Immunology* (7th ed.). Garland Science, London.

Myles, P.R., Hubbard, R.B., Gibson, J.E., Pogson, Z., Smith, C.J.P. and McKeever, T.M. 2009. Pneumonia mortality in a UK general practice population cohort. *European Journal of Public Health* 19 (5): 521–526.

National Institute of Health and Care Evidence, Clinical Knowledge Summaries. 2013. http://cks.nice.org.uk/influenza-seasonal#!topicsummary. Accessed 28 May 2015.

National Institute for Health and Care Excellence. 2008. *National Patient Safety Agency. Technical Patient Safety Solutions for Ventilator Acquired Pneumonia in Adults.* NICE, London.

National Institute for Health and Care Excellence. 2014. *Pneumonia. Diagnosis and Management of Community and Hospital Acquired Pneumonia in Adults. NICE Clinical Guideline 191.* NICE, London.

Neill, A.M., Martin, I.R., Weir, R., Anderson, R., Chereshky, A. and Epton, M.J. 1996. Community-acquired pneumonia: Aetiology and usefulness of severity criteria on admission. *Thorax* 51: 1010–1016.

Nguyen, B., Rivers, E.P., Knoblich, B., Jacobsen, G., Muzzin, A., Ressler, J.A. and Tomlanovich, M.C. 2004. Early lactate clearance is associated with improved outcome in severe sepsis and septic shock. *Critical Care Medicine* 32: 1637–1642.

O'Driscoll, B.R., Howard, L.S. and Davison, A.G. 2008. British Thoracic Society Guideline for emergency oxygen use in adults. *Thorax* 63 (suppl VI): vi1–vi73.

Penack, O., Beinert, T., Bucheidt, D., Einsele, H., Hebart, H., Keihl, M.G., Massenkeil, G. et al. 2010. Management of sepsis in neutropenic patients: Guidelines from the infectious diseases working party of the German Society of Haematology and Oncology. *Annals of Hematology* 85: 424–433.

Perry, M. 2012. How signs and symptoms of common infections vary with age. *Practice Nursing* 23 (4): 176–182.

Podolsky, S.H. 2005. The changing fate of pneumonia as a public health concern in 20th century America and beyond. *American Journal of Public Health* 95 (12): 2144–2154.

Poeze, M., Ramsay, H., Gerlach, H., Rubulotta, F. and Levy, M. 2004. An international sepsis survey: A study of doctors' knowledge and perception about sepsis. *Critical Care* 8 (6): R409–R413.

Public Health England. 2013. Pneumococcal.: In: Salisbury, D., Ramsay, M. and Noakes, K. (eds.). *The Green Book*. PHE, London, Chapter 25, pp. 295–314.

Public Health England. 2014. Pneumococcal disease: Guidance, data and analysis. https://www.gov.uk/government/collections/pneumococcal-disease-guidance-data-and-analysis

Public Health England. 2015. *Flu Plan 2015/2016*. PHE, London.

Quinn, B., Baker, D.L., Cohen, S., Stewart, J.L., Lima, C.A. and Parise, C. 2014. Basic nursing care to prevent nonventilator hospital acquired pneumonia. *Journal of Nursing Scholarship* 46 (1): 11–19.

Raghavendran, K., Mylotte, J.M. and Scannapieco, F.A. 2007. Nursing home-associated pneumonia, hospital acquired pneumonia and ventilator-associated pneumonia: The contribution of dental biofilms and periodontal inflammation. *Periodontology 2000* 44: 164–177.

Rello, J., Afonso, E., Lisboa, T., Ricart, M., Balsera, B., Rovira, A., Valles, J. and Diaz, E. 2013. A care bundle approach for prevention of VAP. *Clinical Microbiology and Infection* 19 (4): 363–369.

Rivers, E., Nguyen, B., Havstad, S., Ressler, J., Muzzin, A., Knoblich, B., Peterson, E. and Tomlanovich, M. 2001. Early goal directed therapy in the treatment of severe sepsis and septic shock. *New England Journal of Medicine* 345: 1368–1377.

Robson, W., Beavis, S. and Spittle, N. 2007. An audit of ward nurses' knowledge of sepsis. *Nursing in Critical Care* 12 (2): 86–92.

Robson, W.P. and Daniels, R. 2008. The sepsis six: Helping patients survive sepsis. *British Journal of Nursing* 17 (1): 16–21.

Schultz, T.R. 2003. On the trail of community acquired pneumonia. *Nursing Management* 34 (2): 27–32.

Singanayagam, A., Chalmers, J.D. and Hill, A.T. 2009. Severity assessment in community acquired pneumonia: A review. *Quarterly Journal of Medicine* 102: 379–388.

Suh, E.S. and Hart, N. 2012. Respiratory failure. *Medicine* 40 (6): 293–297.

Tang, C.M. and Macfarlane, J.T. 1993. Early management of young adults dying from community-acquired pneumonia. *Respiratory Medicine* 87: 289–294.

The Sepsis UK Trust. 2013. http://sepsistrust.org/. Accessed 26 November 2013.

Tortora, G.J. and Derrickson, B. 2012. *Principles of Anatomy and Physiology* (13th ed.). John Wiley and Sons Inc, Hoboken, New Jersey.

van der Poll, T. 2011. Management of serious pneumococcal pneumonia- Pathogenesis. *Reanimation* 20: S318–S521.

van der Poll, T. and Opal, S.M. 2008. Host-pathogen interactions in sepsis. *The Lancet* 8: 32–43.

Ward, J. J. 2013. High flow oxygen administration by nasal cannula for adult and perinatal patient. *Respiratory Care* 58 (1): 98–122.

World Health Organisation. 2013. Pneumonia. Fact Sheet No 331. Available at: http://www.who.int/mediacentre/factsheets/fs331/en/. Accessed 9 July 2014.

Lung cancer

11

GILLIAN WALTON

LEARNING OBJECTIVES

Upon completion of this chapter the reader should be able to:

- Discuss the prevalence of lung cancer in the United Kingdom and provide a definition of the disease classifications
- Appraise the challenges associated with the prevention and early detection of lung cancer
- Discuss current diagnostic approaches
- Discuss the importance of staging
- Develop an understanding of contemporary treatments in lung cancer
- Consider the psychological and social impact through a patient case study

INTRODUCTION

Lung cancer is the second most common cancer diagnosis in the United Kingdom (UK) after breast cancer. It is a devastating disease accounting for 41,500 new diagnoses per year (Roy Castle Lung Cancer Foundation [RCLCF], 2014), which accounts for approximately 120 people every day (Cancer Research United Kingdom [CRUK], 2014). The disease has an enormous impact on national mortality and currently accounts for 6% of all deaths and 22% of all deaths from cancer in the UK (National Cancer Intelligence Network [NCIN], 2008). It has the highest mortality rate worldwide than any other cancer (Siegel et al., 2012). It is the most common cause of cancer death in the UK, accounting for approximately 35,000 deaths from the disease in 2011 (CRUK, 2014): more than for breast cancer and colorectal cancer combined (Siegel et al., 2012). Lung cancer is a complex disease, and despite state-of-the-art contemporary treatments, unfortunately outcomes remain poor. Approximately 80% of patients will have advanced disease at presentation (Dela Cruz et al., 2011).

This chapter aims to provide the reader with an overview of the management of lung cancer and will include: the signs and symptoms of the disease, diagnostics, staging, treatment options and palliative care. A case study will be used to demonstrate the complex nature of the disease and the challenges faced by patients and practitioners.

PREVALENCE

Lung cancer has one of the lowest survival outcomes of any cancer because over two-thirds of patients are diagnosed at a late stage when curative treatment is no longer possible. The overall 5-year survival rate for non-small cell lung cancer (NSCLC) remains at less than 15% and has continued unchanged despite advances in oncology. Public awareness of signs and symptoms remains poor, and therefore earlier diagnosis and access to appropriate treatment options remains a focal concern (RCLCF, 2014). Unlike the majority of cancers, and despite state-of-the-art new treatment options, relative survival for lung cancer has not showed much improvement since the early 1970s compared with some North American and European countries (National Institute of Health and Care Excellence [NICE], 2011), furthermore there is evidence that outcomes differ within the UK, which may be explained by variations in care (RCLCF, 2011).

Cancer of the lung is rare in people under the age of 40 and is generally a disease of old age, the average age at onset being 60–70 years and the fact that many of the elderly population have co-morbidities consequently influences survival rates. It has been suggested that approximately 80% of people present late (Tod et al., 2008). Corner et al. (2005) identified that delays of up to a year following the onset of worrying symptoms were not unusual before patients decided to pursue medical help, confirming that individuals failed to recognise serious symptoms prior to diagnosis. As a result, survival rates are poor with only 30% of cases surviving one year or more and the overall 5-year survival rate remaining low at approximately 8% (RCLCF, 2014).

The link between lung cancer incidence and tobacco was established over 50 years ago (Peto et al., 2000), therefore it is widely recognised that the majority of lung cancers are caused by smoking (approximately 90%). Other known sources include exposure to workplace and environmental hazards such as asbestos and arsenic, radon gas, exhaust fumes and inherited genome susceptibility (Leary, 2012). Incidence of lung cancer is greater in lower socio-economic groups and in areas of high deprivation. This is attributed to poorer health-seeking behaviour, leading to late presentation, which contributes to poor outcomes. Evidence suggests a strong association between lung cancer mortality and deprivation for both males and females in England. Incidence in males was once greater, but changes in smoking habits have seen a steep rise in female prevalence (NCIN, 2008). Lung cancer rates in Scotland are the highest in the world, reflecting the high incidence of smoking (CRUK, 2014). It is now the leading cause of cancer death in women (NICE, 2011).

Although most lung cancers are a consequence of smoking, approximately 25% of lung cancer cases worldwide occur in patients with no history of tobacco use (World Health Organisation, 2010), accounting for over 300,000 deaths each year (Sun et al., 2007). Patients who have smoked less than 100 cigarettes during their lifetime are considered as 'never-smokers', whereas people who have smoked more are considered as 'ever-smokers'. There is increasing evidence that lung cancer is a heterogeneous disease and occurrences in never-smokers differ from those in smokers in their molecular profile and response to targeted therapy (Rudin et al., 2009). Factors closely linked to lung cancer in never-smokers include exposure to known and suspected carcinogens, second-hand tobacco smoke and other air pollutants. However, a high proportion of cases cannot be related to obvious known environmental exposure. Women appear to be more susceptible and the reason for this is still uncertain; however, hormones, genetic susceptibility and the fact that twice as many women as men are never-smokers and that this difference increases with age may be significant (Etzel et al., 2006).

CATEGORISATION OF LUNG CANCER

Lung cancer can be categorised broadly into two subtypes, small cell (SCLC) and non-small cell (NSCLC), which have considerably different diagnostic and management plans. SCLC accounts for approximately 10%–15% of all diagnoses (CRUK, 2016). It is a highly proliferating cancer and metastatic disease is often present at diagnosis. It is significantly associated with smoking with approximately 90% of patients being current or past heavy smokers. The risk rises with increasing duration and intensity of smoking (Rothschild et al., 2010). Patients often present with rapid-onset symptoms that can occur within 8–12 weeks (van Meerbeeck et al., 2011). Prognosis in SCLC is poor with median survival without treatment being 2–4 months depending upon the extent of the disease at diagnosis. In view of the rate of growth and extent of local and regional spread, accurate staging of the disease is important to define metastatic disease. Around two-thirds of patients present with clinically obvious metastatic disease (van Meerbeeck et al., 2011); therefore, the majority of patients are palliative at diagnosis.

The NSCLC can then be classified into three subgroups: squamous cell, adenocarcinoma and large cell. Squamous cell cancer arises from the bronchial squamous epithelium. It is the commonest form of NSCLC and is closely associated with smoking. Adenocarcinoma arises from the glandular, mucous-producing cells located in the epithelium lining the bronchi. The incidence of adenocarcinoma continues to rise and is the most common form of lung cancer in women (Leary, 2012). Although adenocarcinoma is related to smoking and the increase in incidence could be attributed to filtered low-tar cigarettes, which lead to deeper inhalation of nicotine and other harmful substances, it is becoming more common in non-smokers (D'Addario et al., 2010). Large cell carcinoma is composed of large cells that are anaplastic and therefore tends to proliferate more quickly than the other types of NSCLC.

PRESENTATION

Lung cancer is a complex disease and may present in many ways; however, some patients typically present with local symptoms related to the primary cancer, which include cough, breathlessness, chest pain, haemoptysis and hoarseness of voice (Teh and Belcher, 2014). Cough is present in up to 75% of patients with lung cancer, and can often be a distressing symptom having an impact on quality of life and functioning (Doyle et al. 2004). More than 25% have a productive cough. Many lung cancers occur in central airways and may lead to post-obstructive

pneumonia and breathlessness. Breathlessness is the most commonly reported symptom in lung cancer, with 10% to 15% of patients having breathlessness at diagnosis, and 65% having this symptom at some point during their illness (Twycross and Lack, 1986).

Individuals may present with systemic or non-specific symptoms such as fatigue, anorexia and cachexia, which contribute to late presentation. Cytokines are molecular messengers and are produced by a broad range of cells, including immune cells. They are released in response to infection, inflammation and immunity. They can function to inhibit tumour development and progression; however, cycling cytokines contributes to production of paraneoplastic syndromes, which is a disease or symptom of some cancers including SCLC. These syndromes such as hypercalcaemia and Cushing's syndrome, syndrome of inappropriate antidiuretic hormone secretion which leads to hyponatremia, are common presenting symptoms in patients with SCLC. Metastatic disease is common and patients may present with bone pain or pathological fracture, neurological symptoms from brain metastases or jaundice. Because of the varied symptom pathology, patients may be referred via a number of different pathways such as via the orthopaedic route with spinal metastases, or neurology with symptoms of brain metastases. NICE (2011) recommends that people reporting one or more symptoms suggesting lung cancer are referred within one week of presentation for a chest X-ray or directly to a chest physician who is a core member of the lung cancer multidisciplinary team. Despite this, a large proportion of patients present as an emergency through an Emergency Department (NCIN, 2010). Rapid and timely access to services is essential and many initiatives and directives such as the 'two-week cancer wait' have been enforced to enable this and ensure the patient starts on the appropriate care pathway (NICE, 2005).

All patients with a confirmed or suspected lung cancer should be referred to a member of the lung cancer multidisciplinary team (MDT), usually a chest physician (NICE, 2005). Since the inception of the Calman–Hine Report, MDT working has been endorsed as the principle way of managing all cancer care in the UK (DH, 1995). MDTs deal specifically with one type of cancer or group of cancers, and consist of the relevant healthcare professionals including lung cancer clinical nurse specialists with expert knowledge of diagnosis and treatment. There is a growing evidence base to suggest that clinical nurse specialists (CNS) enhance the cancer patient's experience of care (DH, 2013). Patients who have a CNS are more likely to be positive about their care and treatment than patients who do not. Having a lung CNS involved in the lung cancer patient's care has an impact on treatment access and is described by Tod et al. (2013) as key to the delivery of care and the efficiency of the related systems and processes. Patients with lung cancer should be allocated a 'key worker', usually the lung cancer nurse specialist (LCNS), to help patients to navigate their way around the complexities of diagnosis and treatment as well as managing the information needs. All patients with a suspected or confirmed lung cancer should be discussed at a regular MDT meeting where a treatment plan will be formulated. Current National Lung Cancer audit data suggest that 95% of patients diagnosed are discussed at MDT and this level should be sustained (National Health Service Information Centre [NHSIC], 2012). NICE (2011) guidance states that time from initial referral to the commencement of definitive treatment should be no longer than 62 days, which includes a diagnostic preparation which should be complete within 31 days.

DIAGNOSIS

There is currently no screening programme in the UK for lung cancer because of the lack of a sensitive test and the resources available (CRUK, 2015). However, there is currently a UK lung cancer trial reviewing the use of spiral CT scans and fluorescent bronchoscopy as well as a study to detect biomarkers in high-risk groups, which could indicate lung cancer prior to the development of symptoms (CRUK, 2015). Presently the main message to the public is to promote awareness of signs and symptoms of lung cancer and encouragement to seek advice and timely referral to specialist services. Smoking cessation is also a key message.

The pathway to investigations and eventual diagnosis of lung cancer can be complex. Thirty-eight percent of patients will present as an emergency (NCIN, 2010); the relative one-year survival rate is significantly lower in those patients presenting via this route and therefore early recognition and intervention is paramount. All patients with a history of cough lasting more than three weeks should have a chest X-ray and referral to the specialist MDT within 2 weeks (DH, 2005; NICE, 2011). A number of diagnostic tests are available and NICE (2011) guidance suggests that tissue diagnosis should be the gold standard. A contrast computerised tomography (CT) scan of the chest with further imaging with positron emission tomography (PET) scanning for those patients to be treated radically is advised to accurately stage the extent of the disease. A contrast CT scan of the thorax will give accurate structural evidence on areas of high suspicion such as the mediastinal lymph nodes and will be used as a guide to select the most appropriate area for histological biopsy. Investigations that give the most information about diagnosis and staging with least risk to the patient should then be initiated (NICE, 2011). A fibre optic bronchoscopy may be performed on patients who have a central lesion visualised on CT so histological diagnosis through transbronchial needle aspiration can be obtained. CT-guided transthoracic needle biopsy can be used for patients with peripheral lung lesions. Mediastinoscopy carried out under general anaesthesia was the preferred standard treatment to determine the presence of nodal metastases in the mediastinum. However, endobronchial ultrasound-guided transbronchial needle aspiration (EBUS-guided TBNA) is an alternative less invasive technique used for guided transbronchial needle aspiration and histological sampling of the lymph nodes. EBUS-TBNA offers a minimally invasive alternative to mediastinoscopy with additional access to the hilar nodes with a better safety profile (Medford et al., 2010). The procedure is carried out under local or sometimes general anaesthetic and as an outpatient. A small bronchoscope with an ultrasound probe attached can image the mediastinum and will visualise and sample adequate tissue biopsy. Once pathology is confirmed with an adequate tissue sample, histological examination will be carried out by a thoracic pathologist to determine the differential diagnosis of lung cancer. If the tissue is classified as a NSCLC, further molecular pathology of the specimen will be undertaken.

MOLECULAR BIOMARKERS

Molecular biomarkers are distinctive gene mutations that are present within the cell and are over expressed in certain cancers. A gene mutation is a fault in the DNA sequence of a gene. NSCLC can be divided into specific molecular subsets based on specific biomarkers or mutations. Epidermal growth factor receptor (EGFR) is a protein that is found on the surface of cells. It produces tyrosine kinase, which acts as a signal that regulates cell growth. A mutation known as KRAS has also been detected which stimulates cell signalling. This discovery has led to the development of a group of drugs named tyrosine kinase inhibitors (TKI). A subgroup of patients with non-squamous cell NSCLC have specific mutations in the EGFR gene, which leads to increased growth factor signalling and uncontrolled cell division (Lynch et al., 2004). A further 2.5%–5% of patients have been found to have rearrangement in a gene called anaplastic lymphoma kinase (ALK). This gene mutation is most commonly seen in young adults (50 years or under), none or light smokers, females and adenocarcinoma subtype. A patient's EGFR, KRAS and ALK mutation status can be confirmed via a diagnostic test using a tissue sample. EGFR mutations are more common in people who have adenocarcinoma, are never-smokers, female, or of Asian descent (Rosell et al., 2009). The EGFR mutation plays an important role in the management of NSCLC and has introduced personalised treatment to this group of patients using targeted therapy, which will be discussed in more detail under treatment options.

STAGING

All NSCLC are staged using the tumour, node metastases (TNM) International Association for the Study of Lung Cancer (IASLC) classification. The T defines the extent of the primary tumour, the N describes the extent of involvement of regional lymph nodes and the M the extent of metastatic spread to distant sites (Goldstraw et al., 2007) The two most common types of stage assessment are clinical staging (the stage determined using all information available prior to any treatment). This would include chest X-ray, CT and PET scanning and EBUS and pathologic staging, which could include nodal sampling through mediastinoscopy or video-assisted thoracoscopic surgery (VATS) or will be definite after a resection has been carried out. The TNM classification is then broken down into the size of the tumour T1, where the tumour is less than 3 cm to T4 where the tumour could be of any size but is invading the mediastinum, heart, great vessels and trachea. A description of the nodal involvement would be N0 (no regional lymph node metastases) to N3 (contralateral mediastinal, contralateral hilar, ipsilateral or contra lateral scalene or supraclavicular lymph nodes). The metastatic spread would be measured from M0 (no distant metastases) to M1b (distant metastases): hence, staging is crucial when planning optimum care and is used as a prognostic indicator (Goldstraw et al., 2007). IASLC lung cancer staging guidelines are also described using staging from 0 to 5 based on the TNM classification and 5-year survival is indicated using this (CRUK, 2016). The five year survival rate for Stage 1V NSCLC is could not be calculated in the most recent CRUK statistics due to the small number of people surviving more than two years (CRUK, 2016).

SCLC is often staged as limited or extensive disease based on the extent of the disease on imaging. Limited stage was characterised by a tumour volume covered in one radiation threshold; all other disease spread was classified as extensive stage. The IASLC recommend that the TNM classification system should be used for SCLC as well as for NSCLC (Shepherd et al., 2007). As disease extent is the major prognostic factor, staging aims to identify whether the tumour has metastasised.

Once tissue histology is confirmed and the disease is adequately staged, all patients should be discussed by the MDT, who will offer an individual treatment plan based on the available evidence and the patient's current performance status. Many patients with lung cancer have other co-morbidities such as heart disease, chronic obstructive pulmonary disease, diabetes and osteoarthritis, and these will influence the ultimate treatment plan. The Eastern Cooperative Oncology Group (ECOG)/World Health Organisation (WHO) scale of performance status (PS) is used to assess the individual's current functioning and how the disease and symptom burden

Table 11.1 The Eastern Cooperative Oncology Group/World Health Organisation scale of performance status

Performance status	Activity
0	Normal activity
1	Strenuous activity restricted, ambulatory, can do light work
2	Up and about more than 50% of waking hours. Limited self-care
3	Confined to bed or chair for more than 50% of waking hours, limited self-care
4	Confined to bed or chair. No self-care, completely disabled
5	Dead

have affected this. The PS is an assessment scale of 0–5 and is an important prognostic factor. It should be recorded at various stages throughout the patient pathway and is a significant consideration when determining appropriate treatment (see Table 11.1).

TREATMENT

Once the histological diagnosis is ascertained, treatment options will be considered by the respiratory team and the wider MDT. The patient's individual needs, performance status and personal preferences must also be considered to achieve the best outcome. The treatment options for NSCLC include one or more of the following:

- Surgery is available for those patients who have resectable disease and a good performance status
- Radiotherapy
- Chemotherapy
- Best supportive care

Surgical resection should always be considered for those patients with NSCLC who are medically fit and suitable for treatment with curative intent (NICE, 2011). Surgery for early-stage NSCLC remains the mainstay curative treatment. The patient's disease stage, lung function, co-morbidities and PS should be evaluated prior to any surgical intervention. Lobectomy is the operation of choice

if this is possible; however, for those people who are deemed to have borderline fitness but do have smaller tumours, where thorough resection may be achieved, a lung segmentectomy or wedge resection may be elected to preserve as much lung function as possible (NICE, 2011). Surgical resection does not come without dangers and it is important that the patient is given the appropriate information regarding risk of mortality to ensure they have an informed choice. Currently the 30-day mortality rate in Great Britain and Ireland following lobectomy is 2.3% and 5.8% following pneumonectomy (Teh and Belcher, 2014).

For those patients who are not fit for surgical intervention, radical radiotherapy is indicated for patients who have good performance status (PS 0–1) and when the lung cancer can be captured in a radiotherapy treatment volume without the risk of damage to the surrounding normal tissue (NICE, 2011). Radiotherapy is the treatment of cancer with radiation to damage DNA, leading to apoptosis or programmed cell death. Radical radiotherapy is given in higher doses or a longer period of time to maximise cell kill. However, treatment times are long and often debilitating for patients. Advances in radiotherapy techniques have led to greater efficiency and fewer side effects. Stereotactic body radiotherapy (SBRT) can deliver high-dose fractionated radiotherapy to a precise target with limited damage to the surrounding tissues, thus improving side effects and treatment outcomes (Palma et al., 2010). Radiotherapy is also used for locally advanced (LA) disease and can be combined with chemotherapy. This approach remains the commonest used treatment for LA disease (McCloskey et al., 2013). Palliative radiotherapy is given in limited doses with the intent to improve symptom management, for instance in the management of bone pain or haemoptysis. Palliative radiotherapy for symptom management remains one of the most common treatment modality in the elderly lung cancer patient (Turner et al., 2007).

Traditional systemic chemotherapy can be given orally or intravenously with the aim of interrupting the cell cycle and killing cancer cells. Recent advances in targeted therapies have been developed in lung cancer owing to an increased knowledge of genetic mutations and are now available to a distinct group of the population. Most patients with NSCLC present at an advanced stage in their disease and therefore the aim of chemotherapy is to prolong life or palliate symptoms. A number of clinical studies indicated some time ago that chemotherapy, mainly platinum-based regimens, had a modest advantageous influence on survival (Non-Small Cell Collaborative Group [NSCCG], 1995). Many new chemotherapy agents are now available; however, based on this evidence and recent clinical trials, NICE (2011) recommend a regime of one of the newer chemotherapeutic agents and to include a platinum-based compound. Chemotherapy drugs have toxic side effects so consideration of quality of life is vital as the intent is not to cure the disease but to improve overall survival and palliate symptoms. Chemotherapy should only be offered to patients who are considered fit and with a PS of 2 or below.

The major advances in the treatment of NSCLC during the last 6 years are attributable to the discovery of activating EGFR mutations and the development of drugs that can treat these mutations (Cufer et al., 2013). Patients who over express EGFR or ALK and have non-squamous cell histology are now gene tested to ensure that the one-size-fits-all approach to the management of NSCLC is finally changing (Cufer et al., 2013). A greater understanding of molecular biology signifies a major advancement in the treatment of the disease. The drugs have a more tolerable side effect profile and have now been recommended by NICE (2010) as first-line treatment in these patients for locally advanced disease. Those patients who test positive for EGFR mutations will be offered oral tyrosine kinase inhibitors as first-line treatment. Other advances in NSCLC have enabled chemotherapy drugs to be given depending on histological subtype, as an adjuvant pre-surgery to downgrade the cancer or as neo-adjuvant post-surgery to increase the chance of overall 5-year survival or maintenance therapy for those people who have a good response to initial treatment (Cufer et al., 2013).

When patients are not suitable for treatment or make an informed choice not to have any, they should be offered referral to the palliative care team. Over two thirds of people with lung cancer present with advanced disease at diagnosis and therefore good communication between all professionals and

the patient's GP is imperative (CRUK, 2014). The lung cancer clinical nurse specialist is pivotal in the patient pathway and provides holistic care from diagnosis through to treatment, survivorship and end-of-life care and can co-ordinate any referrals, interventions and offer expert advice and guidance to the patient, carers and other health professionals involved in the patient's care (National Cancer Action Team [NCAT], 2007). Patients may require radiotherapy for symptoms such as haemoptysis or brain or bone metastases or specialist palliative interventions for symptoms such as pain and breathlessness, so good MDT care is imperative.

Treatment for SCLC includes chemotherapy, radiotherapy or a combination of both. It has been reported that prognosis of SCLC without treatment is poor, with median survival being 4 months (NICE, 2011). SCLC tends to disseminate earlier in its natural history and displays more multifaceted clinical signs. SCLC has been classified as a neuroendocrine cancer because of the development of paraneoplastic syndromes such as Eaton Lambert syndrome and syndrome of inappropriate secretion of antidiuretic hormone. It is thought that the tumour has a growth response to the secreted neuropeptide (Haddadin and Perry, 2011). Disease extent is the most important prognostic factor and staging aims to identify metastases. Around two thirds of patients present with clinically evident metastatic disease (van Meerbeeck et al., 2011). As most patients present late, surgery is rarely an option owing to the risk of distant metastases in the brain, liver, bone or lung. Although no absolute cure has been found for SCLC, combined chemotherapy remains the recommended treatment and can improve overall median survival to 15–20 months in limited disease (van Meerbeeck et al., 2011).

Treatment is dependent on the stage of the cancer. SCLC is very chemo sensitive because of the rapid proliferation of cells and therefore is the treatment of choice in limited and extensive disease if the patient's performance status allows. Treatment should be initiated within 2 weeks of diagnosis (NICE, 2011). Those with limited disease and good performance status (PS 0–1) will be offered concurrent chemo radiation if the cancer can be encompassed in the radiotherapy field (NICE, 2011). This is the use of chemotherapy and radiotherapy given together usually starting at the second cycle of chemotherapy to maximise cell kill. For patients with extensive-stage disease SCLC, thoracic radiotherapy should be considered after chemotherapy if there has been a complete response or at least a good partial response within the chest (NICE, 2011). Patients with a good response to treatment will be offered prophylactic cranial irradiation (PCI). It has been documented that patients who do not receive PCI go on to develop brain metastases with up to 50% of people developing brain metastases within 2 years (Gregor, 1997). The use of radiotherapy to the brain (PCI) reduces the development of brain metastases and prolongs survival in patients with both limited-stage and extensive-stage disease who have responded to chemotherapy (Goldberg et al., 2013). PCI does not come without risks and it has been reported that neuro cognitive function can be affected post whole-brain radiation. The reduction in the risk of brain metastases, and the associated survival advantage, is clear in this population (Wright and Wolfson, 2012). However, quality of life and patient age and preference must be taken into consideration. Despite current treatments and high initial response rates, the prognosis for SCLC remains poor and patients ultimately relapse (van Meerbeeck et al., 2011). Palliative care is an important aspect in the patient's care and the CNS will play an integral role in the co-ordination of services and assessment of symptoms and quality of life.

CASE STUDY

Joe Brown, a 72-year-old man had been referred to a chest clinic with an abnormal chest X-ray with a possible diagnosis of lung cancer. Joe had had a chest infection and cough for six weeks which had not resolved with antibiotic therapy prescribed by his GP. He also had chronic obstructive pulmonary disease (COPD) and often had exacerbations which responded to antibiotics and steroids. However, on this occasion he said that he felt this was different as the cough would not go away. The GP ordered a chest X-ray that revealed an opacity in the left upper lobe, which could suggest a diagnosis of lung cancer, so an urgent referral to a chest physician was made under the two-week rule.

On examination, Joe looked cachexic having lost 10 kg in weight over the last year. He also complained of loss of appetite and fatigue. Chest crackles were audible on examination and he was visibly breathless, which he said was much worse than normal. Observations revealed a respiratory rate of 20 bpm, blood pressure 160/90 mmHg and temperature 37°C, pulse 92 bpm, oxygen saturation was 95% on room air. Full blood count with urea and electrolyte screen was ordered and spirometry was used to measure the extent of Joe's COPD. The chest X-ray revealed a large opacity obliterating the left hilum. It was associated with some volume loss in the left hemithorax and what appeared to be a small pleural effusion. A trans-bronchial ultra sound was ordered to obtain histological diagnosis. This later revealed a non-small cell squamous cell lung cancer. Positron emission tomography (PET) and computed tomography (CT) scan was performed as an outpatient within the 32-day target, which revealed a large upper lobe mass measuring 3 cm x 2 cm with ipsilateral mediastinal nodal involvement.

Joe had a past history of COPD which he managed with bronchial dilators and occasional steroids and antibitoics. He had mild hypertension controlled with medication. Joe's father died at an early age of heart disease and his mother died aged 77 of a stroke, there was no other significant family history. Joe lived with his wife Bella and they had three children who were married and lived away from home. Joe worked in the ship yards as a welder for most of his life until he had to take early retirement due to his chest condition. Joe and Bella lived in an upstairs flat and Joe was finding it increasingly difficult to get up the stairs due to breathlessness, he was becoming increasingly lethargic and 'worn out'. Joe was an occasional drinker of alcohol and an ex-smoker, he had smoked 20 cigarettes per day since the age of 13 up until he was diagnosed with COPD five years ago. Joe was taking medications, which include tiotropium bromide inhaler, salbutamol inhaler, budesonide and formoterol turbuhaler and amoxicillin.

Unfortunately, Joe was diagnosed with in-operable non-small cell lung cancer. Joe and Bella were invited to an outpatient clinic appointment where the diagnosis was discussed with them. Joe and Bella were obviously shocked and spent some time with the cancer nurse specialist (CNS) who provided support and information regarding the ongoing management and carried out a holistic assessment of Joe's needs. The CNS acted as Joe's key worker and assessed his psychological, social and spiritual concerns and co-ordinated care to ensure that Joe's treatment plan was patient centred. Joe was referred to the district nursing team for assessment of ongoing needs in the community. Two weeks later Joe was admitted as an emergency via the medical admissions ward with breathlessness and general deterioration. Bella was finding it difficult to look after Joe and she had rang the GP who arranged admission. However, Joe and Bella decided that with good community support they would like Joe to be cared for at home. Joe's symptoms were managed by the CNS and palliative care team. The CNS and the ward staff liaised with the community team and GP to ensure Joe was discharged home with adequate supportive care in the community. Joe died two days later at home with Bella at his side.

CASE STUDY DISCUSSION

Joe's lung cancer was staged using the TNM staging as T2, N2, M1; stage 1V demonstrating a large tumour with spread. The treatment for advanced stage non-small cell lung cancer is to prolong life and optimise quality of life through good symptom control, palliative care and end-of-life care. Accurate staging for Joe using CT PET scan revealed involvement of the mediastinal lymph nodes and probable adrenal metastasis, rendering operative resection impossible. Joe's performance status was deteriorating and he had marked breathlessness and a number of other symptoms. Spirometry revealed a decline in pulmonary function and Joe's main problems were breathlessness and fatigue. Joe's case was discussed along with all the diagnostic and histological evidence at an MDT meeting (DH, 2005). The team decided that because of Joe's symptoms of anorexia, weight loss and fatigue which are indicators of poor prognosis in advanced disease (Mussi et al., 1996), and the fact that Joe's cancer was in-operable, the best form of treatment would be symptom management and good palliative care. The oncologist discussed having palliative chemotherapy as this could help relieve symptoms and also improve outcome. However, declining performance status would contraindicate this (NICE, 2011). Joe's performance status was calculated at 3–4 and he appeared to be more breathless and sleepy.

The psychological impact of the diagnosis and prognosis of lung cancer requires co-ordinated care by many members of the MDT (RCLCF, 2011). The national end of life care strategy (DH, 2008) recommends that healthcare professionals involve patients approaching end of life, and their carers, in discussions about preferred place of death in order to identify and meet their wishes. It was clear from examination that Joe was reaching the end of his life and the CNS had a discussion with Joe and Bella about his preference for place of care which resulted in Joe being transferred back home to die (DH, 2008).

SUMMARY

Despite advances in the diagnosis, management and state-of-the-art treatment modalities, lung cancer remains the most common cause of cancer death in the UK. Detection and public awareness of signs and symptoms remain problematic. Unlike the majority of cancers, survival for lung cancer has not shown much improvement since the early 1970s (CRUK, 2014).

The route to diagnosis can be challenging and complex and patients often present in the later stages of the disease, making this devastating illness difficult to cure. Symptom management and quality-of-life issues are paramount as the period from diagnosis to end-of-life care can be short. The role of the multidisciplinary team is crucial in the management of lung cancer and all patients with a suspected or definitive diagnosis should be referred to a chest physician (NICE, 2005). Nurses play a crucial role in the diagnostic pathway to ensure patients presenting in primary or secondary care with symptoms suspicious of lung cancer are assessed and referred as early as possible and that they are supported throughout their care.

New agents such as EGFR inhibitors and targeted therapies, radiotherapy advances and more contemporary diagnostic tools are all promising in the ongoing treatment of the disease and new treatment options in radiotherapy and surgical techniques are evolving to improve patient outcomes.

REFERENCES

Cancer Research UK. 2014. *Lung Cancer Statistics Key Facts*. http://publications.cancerresearchuk.org/downloads/Product/CS_KF_LUNG.pdf. Accessed 15 April 2015.

Cancer Research UK. 2015. A study to see if a new type of CT scan can help improve radiotherapy outcomes for non small cell lung cancer. http://www.cancerresearchuk.org/about-cancer/find-a-clinical-trial/a-study-to-see-if-a-new-type-of-ct-scan-can-help-improve-radiotherapy-outcomes-for-non-small-cell-lung-cancer. Accessed 26 March 2015.

Cancer Research UK. 2016. http://www.cancerresearchuk.org/health-professional/cancer-statistics/statistics-by-cancer-type/lung-cancer/survival#heading-Three. Accessed 9 June 2016.

Corner, J., Hopkinson, J., Fitzsimmons, D., Barclay, S. and Muers, M. 2005. Is late diagnosis of lung cancer inevitable? Interview study of patients' recollections of symptoms before diagnosis. *Thorax* 60 (4): 314–319.

Cufer, T., Ovcaricek, T. and O'Brien, M. 2013. Systemic therapy of advanced non-small cell lung cancer: Major developments of the last 5-years. *European Journal of Cancer* 49 (6): 1216–1225.

D'Addario, G., Fru, M., Reck, M., Baumann, P., Klepetko, W. and Felip, E. 2010. Metastatic non-small-cell lung cancer: ESMO Clinical Practice Guidelines for diagnosis, treatment and follow-up. *Annals of Oncology* 21 (Suppl 5): v116–v119.

Dela Cruz, C.S., Tanoue, L.T. and Matthay, R.A. 2011. Lung cancer: Epidemiology, aetiology and prevention. *Clinics in Chest Medicine* 32 (4): 605–644.

Department of Health (DH). 1995. *A Policy Framework for Commissioning Cancer Services: A Report by the Expert Advisory Group on Cancer to the Chief Medical Officers of England and Wales*. Department of Health, London.

Department of Health (DH). 2008. *End of Life Care Strategy: Promoting High Quality Care of All Adults at the End of Life*. Department of Health, London.

Department of Health (DH). 2013. *Cancer Patient Experience Survey National Report*. http://www.quality-health.co.uk/resources/surveys/national-cancer-experience-survey-reports/301-2013-national-cancer-patient-experience-survey-programme-national-report/file. Accessed 26 March 2015.

Doyle, D., Hanks, G.W.C., MacDonald, N. (eds.) 2004. *Oxford Textbook of Palliative Medicine*. Oxford University Press, Oxford.

Etzel, C.J., Lu, M., Merriman, K., Liu, M., Vaporciyan, A. and Spitz, M.R. 2006. An epidemiologic study of early onset lung cancer. *Lung Cancer* 52 (2): 129–134.

Goldberg, S., Willers, H. and Heist, R.S. 2013. *Multidisciplinary Management of Small Cell Lung Cancer*. W B Saunders Co-Elsevier Inc., Philadelphia.

Goldstraw, P., Crawley, J., Chanskey, K., Giroux, D. J., Groome, P.A., Rami-Porter, R., Postmus, P.E., Rusch, V. and Sobin, L. 2007. The IASLC lung cancer staging project: Proposals for the revision of the TNM stage groupings in the forthcoming (seventh) edition of the TNM classification of malignant tumours. *Journal of Thoracic Oncology* 2 (8): 706–714.

Gregor, A. 1997. Prophylactic cranial irradiation in small cell lung cancer (SCLC) makes a comeback. *Clinical Oncology* 9 (3): 148–149.

Haddadin, S. and Perry, M.C. 2011. History of small cell lung cancer. *Clinical Lung Cancer* 12 (2): 87–93.

Leary, A. 2012. *Lung Cancer: A Multidisciplinary Approach*. Wiley Blackwell Publishing, Oxford.

Lynch, T.D., Bell, D.W., Sordella, R., Gurubhagavatula, S., Okimoto, R.A., Brannigan, B.W., Harris, M.S. et al. 2004. Activating mutations in the epidermal growth factor receptor underlying responsiveness of non-small-cell lung cancer to Gefitinib. *New England Journal of Medicine* 350 (21): 2129–2139.

McCloskey, P., Balduyck, B., Van Schil, P.E., Faivre-Finn, C. and O'Brien, M. 2013. Radical treatment of non-small cell lung cancer during the last 5 years. *European Journal of Cancer* 49 (7): 1555–1564.

Medford, A.R., Bennett, J.A., Free, C.M. and Agrawal, S. 2010. Endobronchial ultrasound guided transbronchial needle aspiration. *Post Graduate Medical Journal* 86 (1012): 106–115.

Mussi, A., Pistolesi, M., Lucchi, M., Janni, A., Chella, A., Parenti, G., Rossi, G. and Angeletti, C.A. 1996. Resection of single brain metastasis in non-small-cell lung cancer: Prognostic factors. *Journal of Thoracic and Cardiovascular Surgery* 112 (1): 146–153.

National Cancer Action Team (NCAT). 2007. *Holistic Common Assessment of Supportive and Palliative Care Needs for Adults with Cancer – Assessment Guidance.* NCAT, London.

National Cancer Intelligence Network (NCIN). 2008. *Cancer Incidence by Deprivation England, 1995–2004.* http://tinyurl.com/oydhhhv. Accessed 26 March 2015.

National Cancer Intelligence Network (NCIN). 2010. *Routes to Diagnosis Project.* http://ncin.org.uk/publications/routes_to_diagnosis.aspx. Accessed 30 March 2015.

National Institute for Health and Care Excellence (NICE). 2005. *Clinical Guideline 24, Lung Cancer: Diagnosis and Treatment.* NICE, London. https://www.nice.org.uk/guidance/cg27. Accessed 30 March 2015.

National Institute for Health and Care Excellence (NICE). 2010. *Technology Appraisal Guidance 192, Gefitinib for the First Line Treatment of Locally Advanced Metastatic Non-small Cell Lung Cancer.* http://guidance.nice.org.uk/TA192. Accessed 15 April 2015.

National Institute for Health and Care Excellence (NICE). 2011. *Clinical Guideline 121, The Diagnosis and Treatment of Lung Cancer.* http://www.nice.org.uk/guidance/CG121. Accessed 16 March 2015.

NHS Information Centre (NHSIC). 2012. *National Lung Cancer Audit Report 2012: Report for the Audit Period 2011.* NHSIC, UK.

Non-small Cell Collaborative Group (NSCCG). 1995. Chemotherapy in non-small cell lung cancer: A meta-analysis using updated data on individual patients from 52 randomised clinical trials. *British Medical Journal* 311 (7010): 899–909.

Palma, D., Visser, O., Lagerwaard, F.J., Belderbos, J., Slotman, B.J. and Senan, S. 2010. Impact of introducing stereotactic lungradiotherapy for elderly patients with stage I non-small-cell lung cancer: A population-based time-trend analysis. *Journal of Clinical Oncology* 28 (35): 5153–5139.

Peto, R., Darby, S., Harz, D., Silcocks, P., Whitley, E. and Doll, R. 2000. Smoking, smoking cessation, and lung cancer in the UK since 1950: Combination of national statistics with two case–control studies. *British Medical Journal* 321 (7257): 323–329.

Rosell, R., Moran, T., Queralt, C., Porta, R., Cardenal, F. and Camps, C. 2009. Screening for epidermal growth factor receptor mutations in lung cancer. *New England Journal of Medicine* 361 (10): 958–967.

Rothschild, S.I., Gautsch, O., Haura, E.B. and Johnson, F. 2010. SRC inhibitors in lung cancer: Current status and future directions. *Clinical Lung Cancer* 11 (4): 238–242.

Roy Castle Lung Cancer Foundation (RCLCF). 2011. *Explaining Variations in Lung Cancer in England.* http://www.roycastle.org/how-we-help/our-campaigns/improving-treatment-and-care/mapping-a-picture-of-lung-cancer-in-england-and-scotland. Accessed 19 August 2015.

Roy Castle Lung Cancer Foundation (RCLCF). 2014. *Lung Cancer Facts and Figures.* http://www.roycastle.org/lung-cancer/Lung-Cancer-Facts-and-Figures. Accessed 26 July 2014.

Rudin, C., Tang, E.A. and Samet, M. 2009. Lung cancer in never smokers: A call to action. *Clinical Cancer Research* 15 (18): 5622–5625.

Shepherd, F.A., Crowley, J., Van Houtte, P., Postmus, P., Carney, D., Chansky, K., Shaikh, Z. and Goldstraw, P. 2007. The International Association for the Study of Lung Cancer Lung Cancer Staging Project: Proposals regarding the clinical staging of small cell lung cancer in the forthcoming (seventh) edition of the tumour, node, metastasis classification for lung cancer. *Journal of Thoracic Oncology* 2 (12): 1067–1077.

Siegel, R., Naishadham, D. and Jemal, A. 2012. Cancer statistics 2012. *CA: A Cancer Journal for Clinicians* 62 (1): 10–29.

Sun, S., Schiller, J.H. and Gazdar, A.F. 2007. Lung cancer in never smokers – A different disease. *Nature Reviews Cancer* 7 (10): 778–790.

Teh, E. and Belcher, E. 2014. Lung cancer: Diagnosis, staging and treatment. *Surgery* 32 (5): 242–248.

Tod, A.M., Craven, J. and Allmark, P. 2008. Diagnostic delay in lung cancer: A qualitative study. *Journal of Advanced Nursing* 61 (3): 336–343.

Tod, A.M., McDonnell, A. and Redman, J. 2013. *Opening Doors to Treatment: Exploring the Impact of Lung Cancer Specialist Nurses on Access to Anti-cancer Treatment, an Exploratory Case Study.* Available from Sheffield Hallam University Research Archive (SHURA) at: http://shura.shu.ac.uk/7921/. Accessed 26 March 2015.

Turner, N.J., Muers, M.F., Haward, R.A. and Mulley, G.P. 2007. Psychological distress and concerns of elderly patients treated with palliative radiotherapy for lung cancer. *Psycho-Oncology* 16 (8): 707–713.

Twycross, R.G. and Lack, S.A. 1986. *Therapeutics in Terminal Cancer.* Churchill Livingstone, Edinburgh.

van Meerbeeck, J.P., Fennell, D.A. and De Ruysscher, D.K. 2011. Small cell lung cancer. *The Lancet* 78 (9804): 1741–1755.

World Health Organization. 2010. *World Health Statistics 2010* [Internet]. WHO, Geneva. Available at: http://www.who.int/whosis/whostat/2010/en/. Accessed 24 July 2014.

Wright, J. and Wolfson, A. 2012. Prophylactic cranial irradiation: Do benefits outweigh neurocognitive impact? *Current Problems in Cancer* 36 (3): 106–116.

Bronchiectasis

12

GILLIAN MAW

LEARNING OBJECTIVES

Upon completion of this chapter, the reader of this should be able to:

- Provide a definition of bronchiectasis
- Identify causative factors and associated symptoms
- Discuss key aspects of investigation and care management
- Apply the knowledge and key practice issues to a patient exhibiting symptoms of bronchiectasis

INTRODUCTION

This chapter aims to provide an overview of bronchiectasis and will include: a definition, classification of the disease, causes, signs and symptoms, and the management of bronchiectasis. The presenting symptoms of bronchiectasis can reflect many respiratory diseases, but this chapter aims to heighten awareness of key factors leading to diagnosis and how understanding the pathophysiology of the disease can influence the management and quality of life experienced for individuals diagnosed with bronchiectasis.

Bronchiectasis is uncommon and recent statistics suggest 1:1000 adults within the United Kingdom (UK) are diagnosed with the condition (National Institute of Health and Care Excellence [NICE], 2015). It can occur at any age, but generally symptoms

develop around middle age (Loebinger et al., 2009). It is estimated that there were 16,000 hospital admissions related to exacerbations of bronchiectasis in 2011/12 with over 12,000 patients admitted being 60 years or over. The incidence of bronchiectasis varies between populations, but more recently a decline in the disease has been recognised and is thought to be related to mass immunisation programmes and the appropriate prescribing of antibiotics (Chang et al., 2009). The incidence of bronchiectasis increases with age, but is demonstrably higher in older females, and generally more women are affected than men (Chung and Pavord, 2008). A more recent study by Goeminne et al. (2012) considers this 'female' trend, but the causative factors remain a mystery.

A case study will be presented that illustrates the challenges of diagnosing bronchiectasis and the importance of adequate clinical history and assessment skills to both ensure an accurate diagnosis, appropriate management and ultimately improvement to an individual's quality of life.

DEFINITION

Pasteur et al. (2010, i7) defines bronchiectasis as:

> Bronchiectasis is a persistent or progressive condition characterised by dilated thick-walled bronchi. The symptoms vary from intermittent episodes of expectoration and infection localised to the region of the lung that is affected to persistent daily expectoration often of large volumes of purulent sputum

The dilation of the bronchi results in 'floppy' airways, which are prone to collapse, consequently effecting airflow (Lane, 2003). The extent of the disease can vary considerably from person to person; for example, one section of one airway can be widened and abnormal as compared with an extreme presentation where many airways are involved (O'Brien et al., 2000). If infection develops, bronchi may become more damaged, more mucus gathers and the risk of repeated infection increases (O'Donnell, 2008) (see Figure 12.1). The cyclical nature of the disease gradually perpetuates the progression of the disease over a person's life span (Lane, 2003).

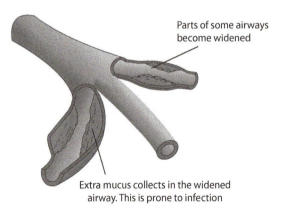

Parts of some airways become widened

Extra mucus collects in the widened airway. This is prone to infection

Figure 12.1 Bronchiectasis: The process of damage to the bronchi. (Reproduced with permission of Chest Heart & Stroke Scotland, http://www.chss.org.uk.)

DISEASE CLASSIFICATION

The disease can be classified into three forms:

1. *Cylindrical bronchiectasis*: The bronchi are enlarged and cylindrical.
2. *Varicose bronchiectasis*: The bronchi are irregular with areas of dilation and constriction.
3. *Saccular or cystic bronchiectasis*: The dilated bronchi form clusters of cysts. This is the most severe form of bronchiectasis and is most commonly associated with cystic fibrosis (King et al., 2006).

CAUSES OF BRONCHIECTASIS

The causes of bronchiectasis are complex and in approximately 50% of adults and 25% of children diagnosed with the disease, no underlying cause can be identified and it is referred to as idiopathic bronchiectasis (O'Donnell, 2008). The complex nature of the disease requires the healthcare professionals to have a robust knowledge of causative factors to ensure excellent clinical reasoning and patient management. Bronchiectasis develops when tissue and muscle surrounding bronchi become damaged, but the reasons for this can be very complex.

Potential causative factors are:

- Childhood lung infections, for example pneumonia, tuberculosis, whooping cough and measles.
- Underlying pathology of the immune system which results in the bronchi becoming more susceptible to damage and can be associated with immunosuppression, allergy, human immunodeficiency virus (HIV) and genetic disorders.
- Allergic bronchopulmonary aspergillosis (ABPA), which is an allergy to the fungi 'aspergillus' which inflames the bronchi if the fungal spores are inhaled. Statistics suggest this accounts for 1/14 diagnoses of bronchiectasis.
- Aspiration, where the contents of the stomach accidentally pass into the lungs rather than the

gastrointestinal tract. This accounts for 1/25 cases of bronchiectasis.

- Cilia abnormality, when the cilia become damaged, this can lead to bronchiectasis. For example, Young's disease is a rare condition only affecting males but accounting for 1/33 cases of bronchiectasis. A further rare condition is primary ciliary dyskinesia, which is genetically inherited and is thought to account for 1/100 diagnoses of bronchiectasis.
- Inflammatory diseases which lead to the immune system 'attacking' healthy tissue can lead to bronchiectasis and classic examples include: rheumatoid arthritis, ulcerative colitis, Crohn's disease, coeliac disease and systemic lupus erythematosus.
- Bronchial obstruction where inhaled objects such as pen tops and peanuts can lead to local damage of the bronchi. Similarly, the same effect can be caused by tumour or lymphadenopathy.
- Congenital defects such as cystic fibrosis, alpha 1 antitrypsin deficiency and 'yellow nail' syndrome, which is a rare disorder in which there is a triad of nail discolouration and nail dystrophy, lymphoedema and chronic respiratory disorders.
- Inhalations of irritants such as smoking, paint fumes, gases and flour.

- Many people with bronchiectasis may also have asthma and this is associated with non-responsive or poorly controlled asthma.
- Ehlers–Danlos syndrome and Marfan's syndrome are a group of genetic connective tissue disorders characterised by unstable, hypermobile joints, loose, 'elastic' skin and fragile tissues.
- Panbronchiolitis is an idiopathic inflammatory disease that principally affects the respiratory bronchioles. It can result in a progressive suppurative and severe obstructive respiratory disorder. If left untreated, there is progression to bronchiectasis, respiratory failure and eventually death. Owing to a generic predisposition, it is seen mainly in patients of East Asian origin and is well recognised in Japan.

(Pasteur et al., 2000).

SIGNS AND SYMPTOMS

The presence and severity of symptoms correlate to the number of airways affected and how severe the damage is, but the associated signs and symptoms are often varied and complex to evaluate (see Table 12.1).

Unfortunately, many of the presenting symptoms can be confused with other respiratory diseases

Table 12.1 Signs and symptoms of bronchiectasis

Signs and symptoms	Consideration
Cough	90% of patients will present with cough as the major symptom
Unproductive cough	8% of adults affected
Daily productive cough	75% of adults affected
Lethargy	Nutrition, anaemia, low mood, hypoxia
Purulent sputum	Inflammatory process, infection
Breathlessness	83% of adults affected
Chest pain or chest discomfort	31% of adults affected
Haemoptysis	27% of adults affected
Poor concentration	Fatigue, hypoxia
Wheeze	34% of adults affected
Generally feeling unwell	Infection, low mood, hypoxia
Chronic sinusitis	Post nasal drip, excessive mucus production
Finger clubbing	Rarely seen

Source: Adapted from Barker, A.F. 2002., *New England Journal of Medicine*, 346 (18): 1383–1393, 2002; Rosen, M.J. 2006., *Chest*, 129 (Suppl 1): 122S–131S; King, P.T. et al. 2006. *Respiratory Medicine*, 100 (12): 2183–2189.

such as emphysema, bronchitis and asthma. This often leads to misdiagnosis in association with inappropriate prescribing and self-management. The key to the correct diagnosis being made is accurate history taking, coupled with suitable clinical investigations.

REACHING A DIAGNOSIS

When reaching a diagnosis, it is essential that the practitioner engage with a systematic approach to clinical investigation. Detailed history taking (see Chapter 2) can influence the patient experience significantly and this information can supply the healthcare professional with more than enough evidence to support a provisional diagnosis before any investigations are even considered (Ellis et al., 1981). This is only possible if the knowledge base of the healthcare professional is informed and they have the ability to tease out key aspects of the patient's history to reach a successful conclusion (Murray and Hill, 2009).

Of all of the potential investigations listed in Table 12.2, following a detailed clinical history, a CT scan is recommended as the gold standard method of diagnosis for individuals presenting with key symptoms of bronchiectasis (Pasteur et al., 2010).

TREATMENT, INTERVENTIONS AND THERAPY

Treatment pathways are dependent upon the severity of the disease and the disease progression. Fundamental for successful management of the patient is the ability to recognise the 'norm' for them and recognise slight changes for which interventions can be undertaken to prevent an acute exacerbation or indeed treat a resulting episode. There are many aspects of treatment which can be considered, and each individual patient with a diagnosis of bronchiectasis needs to be managed according to their experience and presenting symptoms.

Treatment, interventions and therapies used in the management of bronchiectasis include the following:

BREATHING EXERCISES

Exercises are taught by physiotherapists; this might involve active cycle of breathing techniques (ACBT), which is a process of repeated cyclical breaths (Bott et al., 2009). This includes normal breaths, which are then followed by deep breaths to loosen and encourage mucus to be moved upwards in the respiratory tract, enabling expectoration (Hacken et al., 2007).

Table 12.2 Key investigations to consider in the diagnosis of bronchiectasis

Investigation	Rationale
Presenting symptoms and related problems	
Physical chest examination	*Crackles* heard during chest auscultation are often evident (70% of adults with bronchiectasis) as air passes over excess mucus
Chest X-ray	To eliminate tumour, bullae, or pneumothorax
Sputum for culture and sensitivity	Risk of infection
Spirometry to assess lung function	Forced expiratory volume in 1 second (FEV_1), forced vital capacity (FVC), peak expiratory flow (PEF) and vital capacity (VC)
Computerised tomography (CT)	Imaging enables an accurate diagnosis given the similarities between potential diagnosis and differing management. Gold standard management
Blood sample	Full blood count (FBC), white cell count (WCC), inflammatory markers, autoimmune screening (IgA, IgG, IgM)
Sweat test	If salt content is elevated, indicative of cystic fibrosis
Bronchoscopy	Offers the potential to take tissue and mucus samples for analysis, also potential therapeutic outcome of sputum removal via suction
Allergy testing	For aspergillus fumigatus and aspergillus precipitins

The time scale for undertaking such activity is varied to match the severity of disease, but is a method of management recommended by Pasteur et al. (2010) and easily managed by sufferers.

POSTURAL DRAINAGE

Postural drainage is where the patient's body is positioned so that the trachea is inclined downward and below the affected chest area (Bradley et al., 2002). Postural drainage is again taught by physiotherapists and they enable patients to 'tip' themselves into a position in which the lobe to be drained is uppermost. This is often undertaken at least three times daily for up to 30 minutes per session depending upon disease severity (Bott et al., 2009). There are drainage positions for all segments of the lung and these positions can be modified depending on the patient's condition and ability (Bradley et al., 2002). The treatment is often used in conjunction with a technique for loosening secretions in the chest cavity, called chest percussion. Chest percussion is performed by clapping the back or chest with a cupped hand. Alternatively, a mechanical vibration device may be used in some cases to facilitate loosening of secretions. Postural drainage may be followed by breathing exercises to help expel loosened secretions from the airway as detailed above (Bott et al., 2009).

INHALATION THERAPY

Inhaled treatment varies according to the severity and progression of the disease. The efficacy of the use of some products is questionable as the progression of the disease influences prescribing decisions (Franco et al., 2003; Murray et al., 2011). However, the healthcare professional needs to consider the effect upon daily living and address inhaled treatment accordingly. Key methods of inhalation are metred-dose inhalers used in conjunction with a spacing device and nebulised methods of delivery. Both methods offer greater deposition of the product in the airways and require less inspiratory effort to enable therapeutic use. Both methods are not as convenient as some powder devices, but in relation to deposition, the evidence suggests they offer a better response rate (Sheikh et al., 2001; Goeminne et al., 2012). The main aim of inhaled therapy is to induce bronchodilation and enable expectation of excess mucus (Corless and Warburton, 2000). Salbutamol is often the first drug of choice, which may or may not facilitate an effect. This depends upon beta-receptor sites and how responsive they are. Often anticholinergic inhaled products offer a better response due to the mode of action, tolerance of higher doses and the benefit of reduced or thinner mucus production (Baxter, 2008). Examples of anticholinergic products are ipratropium and tiotropium (Joint Formulary Committee [JFC], 2015).

OTHER DRUG THERAPY

Other medication can be used in conjunction or indeed stand-alone treatments for bronchiectasis, but the response can be unpredictable and not always therapeutic (Baxter, 2008). Mucolytics can facilitate thinning of the excess mucus (Crockett et al., 2002), i.e. carbocisteine, which promotes easier expectoration; however, the effect is not always positive and can cause gastrointestinal bleeding (JFC, 2015). Concordance can also be difficult to achieve when patients are required to take the medication four times daily to achieve a therapeutic response but often in conjunction with inhaled therapy (Baxter, 2008). The introduction of leukotriene receptor agonists was initially thought to be progressive treatment for bronchiectasis by reducing the inflammatory response, but more recently evidence suggests that this may be questionable and indeed disguise the inflammatory reaction and prevent the individual from recognising subtle changes in their condition which may indicate a warning of an exacerbation (Sheikh et al., 2001).

Antibiotics are used extensively for individuals with bronchiectasis; however, a key factor in their use is the early identification of the causative pathogen. If time allows, culture and sensitivity of the causative organism can influence prescribing and prevent both overuse of antibiotics and inappropriate use (Evans et al., 2007). This is particularly important given the risks associated with overuse of antimicrobials, specifically the potential for drug resistance. Antibiotics can be taken orally, but the option to nebulise can enable the product to bypass first-pass metabolism and improve and accelerate the therapeutic effect (Baxter, 2008). This also has the benefit of increasing patient tolerance when side effects can be more problematic than the chest infection (JFC, 2015).

Guidelines supporting the long-term use of antibiotic therapy for bronchiectasis patients have been influenced by the evidence base associated with antibiotic usage for those with cystic fibrosis (Bryskier and Butzler, 2003). NICE (2014) supports the long-term use for individuals with bronchiectasis, but recognises that such therapy does not always have a positive response and many clinicians question the viability of such prescribing. This issue of microbial resistance remains a major concern and using a long-term delivery of such products is not supported with current evidence.

COMPLICATIONS

Bronchiectasis can bring a complex collection of complications because of the systemic effect upon the human body. Some of the classic complications of bronchiectasis include breathing difficulties, fatigue, malaise and poor appetite, but as the disease progresses cardiac involvement often becomes a secondary disease process owing to hypoxic pulmonary vasoconstriction. This in turn subjects the patient to symptoms of right-sided heart failure, which further complicates the management process for the practitioner (Chung and Pavord, 2008).

Depression can be a significant complication of bronchiectasis; consequently an early diagnosis of depression and an awareness of the relationship between depression and the disease process can improve outcomes and future management for patients (Girón Moreno et al., 2013). Key causative factors are self-blame, social stigma, fear and embarrassment. Diagnosis and appropriate care can only be possible if practitioners are adequately trained, motivated and, above all, listen to patients with bronchiectasis (Girón Moreno et al., 2013).

One of the rarely seen, but catastrophic complications is haemoptysis (Lane, 2003). The inflammatory nature of the disease results in engorgement of superficial blood vessels and, when added to a persistent and often aggressive cough, can cause rupture of blood vessels (Lane, 2003). Presenting symptoms can include blood-stained sputum, which can be suggestive of malignancy, but in the context of bronchiectasis could suggest a blood vessel rupture.

CASE STUDY

Mrs Cooper is a 47-year-old lady who was diagnosed with asthma, and as a small child had spent many months in hospital during her childhood. During this time many different procedures were undertaken, some of which were not recorded within medical records and, as she was a child at the time, cannot be recalled for accuracy. Both her mother and father have since died and no accurate record of investigations can be found.

Over the years she has become accustomed to being an asthmatic, her physical exertion limits, what foods to avoid and knowing the particular things that trigger asthma symptoms. She copes by trying to avoid circumstances that will trigger coughing and sputum production, avoiding exertion and general exercise. Generally, she makes her life fit around a respiratory condition that has never been controlled but requires considerable management, prescribing interventions and reliance upon salbutamol via a MDI and spacing device.

In the past few months, persistent chest infections have become more and more problematic. Repeated courses of antibiotics often coupled with oral steroids have been required, with symptoms only to manifest themselves again a few weeks later. An increased cough has become more and more difficult to cope with and engaging in social activities has become impossible. During this time, numerous chest X-rays and general discussion about asthma management were undertaken but the detail of this lady's history was always skimmed over due to the confirmed diagnosis of asthma and a lack of healthcare professionals being able or indeed prepared to look further than the already defined diagnosis.

At her latest visit to her GP practice Mrs Cooper presented with increasing cough, sputum production, shortness of breath and being generally unwell. Her observations were pulse 85 bpm, respiratory rate 17 bpm, temperature 36.6°C, blood pressure 130/80 mmHg, PERF was 260 L/min and SpO_2 was 92% on room air. On examination, peripheral cyanosis was evident on arrival, which resolved with rest. Physically, Mrs Cooper looked exhausted, pale and weary. Chest examination revealed no concerns on inspection and palpation. Percussion revealed dull tones over the mid zones and on auscultation breath sounds were harsh; there were multiple wheezes and poor air entry to both bases.

Mrs Cooper had been diagnosed with asthma as a child. Generally, her health had remained good. However, she did suffer from frequent exacerbations of asthma and frequent chest infections. Mrs Cooper had never smoked and neither had her parents. Both of her parents are deceased but she remembers her mother constantly having a 'bad chest' and her father worked in the mines locally and always coughed. She also remembers a maternal aunt dying due to a respiratory problem, but no specific details were available.

Mrs Cooper lives with her husband and three children but no longer works as she had experienced repeated episodes of sickness. She has had to adapt her lifestyle and her home has been designed to reduce the risk of allergy including no carpets, hypoallergenic bedding, no pets, no central heating and no smoking.

Currently Mrs Cooper is on the following medication:

- Salbutamol MDI (100 mgs), via spacer, two puffs as required.
- Fluticasone MDI (80 mcg), via spacer, four puffs twice daily.
- Salmeterol MDI (25 mcg), via spacer, two puffs twice daily.

Following a detailed history, the healthcare professional was able to ascertain that the experienced symptoms, cough and sputum expectoration were not classically associated with asthma (see Chapter 6). Although recent chest X-rays had not revealed significant abnormalities, the crudeness of the image demanded further investigation for appropriate management to be agreed. Considerations at this point were bronchiectasis, asthma and emphysema. The patient was referred for CT imaging urgently, which revealed extensive bronchiectasis and enabled a new care pathway to be developed.

A diagnosis of bronchiectasis finally gave a name to what had been causing so many problems and leaving Mrs Cooper constantly feeling unwell. Instigation of breathing exercises and review of medication to include mucolytics were the initial steps of improved management and improved health. For many patients, the experience of a 'new' diagnosis can be life changing and very stressful, bringing a whole new range of issues to be managed (Bradley et al., 2002).

DISCUSSION OF CASE STUDY

For a patient presenting with such myriad problems it would be a consideration to involve a multidisciplinary team for guidance and care planning. Physiotherapy is an essential aspect of bronchiectasis care and this cannot be undertaken by other professionals who 'think' they have the knowledge to guide and teach (Flude et al., 2012). Low mood and well-being may already be or indeed become a significant aspect of care for an individual in such circumstances and support from an appropriate healthcare professional, for example GP, practice nurse, district nurse, community mental health nurse, may prove invaluable. Involvement of social workers, if appropriate, can offer support from a more practical perspective and offer guidance in relation to home support, financial aid and indeed care support. When coupled with knowledge from doctors, nurses and other related healthcare professionals, this can empower an individual diagnosed with bronchiectasis to manage the disease and improve their own life considerably. When patients present with repeated episodes of the same symptoms, it is important for healthcare professionals to reconsider the diagnosis, especially if this was made many decades earlier and without the aid of contemporary imaging techniques.

SUMMARY

Bronchiectasis is a life-changing condition, which has variable presentations mainly dependent upon the cause of bronchial damage. Generally, life expectancy is not compromised, but this depends upon management and lifestyle adjustment. Treatment is continually improving, which is encouraging, but the overarching theme is early diagnosis, education, improved health through immunisation and safety management, which means less exposure to irritants, disease processes and ultimately reduction in the disease prevalence.

It is essential that healthcare professionals have the knowledge base to assess patients, achieve an accurate clinical diagnosis and be confident that management is both accurate and appropriate. Patient assessment and clinical judgement are vital in determining the most appropriate environment for treatment. Patient stability, co-morbidities and social circumstances must also be taken into account when deciding on treatment.

As the case study in this chapter demonstrates, a diagnosis is not always accurate and symptoms can be consistent with other disease processes. Reconsidering the original diagnosis is important and the healthcare professional must be a confident and competent practitioner in order to do this.

REFERENCES

Barker, A.F. 2002. Bronchiectasis. *New England Journal of Medicine* 346 (18): 1383–1393.

Baxter, K. 2008. *Stockley's Drug Interactions: A Source Book of Interactions, Their Mechanisms, Clinical Importance and Management* (8th ed.). Pharmaceutical Press, London.

Bott, J., Blumenthal, S. and Buxton, M. 2009. Guidelines for the physiotherapy management of the adult, medical, spontaneously breathing patient. *Thorax* 64 (Suppl 1): i1–i51.

Bradley, J.M., Moran, F. and Greenstone, M. 2002. *Physical Training for Bronchiectasis (Cochrane Review)*. The Cochrane Collaboration. John Wiley & Sons, Ltd, Hoboken, NJ.

Bryskier, A. and Butzler, J.P. 2003. Macrolides. In: Finch, R.G., Greenwood, D., Noorby, S.R. and Whitley, R.J. (eds.). *Antibiotic and Chemotherapy: Anti-Infective Agents and Their Use in Therapy* (8th ed.). Churchill Livingstone, Edinburgh.

Chang, C.C., Morris, P.S. and Chang, A.B. 2009. *Influenza Vaccine for Children and Adults with Bronchiectasis (Cochrane Review)*. The Cochrane Collaboration. John Wiley & Sons, Ltd, Hoboken, NJ.

Chung, K.F. and Pavord, I.D. 2008. Prevalence, pathogenesis, and causes of chronic cough. *Lancet* 371 (9621): 1364–1374.

Corless, J.A. and Warburton, C.J. 2000. *Leukotriene Receptor Antagonists for Non-Cystic Fibrosis Bronchiectasis (Cochrane Review)*. The Cochrane Collaboration. John Wiley & Sons, Ltd, Hoboken, NJ.

Crockett, A., Cranston, J.M., Alpers, J.H. and Latiner, K.M. 2002. *Mucolytics for Bronchiectasis (Cochrane Review)*. The Cochrane Collaboration. John Wiley & Sons, Ltd, Hoboken, NJ.

Ellis, D.A., Thornley, P.E. and Wightman, A.J. 1981. Present outlook in bronchiectasis: Clinical and social study and review of factors influencing prognosis. *Thorax* 36 (9): 659–664.

Evans, D.J., Bara, A. and Greenstone, M. 2007. *Prolonged Antibiotics for Purulent Bronchiectasis in Children and Adults (Cochrane Review)*. The Cochrane Collaboration. John Wiley & Sons, Ltd, Hoboken, NJ.

Flude, L.J., Agent, P. and Bilton, D. 2012. Chest physiotherapy techniques in bronchiectasis. *Clinical Chest Medicine* 33 (2): 351–361.

Franco, F., Sheikh, A. and Greenstone, M. 2003. *Short Acting Beta2-Agonists for Bronchiectasis (Cochrane Review)*. The Cochrane Collaboration. John Wiley & Sons, Ltd, Hoboken, NJ.

Girón Moreno, R.M., Fernandes Vasconcelos, G., Cisneros, C., Gómez-Punter, R.M., Segrelles Calvo, G. and Ancochea, J. 2013. Presence of anxiety and depression in patients with bronchiectasis unrelated to cystic fibrosis. *Archivos de Bronconeumologia* 49 (10): 415–420.

Goeminne, P.C., Scheers, H., Decraene, A., Seys, S. and Dupont, L.J. 2012. Risk factors for morbidity and death in non-cystic fibrosis bronchiectasis: A retrospective cross-sectional analysis of CT diagnosed bronchiectatic patients. *Respiratory Research* 13 (21): 1186–1465.

Hacken, N.H.T., Wijkstra, P.J. and Kerstjens, H.A.M. 2007. Treatment of bronchiectasis in adults. *British Medical Journal* 335 (7629): 1089–1093.

Joint Formulary Committee (JFC). 2015. *British National Formulary* (68th ed.). British Medical Association and Royal Pharmaceutical Society of Great Britain, London.

King, P.T., Holdsworth, S.R. and Freezer, N.J. 2006. Characterisation of the onset and presenting clinical features of adult bronchiectasis. *Respiratory Medicine* 100 (12): 2183–2189.

Lane, D.J. 2003. The clinical presentation of chest diseases. In: Warrell, D.A., Cox, T.M., Firth, J.D. and Benz, E.J. (eds.). *Oxford Textbook of Medicine* (4th ed.). Oxford University Press, Oxford.

Loebinger, M.R., Wells, A.U. and Hansell, D.M. 2009. Mortality in bronchiectasis: A long-term study assessing the factors influencing survival. *European Respiratory Journal* 34 (4): 843–849.

Murray, M.P. and Hill, A.T. 2009. Non-cystic fibrosis bronchiectasis. *Clinical Medicine* 9 (2): 164–169.

Murray, M.P., Govan, J.R. and Doherty, C.J. 2011. A randomized controlled trial of nebulized gentamicin in non-cystic fibrosis bronchiectasis. *American Journal of Respiratory Critical Care Medicine* 183 (4): 491–499.

National Institute of Health and Care Excellence. 2014. Non-Cystic Fibrosis Bronchiectasis: Long term azithromycin, NICE Advice (ESUOM38).

National Institute of Health and Care Excellence. 2015. Clinical Knowledge Summaries. Bronchiectasis. Available at: http://cks.nice.org.uk/bronchiectasis

O'Brien, C., Guest, P.J., Hill, S.L. and Stockley, R.A. 2000. Physiological and radiological characterisation of patients diagnosed with chronic obstructive pulmonary disease in primary care. *Thorax* 55 (8): 635–642.

O'Donnell, A.E. 2008. Bronchiectasis. *Chest* 134 (4): 815–823.

Pasteur, M.C., Bilton, D. and Hill, A.T. 2010. British Thoracic Society Guideline for non-CF bronchiectasis. British Thoracic Society Bronchiectasis (non-CF) Guideline Group. *Thorax* 75 (Suppl 1): i1–i58.

Pasteur, M.C., Helliwell, S.M. and Houghton, S.J. 2000. An investigation into causative factors in patients with bronchiectasis. *American Journal of Respiratory and Critical Care Medicine* 162 (4): 1277–1284.

Rosen, M.J. 2006. Chronic cough due to bronchiectasis: ACCP evidence-based clinical practice guidelines. *Chest* 129 (Suppl 1): 122S–131S.

Sheikh, A., Nolan, D. and Greenstone, M. 2001, *Long-Acting Beta2-Agonists for Bronchiectasis (Cochrane Review).* The Cochrane Collaboration John Wiley & Sons, Ltd, Hoboken, NJ.

Cystic fibrosis

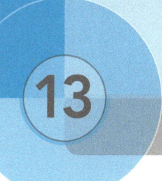

13

LISA PRIESTLEY, CASSANDRA GREEN
AND ZOE ABEL

LEARNING OBJECTIVES

Upon completion of this chapter the reader should be able to:

- Describe the role of the cystic fibrosis transmembrane conductance regulator (CFTR) in the pathophysiology of cystic fibrosis (CF)
- Identify the effects of cystic fibrosis on various organs and systems of the body
- Identify treatment options for short- and long-term CF care

INTRODUCTION

Cystic fibrosis (CF) is the most common life-threatening genetically acquired multisystem disease, affecting 1 in every 2500 live births in the UK, with currently 10,500 people in the UK living with CF (Cystic Fibrosis Trust [CFT], 2015a). Once considered a disease of childhood and adolescence, it has now evolved into a serious long-term, chronic condition with over half of its population aged over 16 years and transitioning into adult healthcare settings (CFT, 2015a).

This chapter aims to provide an overview of CF and will include an explanation of the genetics and pathophysiology associated with CF. Signs and symptoms of an infective exacerbation of CF will be discussed with reference to some of the most common microbiology seen in the CF lung. Treatment options for short- and long-term CF care will be identified. Finally, a case study will be presented that illustrates the challenges associated with the diagnosis of CF.

DEFINITION

CF is a genetic condition that mainly affects the respiratory and digestive systems. CF causes thick, sticky mucous secretions to block the lungs and intestines. The name derives from fibrous tissue that develops in the pancreas. CF affects the ability of the body to move salt and water in and out of cells, which results in thick mucous secretions and provides a perfect environment for bacteria to grow. The mucus also blocks the essential enzymes that break down food and prevents the absorption of nutrients. Consequently, people with CF have to take medication throughout their life to aid digestion of food, to fight infections and reduce the amount of mucus in their lungs.

159

CF was first described in 1938 with a life expectancy of only 6 months (Andersen, 1938). Today's average life expectancy is 40.1 years (CFT, 2015a), but a child born in 2000 is expected to live into their 50s (Dodge et al., 2007). CF is no longer a disease of childhood and healthcare provision has therefore evolved to reflect this: until now, the increasing survival of those with CF has been due to antibiotic therapies, nutrition and physiotherapy. There are now new milestones in CF drug therapy with the introduction of drugs that treat the underlying cause of CF, attempting to correct the defective protein, not just the symptoms (Pettit and Fellner, 2014).

GENETICS

CF is one of the most widespread autosomal recessive diseases in the world, although the incidence varies between ethnic groups (World Health Organisation [WHO], 2015). Within the Caucasian population in the UK 1:25 people are carriers for CF; this reduces with other ethnicities. The CF gene was first found in 1989 (Kerem et al., 1989) following the work by Tsui et al. (1985). The CF mutation is a protein found on the long arm of chromosome 7 and affects the chloride (Cl^-) channel known as the cystic fibrosis transmembrane conductance regulator (CFTR). There are currently five classes of CFTR mutations with approximately 2000 variations identified to date, although the majority are extremely rare, with only 127 CFTR mutations confirmed as CF-causing (Sosnay et al., 2013). CFTR is found in the cells of exocrine glands throughout the body, specifically in the lungs, digestive tract, sweat glands and genitourinary system, making CF a multisystem disease. CFTR disrupts the balance of sodium (Na) and water in the cell, causing decreased chloride (Cl^-) secretion and increased sodium absorption, resulting in abnormal amounts of viscous mucus secretions accumulating in the lungs, pancreas, liver, intestine and reproductive organs. Specific pulmonary complications associated with the CFTR mutation include reduced mucociliary clearance, potential airway obstruction and colonisation with pathogenic bacteria. Recurrent cycles of infection and inflammation can contribute to lung damage and subsequent development of bronchiectasis. See Chapter 12 for further information concerning bronchiectasis.

In the pancreas, the exocrine ducts become blocked by secretions, resulting in pancreatic destruction and pancreatic enzyme insufficiency. This leads to approximately 25% of CF patients developing CF-related diabetes (CFRD) (Mackie et al., 2003).

CF is characterised by a wide variation in disease severity, progression and organ involvement. This is because several factors influence the clinical phenotype: the CFTR genotype and activity, modifier genes and environmental factors such as nutritional status, exposure to pollutants and socio-economic status (Zielenski, 2000; Quittner et al., 2010).

PATHOPHYSIOLOGY

In CF there is hyperabsorption of Na+ into epithelial cells, drawing in the water and Cl− , leaving the mucus or secretions outside the cell dehydrated, resulting in viscous secretions (Donaldson and Boucher, 2007). The widespread presence of CFTR throughout the body helps explain why CF is a multisystem condition affecting multiple organs and systems.

LUNGS

Respiratory disease is the main cause of mortality in the CF population. CFTR dysfunction is associated with the composition and amount of airway surface liquid. The cilia are inhibited by the presence of sticky mucus and dry airways, so cannot help with the cleansing action of moving mucus up and out of the lungs. This provides a perfect environment for bacterial infection to take hold, causing chronic chest infections, which in turn can lead to bronchiectasis.

LIVER

Twenty-five percent of CF sufferers show signs of liver disease. CFTR dysfunction can lead to increased viscosity of bile, obstructing hepatic ducts and causing focal biliary cirrhosis, inflammation, hepatic scarring and fibrosis. Liver disease is associated with increased mortality at an earlier age. CFTR channels line the hepatic bile ducts and gall bladder, leading to gall stones. Dysfunction results in viscous mucus that obstructs hepatic bile ducts.

PANCREAS

In a healthy pancreas, chloride and bicarbonate ions (HCO³) are normally secreted through CFTR channels into the lumen of pancreatic ducts. The alkaline secretions contain digestive enzymes essential to break down carbohydrates, proteins and lipids in the small intestine. Owing to the abnormal CFTR in CF and secretion of Cl⁻ and bicarbonate into the lumen of the pancreatic duct, secretions become acidic and epithelial cells become inflamed and enlarged. This leads to obstruction of ducts by viscous secretions that prevent pancreatic enzymes reaching the gut and functioning at an optimum pH. Over time this can lead to autolysis and inflammation of the exocrine pancreas, and this prevents movement of digestive enzymes into the duodenum. If left untreated this leads to nutrient malabsorption, failure to thrive and progressive damage of the pancreas owing to auto-digestion of pancreatic tissue by enzymes. There is a correlation between disease severity and pancreatic sufficiency. Pancreatic insufficiency sufferers have class 1, 2 or 3 CFTR mutations.

GASTROINTESTINAL TRACT

CFTR is present on the epithelial cells lining the gastrointestinal tract, leading to reduced secretion of chloride and bicarbonate into the intestinal tract and hyperabsorption of water from the gut. This causes accumulation of viscous mucus and faecal material in the terminal ileum, caecum and ascending colon, leading to obstruction by mucofaeculant material. Meconium ileus and distal intestinal obstructive syndrome (DIOS) occur later in life.

REPRODUCTION

Around 98% of men with CF are infertile owing to abnormal development of the vas deferens *in utero*. This congenital absence of the vas deferens (CAVD) prevents transport of spermatozoa from the testes or epididymis to the penis, resulting in azoospermia. CAVD is also characterised by production of low volume of acidic semen and the fertilising capacity is impaired by dysfunctional CFTR channels located on the surface of sperm. Women with CF are able to have children; most fertility problems arise from co-morbidities such as poor nutrition and/or inadequate management of CFRD.

DIAGNOSIS OF CYSTIC FIBROSIS

One in 25 people are carriers for the CF gene (see Figure 13.1). Many people are unaware that they carry the CF gene until they have a child affected with CF or are identified through the national newborn screening programme. Newborn screening uses a bloodspot to measure immunoreactive trypsin, which can also then be assessed for CF gene

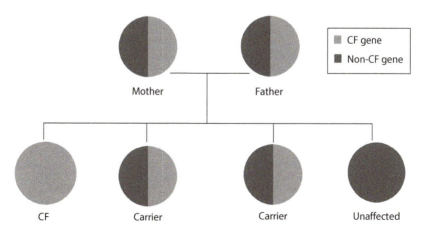

Figure 13.1 Explanation of genetic inheritance.

Table 13.1 List of presenting symptoms for CF

Neonate/infant	Childhood/adolescence	Adult
Routine screening/family history	Recurrent respiratory infections	Recurrent pancreatitis
Failure to thrive	Bowel disturbances/malabsorption	Late-onset bronchiectasis
Meconium ileus	Diabetes symptoms	Unable to conceive
Rectal prolapse	Malnutrition	Nasal polyps/sinus disease
Cough/recurrent chest infections	Sinus disease	Difficult to manage diabetes
	Delayed puberty (due to being underweight)	Arthritis
		Osteopenia/osteoporosis

Note: Diagnosis is made on the presence of two CFTR mutations, a positive sweat test and compatible clinical history.

Table 13.2 Ranges for sweat test results

Sweat test results	Child under 6 months	Over age 6 months (including adults)
CF unlikely	<29 mmol/L	<39 mmol/L
Intermediate (repeat test)	30–59 mmol/L	40–59 mmol/L
CF positive	>60 mmol/L	>60 mmol/L

mutations if necessary (Campbell and White, 2005). The UK CF registry data 2015 have shown that a majority of infants are now diagnosed before the age of 2 months; the most common presentations outside this are failure to thrive and meconium ileus (CFT, 2015a) (see Table 13.1).

Sweat testing and genetic identification are the gold standards for the confirmation of CF as a clinical diagnosis. The salt content of sweat in a CF individual will be high, because of the failure of chloride and sodium reabsorption in sweat ducts with deficient CFTR (Farrell et al., 2008) (see Table 13.2).

TREATMENTS, INTERVENTIONS AND THERAPY

Care of the CF patient is based in hospital and in the community. Regular reviews are required, typically in the outpatient setting in regular clinics. Paediatric patients receive care for their CF through a shared network of providers; visiting local hospitals for regular care and a CF specialist centre once a year for annual reviews. Adult care is organised through attendance of specialist CF centres only. This is due to the increased complexity of adult CF disease.

Clinic reviews involve a multidisciplinary team approach to monitor and assess for signs and symptoms of CF. Clinics are organised so that nosocomial cross-infection between individuals with CF is minimised during hospital visits. Individual segregation is classically used, whereby the CF individual is placed in a clinic room and members of the multidisciplinary team individually assess them. The individual stays in that room for the entirety of their stay. Models of cohorting individuals by microbiology are now being explored to minimise the risk of cross-infection. This is important in CF owing to the high antibiotic use and increasing antibiotic resistance.

While in clinic individuals are assessed and seen by a medical physician with CF expertise, a clinical nurse specialist for CF, respiratory physiotherapist, specialist dietician, psychologist and possibly a social worker.

During a clinic appointment recent chest symptoms or cough, breathlessness, wheeze, sputum production, haemoptysis and recent antibiotics and responses are reviewed. The chest is auscultated; crackles are a typical feature and significant respiratory infection often can occur in the absence of chest signs in patients with CF (see Chapter 2). Wheeze may be audible in those with asthma, with secretions in the airway or with allergic bronchopulmonary aspergillosis (ABPA). Spirometry is performed at each clinic visit and generally plotted in graph form so that loss of function can be more easily interpreted and acted upon.

ANTIBIOTICS

Although antibiotics are the most effective way to treat bacterial infections, they have many complications.

It is important for the patient to be aware of any potential side effects and that they are given specific instructions for the safe administration of any antibiotic prescribed. Photosensitivity may manifest as an exaggerated sunburn reaction, such as blistering of the skin, and patients should be advised to stay out of the sun and where this is not possible to wear a high-factor sunscreen. Most antibiotics have a variety of side effects, such as causing nausea and dizziness, which may be made worse by drinking alcohol (Joint Formulary Committee [JFC], 2015). Alcohol also causes an increase in urination owing to the diuretic effect. This can lead to dehydration, which in CF patients can cause a thickening of secretions.

MICROBIOLOGY OF THE CF LUNG

Bronchopulmonary infection in CF patients is associated with chronic progressive lung disease and episodes of acute exacerbation. Frequent infections in cystic fibrosis are related to the mucus in the airway surface liquid, which is thick and not easily expectorated, trapping bacteria.

Infection is predominantly caused by bacteria, although infections with viruses and fungi may play undervalued roles (see Table 13.3). The organisms infecting a patient will determine the treatment, quality of life, prospects for transplantation and overall survival. The accurate and prompt identification of respiratory pathogens is essential for ensuring timely commencement of eradication treatment for early infection with bacterial pathogens. In addition, the use of appropriate long-term and rescue antibiotics for those with chronic bacterial infection and the application of appropriate infection control measures is essential (CFT, 2010). To ensure each patient has individualised treatment targeting their specific microbiological status, the CFT (2010) recommend that respiratory sampling is undertaken at each hospital visit and at times of respiratory exacerbation. Sputum culture is the recommended specimen for routine sampling and cough swabs are to be used only when the patient cannot expectorate.

REHYDRATION SUPPLEMENTS

Salt (sodium and chloride) depletion may occur in hot weather and during excessive exercise due to an increase in sweating. Salt lost through sweat in CF causes an imbalance in sodium levels in the blood and tissues. This can then decrease the desire to drink, which causes a vicious cycle that can result

Table 13.3 Common organisms associated with pulmonary infection in CF patients

Staphylococcus aureus	Frequently isolated in early infancy but can remain a source of infection in to adulthood. If despite treatment, *S.aureus* continues to be isolated, ensure MRSA not present.
Haemophilus influenza	A natural commensal of the upper respiratory tract and therefore there is the need to distinguish infection from contamination.
Pseudomonas aeruginosa	The most common pathogen in CF with prevalence increasing with age and is associated with a more rapid decline in lung function.
Burkholderia cepacia complex	Usually seen later in the progression of CF and is associated with a significant increase in morbidity and mortality.
Stenotrophamonas maltophilia	Appears intermittently rather than chronically colonising patients; the clinical significance in CF patients is unclear.
Achromobacter xylosoxidans	Clinical significance is unclear but treatment should be considered in chronically colonised patients with deteriorating clinical condition.
Non-tuberculous mycobacteria (NTM)	In particular, *Mycobacterium abscessus* can cause severe disease in CF and are a major therapeutic challenge. Infections with *Mycobacterium avium complex* are also often seen.
Fungal	Infections have become more prevalent in people with CF in recent years. *Aspergillus* infection often presents as allergic bronchopulmonary aspergillosis, which leads to respiratory exacerbations.

Source: Adapted from Chapman, S. et al. 2014. *Oxford Handbook of Respiratory Medicine* (3rd ed.) by permission of Oxford University Press, Oxford.

Table 13.4 PERT dosing summary

Just enough PERT	Normal formed non-greasy stools of normal odour and absence of abdominal pain or excessive and malodorous flatus
Too much PERT	Diarrhoea, offensive stools, soreness around anus
	Constipation may occur occasionally
Increased dose too quickly	Constipation may occur
Too little PERT	Malabsorption (abdominal pain, distension, pale, loose, fatty offensive stool)

in both dehydration and hyponatremia. Patients at risk of dehydration are advised to take salt supplements with an aim to replace depleted salt levels to avoid systemic dehydration and in turn thickened secretions.

PANCREATIC ENZYME REPLACEMENT THERAPY (PERT)

The pancreas produces enzymes that help to break down food into nutrients. In CF most people have exocrine pancreatic insufficiency, so require artificial pancreatic enzymes to improve the digestion of fats, proteins and sugars from food. The dosing of PERT will reflect differing degrees of residual pancreatic function, the type of enzyme preparation and pathophysiological factors such as intestinal pH. Dosing will also be influenced by the patient's bowel habit, which includes bowel opening frequency, character of stool and abdominal symptoms, compared to the fat content of food and satisfactory body weight (see Table 13.4).

PERT should be taken just before and during all fat containing meals, snacks and drinks. In addition, the person with CF will also be prescribed vitamin supplements (including the fat-soluble vitamins A, D, E and K).

NUTRITION

The aim of nutritional care is to achieve and maintain optimum nutritional status and normal weight/

height ratio in infants/children or a body mass index (BMI) above 19.0 kg/m^2 in adults. The effects of pancreatic insufficiency should be controlled with PERT and the patient will have adequate serum levels of fat soluble vitamins (CFT, 2002).

For those with CF, optimum nutritional status is associated with improved growth, weight gain and maintenance of pulmonary function. Achieving nutritional targets can be challenging as the energy and protein intake requirements are raised for CF patients due to a number of reasons which include:

- The impaired absorption of fat, carbohydrate and protein compromises energy balance and nutritional status
- Inadequate diet or anorexia from respiratory disease/chronic infections, abdominal symptoms or clinical depression leads to reduction in energy intake
- The lung disease associated with CF increases energy requirements, because of the increased energy involved in breathing and recurrent lung infections

The dietician will tailor the advice given to the individual's lifestyle, using specific energy equations based on basal metabolic rate, forced expiratory volume in 1 second (FEV_1), age, gender, weight and physical activity level. Patients with poor lung function may require up to 5000 kcal/day to maintain weight, which is difficult with normal diet alone.

Dietetic review will also include PERT dosing, vitamin supplementation, as well as nutritional supplements and/or long-term overnight enteral feeding via naso-gastric or gastrostomy tube.

DISTAL INTESTINAL OBSTRUCTIVE SYNDROME (DIOS)

CF patients are at risk of developing distal intestinal obstructive syndrome (DIOS). This is when abnormally viscid faecal material causes gradual narrowing of the terminal ileum, with partial or complete obstruction. This can be precipitated by dehydration and infection, but occasionally spontaneous obstruction can also occur.

One of the main symptoms is abdominal pain, which is often of gradual onset, colicky, usually referred to the right lower quadrant, which is tender on palpation, and a small mass may be felt. It can occur at any time and may wake people from sleeping. Further symptoms include abdominal distention, nausea, vomiting, loss of appetite and reduction in frequency of bowel movements. Abdominal X-ray may show a foamy gas pattern in the right flank, with possible dilated small bowel loops.

The main management of DIOS includes rehydration, non-opioid analgesia for pain relief and laxatives. Most cases will resolve with conservative management using mild laxatives or with bowel cleansing preparations; surgical intervention is rarely required. Other differential diagnoses of abdominal pain include simple constipation, intussusception or small bowel obstruction owing to adhesions, appendicitis or colonic malignancy. Depending on severity, patients are advised to have a light diet or fluids only while taking bowel treatments to clear any blockage. In acute cases the patient will be 'nil by mouth' and a naso-gastric tube may be necessary. Recurrences of DIOS are common, so patients are advised about hydration, adequate PERT and to consider the daily use of laxatives to help prevent further episodes.

PHYSIOTHERAPY

The main aim of physiotherapy is to prevent further airway damage caused by increased resistance and obstruction from secretions, with the use of airway clearance techniques such as active cycle of breathing technique (ACBT) or autogenic drainage (AD). If pulmonary secretions become more difficult to mobilise, the patient is more at risk of complications associated with retention of secretions. These thickened secretions take more effort for the patient to move, leading to fatigue and further impaired airway clearance. Adjuncts are used in the treatment of these patients to include positive expiratory pressure (PEP) such as PEP mask or Pari-PEP and oscillating PEP technology (Acapella or Flutter devices) to assist in the clearance of the viscous secretions. These devices can help with reducing airway obstruction, improve ventilation, delay progression of respiratory disease and maintain the individual's optimal respiratory function (Association of Charted Physiotherapists in CF [ACPCF], 2011).

The CF physiotherapist will also work with individuals to improve their exercise tolerance, look at specific exercises to target reduced bone mineral density and educate on appropriate airway clearance regimens and optimal timing for inhalation therapies. Additional support may also be provided to those using non-invasive ventilation, whether it is required for exercise, airway clearance, acute respiratory failure or nocturnal ventilation for hypercapnia. Part of the advisory role of the physiotherapist will include posture and thoracic mobility, management of haemoptysis, pneumothorax, pregnancy, post-lung transplant, urinary stress incontinence, as well as support during end-stage disease and end-of-life care (ACPCF, 2011).

LONG-TERM CARE

As CF is a long-term chronic condition, collaborative working with the patient and their families is essential in maintaining standards and improving outcomes (CFT, 2015b). Many people with CF manage their care as outpatients with occasional inpatient admissions, but this may increase with the severity of their condition.

Since the faulty gene that causes cystic fibrosis was identified in 1989, scientists have been involved in international research collaborations to investigate ways to correct the defective gene. In 2012 Ivacaftor (Kalydeco), the first medication to target the underlying cause of CF rather than the symptoms, received Food and Drug Administration (FDA) approval and has gone on to improve the health status of many CF sufferers. This medication is effective in approximately 5.7% of the CF population in the UK who have the G551D mutation in at least one copy of their CFTR gene as it targets one of the most common mutations of the defective gene (CFT, 2015a). Further research is currently being conducted in the hope of developing a similar drug that works on other mutations of the gene. While these developments are exciting and revolutionary, research into other treatment alternatives continues to target the management of symptoms such as sputum retention, airways infection and inflammation. Overall, research continues to seek ways to suppress the progression of the disease process (Ratjen, 2009).

For some patients, disease deterioration is inevitable, and for those patients lung transplantation may become an option. For most patients, the decision to have a transplant is an intensely difficult and personal one. Despite great advances in CF care and treatment, many people will reach a stage where a lung transplant has the potential to be the only viable option to enhance quality of life and prolong life expectancy. The referral for transplantation needs to be started early enough to avoid the patient deteriorating to the point where death on the transplant list becomes likely. Currently, one in three CF patients will die while waiting on the list and will never receive a donor lung (CFT, 2015b).

As patients with CF are living longer and in good health, many women are choosing to become parents. Many pregnancies have been reported in the literature and it is clear that, although the outcome for the baby is generally good and some others do well, others find that their CF complicates the pregnancy or that the pregnancy adversely affects their disease severity (Edenborough et al., 2008). Most women with CF become pregnant without any difficulty. Fertility problems that do occur may be related to general ill health, low weight, or poor control of CF-related diabetes mellitus (Johannesson, 2002; Stallings et al., 2005). Pregnancy in women with CF would ideally involve careful consideration and co-ordination of the CF and obstetric teams with a combined objective to optimise the mother's health. Before conception, consideration should be made of nutritional state, psychosocial issues, genetic issues and the potential effects on the foetus that the current treatment regime may have and drugs may need to be stopped or changed during pregnancy; preconception lung function is recommended to be >60% (Conway et al., 2008) of predicted as lung function lower than this is thought to be a predictor of worse prognosis. During pregnancy, it is expected that the mother will need more intensive input from her CF centre, often requiring IV antibiotics, increased physiotherapy support and nutritional supplements.

CASE STUDY

Emma is a 23-year-old, who attended a routine outpatient appointment 2 days prior to a holiday with friends. Five days prior to her appointment her sputum volume had started to increase, becoming green in colour and more viscous. She had sent a sputum sample in to the hospital via her GP. The results were reviewed at her clinic appointment and this confirmed that she was experiencing a mild exacerbation due to *Pseudomonas aeruginosa* and *Staphylococcus aureus* infections. She was given a 2-week prescription for Flucloxacillin 1 g qds and Ciprofloxacin 750 mg bd to take with her. Advice was given regarding alcohol and antibiotics, as well as the photosensitivity side effect of ciprofloxacin, taking sensible precautions with the use of a high-factor sun cream, wearing a hat and avoiding full sunlight (JFC, 2015). She was also given a prescription for salt (slow sodium) tablets and reminded to drink plenty of water to reduce the risk of dehydration.

Her parents contacted the team, as on day six of her 10-day holiday she was returning home on the next available flight. Emma was brought to the hospital for urgent review.

On arrival, it was obvious she had blistering of the skin, as a result of taking her Ciprofloxacin when sunbathing in direct sunlight. Emma complained of some abdominal pain, bloating and constipation as a result of dehydration. She had been drinking a lot of alcohol and not much water in the hot weather and had been taking her salt supplements sporadically. This had led to a build-up of hard, dehydrated stool in the bowel, which if left untreated could become a surgical emergency. This systemic dehydration also had an effect on her chest secretions. It had led to thick, viscous secretions in the airways, which Emma was finding very difficult to move using her usual physiotherapy airway clearance techniques.

Emma was reviewed by the multidisciplinary team (MDT) and the treatment regime required input from the nursing and physiotherapy teams, the dietitian, doctors and the pharmacist. The decision was made to admit her to the CF/respiratory ward to administer intravenous (IV) fluids, IV antibiotics and medications to help with the skin blistering and also to assist the passing of the hardened stool, while observing for signs of DIOS. After 3 days in hospital Emma returned home to complete her 2-week course of IV antibiotics, with weekly reviews by the nurse and physiotherapist. Emma's bowel symptoms resolved with mild laxatives and increased fluids. The dietician spent time with her, reviewing her PERT dosing with her usual diet and plans for her to complete a diet and dosing diary, so they could review her actual enzyme dosing requirements.

CASE STUDY DISCUSSION

The above case is an example of how one CF patient could require multiple members of the CF team to assist in the general maintenance and management of their acute and ongoing care. CF is a complex disease, which requires a multidisciplinary approach and this case confirms the importance of working within a knowledgeable and skilled MDT. This involves utilising knowledge, skills and best practice from across service providers to reach solutions based on an improved collective understanding of patients' complex needs. To enable CF teams to provide improved health and well-being outcomes for patients through co-ordinated care delivery, the MDT attends ward rounds and meet weekly to discuss patients' care, each member of the MDT contributing their specialist area of expertise to ensure a well-rounded approach to care.

SUMMARY

Cystic fibrosis is a common genetic condition that leads to disruption of salt and water transfer in and out of cells. It can affect numerous organs in the body, but major effects are seen on the respiratory and digestive systems where thick mucus and secretions can block the lungs and intestines. CF was once considered a disease of childhood, but over half of sufferers with CF now live on into adulthood and therefore require expert adult services to help them manage their disease. People affected by CF will require life-long medications, supplements and follow up and may suffer from a number of complications of the disease. An expert MDT is essential in the care of patients with CF. Newer medications that target the defective gene have recently become available and it is hoped that developments in this type of therapy will continue. In the meantime, treatment aims to target the management of symptoms, prevent infection and other complications and maintain a healthy weight.

REFERENCES

Andersen, D.H. 1938. Cystic fibrosis of the pancreas and its relation to celiac disease: A clinical and pathological study. *American Journal of Diseases of Children* 56 (2): 344–399.

Association of Chartered Physiotherapist in Cystic Fibrosis (ACPCF). 2011. *Standards of Care and Good Clinical Practice for the Physiotherapy Management of Cystic Fibrosis* (1st ed.). Cystic Fibrosis Trust, Bromley.

Campbell III, P.W. and White, T.B. 2005. Newborn screening for cystic fibrosis: An opportunity to improve care and outcomes. *Journal of Pediatrics* 147 (3): S2–S5.

Chapman, S., Robinson, G., Stradling, J., West, S. and Wrightson, J. 2014. *Oxford Handbook of Respiratory Medicine.* (3rd ed.). Oxford University Press, Oxford.

Conway, S.P., Brownlee, K.G., Peckham, D.G. and Lee, T.W.R. 2008. *Cystic Fibrosis in Children and Adults. The Leeds Methods of Management* (7th ed.). St. James's & Seacroft University Hospitals Leeds Teaching Hospitals Trust, Leeds.

Cystic Fibrosis Trust (CFT). 2002. *Nutritional Management of Cystic Fibrosis.* Cystic Fibrosis Trust, Bromley.

Cystic Fibrosis Trust (CFT). 2010. *Laboratory Standards for Processing Microbiological Samples from People with Cystic Fibrosis (CF)* (1st ed.). Cystic Fibrosis, Bromley.

Cystic Fibrosis Trust (CFT). 2015a. *UK Cystic Fibrosis Registry Annual Data Report 2014.* Cystic Fibrosis Trust, Bromley.

Cystic Fibrosis Trust (CFT). 2015b. *Transplants in Cystic Fibrosis*. Cystic Fibrosis Trust, Bromley.

Dodge, J.A., Lewis, P.A., Stanton, M. and Wilsher, J. 2007. Cystic fibrosis mortality and survival in the UK: 1947–2003. *European Respiratory Journal* 29: 522–526.

Donaldson, S.H. and Boucher, R.C. 2007. Sodium channels and cystic fibrosis. *Chest* 132 (5): 1631–1636.

Edenborough, F.P., Borgo, G., Knoop, C., Lannefors, L., Mackenzie, W.E., Madge, S., Morton, A.M. et al. 2008. Guidelines for the management of pregnancy in women with cystic fibrosis. *Journal of Cystic Fibrosis* 7 (Suppl. 1): S2–S32.

Farrell, P.M., Rosenstein, B.J., White, T.B., Accurso, F.J., Castellani, C., Cutting, G.R., Durie, P.R. et al. 2008. Guidelines for diagnosis of cystic fibrosis in newborns through older adults: Cystic Fibrosis Foundation Consensus Report. *Journal of Pediatrics* 153 (2): S4–S14.

Johannesson, M. 2002. Effects of pregnancy on health: Certain aspects of importance for women with cystic fibrosis. *Journal of Cystic Fibrosis* 1 (1): 9–12.

Joint Formulary Committee (JFC). 2015. *British National Formulary* (68th ed.). British Medical Association and Royal Pharmaceutical Society of Great Britain, London.

Kerem, B.S., Rommens, J.M., Buchanan, J.A., Markiewicz, D., Cox, T.K., Chakravarti, A., Buchwald, M. and Tsui, L.C. 1989. Identification of the cystic fibrosis gene: Genetic analysis. *Science* 245 (4922): 1073–1080.

Mackie, A.D.R., Thornton, S.J. and Edenborough, F. 2003. Cystic fibrosis related diabetes. *Diabetes Medicine* 20 (6): 425–436.

Pettit, R.S. and Fellner, C. 2014. CFTR modulators for the treatment of cystic fibrosis. *Pharmacy and Therapeutics* 39 (7): 500–511.

Quittner, A.L., Schechter, M.S., Rasouilyan, L., Haselkorn, T., Pasta, D.J. and Wagener, J.S. 2010. Impact of socioeconomic status, race and ethnicity on quality of life in patients with cystic fibrosis in the United States. *Chest* 137 (3): 642–650.

Ratjen, F.A. 2009. Cystic fibrosis: Pathogenesis and future treatment strategies. *Respiratory Care* 54 (5): 595–601.

Sosnay, P.R., Siklosi, K.R., Van Goor, F., Kaniecki, K., Yu, H., Sharma, N., Ramalho, A.S. et al. 2013. Defining the disease liability of variants in the cystic fibrosis transmembrance conductance regulator gene. *Nature Genetics* 45 (10): 1160–1167.

Stallings, V.A., Tomezsko, J.L., Schall, J.I., Mascarenhas, M.R., Stettler, N., Scanlin, T.F. and Zemel, B.S. 2005. Adolescent development and energy expenditure in females with cystic fibrosis. *Clinical Nutrition* 24 (5): 737–745.

Tsui, L.C., Buchwald, M., Barker, D., Braman, J.C., Knowlton, R., Schumm, J.W., Eiberg, H., Mohr, J., Kennedy, D. and Plavsic, N. 1985. Cystic fibrosis locus defined by a genetically linked polymorphic DNA marker. *Science* 230 (4729): 1054–1057.

World Health Organisation (WHO). 2015. Genes and human disease. http://www.who.int/genomics/public/geneticdiseases/en/index2.html#CF. Accessed 26 April 2015.

Zielenski, J. 2000. Genotype and phenotype in cystic fibrosis. *Respiration* 67 (2): 117–133.

Thoracic surgery

14

JENNY MITCHELL

LEARNING OBJECTIVES

Upon completion of this chapter the reader should be able to:

- Describe common types of thoracic surgical operation
- Describe the reasons for performing thoracic surgery
- Identify the assessment required to evaluate a patient's fitness for thoracic surgery
- Understand the pre-operative assessment and education required by thoracic surgery patients
- Describe the important issues and their management when caring for patients after thoracic surgery

INTRODUCTION

Thoracic surgery refers to surgery on any structure in the thorax excluding the heart. Surgery aims to treat diseases and anomalies of the neck, oesophagus, trachea, chest wall, diaphragm, mediastinum, pleura, lung and airways. It can be diagnostic, curative, cosmetic or palliative for chronic or acute conditions or diseases. In the United Kingdom (UK) and Ireland 60% of thoracic surgical procedures are carried out for treatment of primary lung cancer (The Society for Cardiothoracic Surgery in Great Britain and Ireland [SCTS], 2011). In the UK, patients with primary lung cancer follow defined pathways for diagnosis and treatment; these pathways include guidance on referral for thoracic surgery based on clinical evidence (National Institute for Health and Care Excellence [NICE], 2011). The remaining 40% of surgical procedures are for other malignancies or benign conditions (SCTS, 2011). This chapter focusses on surgery for common respiratory conditions (lung cancer, pneumothorax, empyema, chronic obstructive pulmonary disease [COPD]). Key learning points are illustrated with a case study.

TYPES OF THORACIC SURGERY

Traditionally, lung resection has been carried out with a thoracotomy approach. More recently video-assisted thoracoscopic surgery (VATS) has been used for an increasing number of surgical interventions. In addition, other surgical approaches such as median sternotomy, suprasternal incisions, anterior mediastinotomy and vertical axillary thoracotomy may be used in appropriate circumstances (Deslauriers and Mehran, 2005).

THORACOTOMY

A thoracotomy incision is the standard incision for thoracic surgery and is used to give access to the structures on one side of the chest (Marshall, 2006). A posterolateral thoracotomy starts at the mid auxiliary line over the fifth or sixth intercostal space and runs posteriorly following the intercostal space (Urschel and Cooper, 1995). In a muscle-sparing thoracotomy the same incision is used but the latissimus dorsi is mobilised and retracted rather than being divided (Deslauriers and Mehran, 2005). A muscle-sparing thoracotomy causes less pain and loss of muscle function post-operatively, but provides poorer access to the chest in comparison to the standard incision (Li et al., 2014; Uzzaman et al., 2014).

VIDEO-ASSISTED THORACOSCOPIC SURGERY (VATS)

VATS surgery has developed with the introduction and development of new technologies in surgical light and instrument design (Begum et al., 2014). In the UK 35% of all thoracic surgical operations are carried out using a VATS technique (SCTS, 2011); across Europe this figure is 25% (European Society of Thoracic Surgeons [ESTS] Database Committee, 2014).

VATS surgery involves two to four incisions – one for the camera, held by the first assistant, and additional ports for the instruments used by the surgeon. Monitors are used for visualisation of the operative field (Leao, 2006). The advantages of a VATS approach over a more traditional thoracotomy are less pain post-operatively, less post-operative dyspnoea and earlier return to normal daily activities (Demmy and Curtis, 1999; Andreetti et al., 2014). In addition, patients undergoing VATS resection for primary lung cancer are able to start adjuvant therapy earlier than those having resection via thoracotomy (Teh et al., 2014). Most of the surgical procedures performed by thoracic surgeons can now be performed using a VATS technique and some surgeons argue that this should be the approach of choice in all suitable patients due to the demonstrated benefits (Begum et al., 2014).

LUNG RESECTION

Surgical removal of part or whole of a lung is most commonly performed as treatment for cancer. In the UK 60% of all lung resections performed in 2010 were for primary lung cancer (SCTS, 2011) (see Chapter 11 for detailed information on diagnosis and treatment of primary lung cancer).

Lung resection may also be performed to remove neuroendocrine tumours, metastatic disease and benign lesions. Surgery is performed to remove lung metastases if the primary tumour is controlled, metastatic disease is confined to the lungs and can be completely removed by surgery, and the patient is fit for surgery (Deslauriers and Mehran, 2005; Younes et al., 2009). Patients with primary colorectal carcinoma represent the largest group undergoing pulmonary metastasectomy (Treasure et al., 2008).

Neuroendocrine tumours are malignancies arising from neuroendocrine cells; the most common sites for tumours to occur are the gastrointestinal and pulmonary systems (Fisseler-Eckhoff and Demes, 2012). Typical and atypical carcinoid tumours are low and intermediate grade neuroendocrine malignancies (Litzky, 2010). They are classified using lung cancer tumour node metastases (TNM) staging (Travis et al., 2008; Gridelli et al., 2013), please see Chapter 11 for more information on lung cancer staging. Surgical removal is the treatment of choice for localised neuroendocrine tumours, with the aim of preserving as much normal lung tissue as possible (Oberg et al., 2010; Gridelli et al., 2013).

FITNESS FOR THORACIC SURGERY

Fitness for surgery is assessed using a number of clinical measures (Brunelli et al., 2009; Lim et al., 2010; NICE, 2011):

- Thoracoscore is a risk assessment tool that is used to predict the risk of death in patients being considered for lung resection. It uses nine variables to predict the risk of in-hospital death based on data from a large study cohort (Falcoz et al., 2007) (see Table 14.1). A number

Table 14.1 Thoracoscore

Category	Variables
Sex	Male
	Female
Age	Below 55 years
	Between 55 and 64 years
	Over 64 years
American Society of Anaesthesiologists (ASA) score	1. Is healthy
	2. Has a moderate systemic disease
	3. Is limited but not incapacitated
	4. Has a life-threatening disease
	5. Has a life expectancy <24 hours
WHO performance status (PS)	0. Is normally active
	1. Cannot carry out heavy physical tasks
	2. Is active >50% of the time
	3. Is at rest >50% of the time
	4. Is at rest 100% of the time
Medical Research Council (MRC) dyspnoea score	0. No dyspnoea
	1. Dyspnoea after going up 2 flights of stairs
	2. Dyspnoea after going up 1 flight of stairs
	3. Dyspnoea when walking on the level
	4. Dyspnoea when walking slowly
	5. Dyspnoea at the slightest effort
Priority for surgery	Scheduled
	Urgent
	Emergency
Procedure	Pneumonectomy
	Other
Diagnosis group	Benign
	Malignant
Number of co-morbidities	0
	1 or 2
	Over 2

Source: Adapted from Falcoz, P.E. et al. 2007. *The Journal of Thoracic and Cardiovascular Surgery* 133 (2): 325–332.

of internet and mobile application tools are available to calculate the score.

- Lung function should be assessed in all patients being considered for thoracic surgery. Forced expiratory volume in 1 second (FEV_1) should be greater than 30% unless the patient has significant heterogeneous emphysema in the resection target when the lung volume reduction effect of surgery will allow patients with a lower FEV_1 to be considered as surgical candidates. Carbon monoxide transfer factor (T_{LCO}) should be measured in all patients; a reading below 30% indicates a high-risk candidate for surgery. Patients with a FEV_1 or T_{LCO} less than 30% can be offered surgery if they understand and are willing to accept the risk of post-operative dyspnoea.

- Exercise tolerance is assessed using a standardised symptom limited stair climbing test where the patient should achieve 22 metres or shuttle walk test with a minimum walk of 400 metres.

- Patients with a history of cardiac disease or with new cardiac symptoms and those unable to climb two flights of stairs on testing should be referred for cardiac assessment. Surgery can be considered once intervention for cardiac conditions is complete or medical therapy is optimised.
- Smoking cessation prior to surgery, for a minimum of 2–4 weeks, is recommended to reduce the post-operative complications associated with a sudden cessation of smoking at the time of surgery (Nakagawa et al., 2001).

WEDGE RESECTION

A small wedge of lung containing a tumour or abnormal area is removed. This is most commonly performed with a stapler that seals and cuts the lung tissue. A wedge resection can be performed to biopsy an area of diseased lung in order to gain a diagnosis or to remove a tumour. Patients with lung metastases who are suitable for surgery commonly have a wedge resection. Wedge resections are also performed for primary lung cancer where the patient is not suitable for a lobectomy (NICE, 2011).

LOBECTOMY

A lobectomy is the removal of one or more of the five lobes of the lungs. This is the gold standard treatment for lung cancer (Brunelli et al., 2009). A segmental resection is a sub-lobar resection along anatomical boundaries. A sub-lobar resection may be performed in patients with poor lung function who would not tolerate a lobectomy (NICE, 2011).

PNEUMONECTOMY

A pneumonectomy is removal of a whole lung. This operation is performed to remove disease that involves all of the lobes of the lung on one side of the chest or the proximal airway. Pneumonectomy is associated with high morbidity (30.4%) and mortality (5.6%) rates and is only performed where other surgical approaches would not give complete removal of disease (Shapiro et al., 2010; NICE, 2011). Post-operative complications include cardiac arrhythmias, chest infection, respiratory failure, pulmonary embolism and broncho-pleural fistula and are a consequence of

the removal of the lung along with its associated circulation (Shapiro et al., 2010; Pricopi et al., 2015).

SLEEVE RESECTION

A sleeve resection is the removal of a lobe of the lung along with part of the bronchus that attaches to it; usually for disease that involves part of the proximal airway. The remaining lobe(s) is then reconnected to the remaining segment of the bronchus (Deslauriers and Mehran, 2005; Kaiser, 2006). This procedure preserves part of the lung and is an alternative to removing the whole lung. Patients require careful respiratory assessment post-operatively as they have a suture line in their airway.

CHEST WALL RESECTION AND RESECTION OF OTHER CHEST STRUCTURES

Resection of other major structures within the thorax (such as the major blood vessels, diaphragm, thymus gland or oesophagus) may be performed along with lung resection when a tumour invades these adjacent structures. The resected area will be reconstructed with appropriate materials (Deslauriers and Mehran, 2005).

SURGERY TO TREAT PNEUMOTHORAX

The aim of surgery in patients who have had a pneumothorax is to achieve lung expansion and pleurodesis (adhesion of the pleural surfaces). Procedures are normally carried out using a VATS approach, although some patients may require open surgery via a thoracotomy incision (see Chapter 8 for more details regarding types and causes of pneumothorax). The components of a surgical approach to preventing further pneumothorax can involve:

BULLECTOMY

Bulla and blebs are removed by staple excision (Shaikhrezai et al., 2011). Bullectomy will be performed where bulla or blebs are present on inspection during surgery (MacDuff et al., 2010).

PLEURECTOMY

The parietal pleura is removed; this causes adhesions to form between the visceral pleura and the chest wall preventing further pneumothorax (Rena et al., 2008).

CHEMICAL PLEURODESIS

A substance is insufflated into the pleural cavity with the aim of causing pleural irritation and inflammation, which leads to formation of adhesions between the two membranes, preventing further pneumothorax (Light, 2003; Shaikhrezai et al., 2011). British Thoracic Society (BTS) guidelines recommend the use of medical-grade sterile talc as the agent of choice for surgical chemical pleurodesis (MacDuff et al., 2010).

SURGERY TO TREAT PLEURAL INFECTION/EMPYEMA

Patients who have failed to respond to treatment of pleural infection after 5–7 days should be considered for surgery (Davies et al., 2010; Kwon, 2014) (see Chapter 8 for more detail concerning pleural infection). Surgical treatment aims to clear infection from the pleural cavity, allowing lung expansion. If a thickened wall has developed around the infection this will be removed (decortication) (Molnar, 2007). In the fibrinopurulent stage of empyema development VATS debridement/decortication of the infected pleural space is an effective treatment with reduced length of stay post-operatively and a reduction in the complication rate compared to thoracotomy (Chambers et al., 2010). In the chronic stage of empyema, a thoracotomy and decortication is the treatment of choice. This will improve pulmonary function in symptomatic patients but functional lung damage resulting from the pleural infection will leave the patient with long-term impairment in pulmonary function (Molnar, 2007).

LUNG VOLUME REDUCTION PROCEDURES FOR TREATMENT OF COPD

See Chapter 5 for information on the medical management of COPD. Lung volume reduction surgery aims to remove the least functional part of a COPD

patient's lung, allowing increased ventilation in the remaining healthier lung (Fishman et al., 2003; NICE, 2005; Clark et al., 2014). This can be performed using a VATS approach, by thoracotomy or median sternotomy (NICE, 2005). A large multicentre randomised trail comparing lung volume reduction surgery to medical therapy for COPD demonstrated improved exercise capacity, quality of life, lung function and dyspnoea in patients with upper lobe predominant emphysema and a pre-operative FEV_1 >20%. These benefits persisted for up to 2 years but came with a higher initial mortality than the medical therapy group (30-day mortality 2.2% for surgery compared to 0.2% for the medical therapy group). Over the 2-year trial the mortality per-person-year was not significantly different (0.09% in the surgery group compared to 0.10% in the medical therapy group) (Fishman et al., 2003). It is important that a multidisciplinary team approach is used to ensure appropriate patient selection and management in this high-risk group of patients (Aziz et al., 2010; Clark et al., 2014).

Endobronchial valves are one-way valves that are placed into airways leading to hyperinflated areas of the emphysematous lung. They allow air and secretions to exit the alveoli distal to the valve and prevent air from entering. This leads to collapse of the hyperinflated lung distal to the valve and improves ventilation in the remaining lung. They are placed using a flexible bronchoscope under either sedation or general anaesthetic (Du Rand et al., 2011). Patient selection requires a multidisciplinary approach to ensure patients are suitable for this treatment, in particular that they have heterogeneous emphysema suitable for targeting with valves. A randomised control trial of one of the valves available has demonstrated improvements in lung function, exercise tolerance and symptoms but is associated with an increase in haemoptysis and COPD exacerbations (Sciurba et al., 2010).

PATIENT CARE

PRE-OPERATIVE ASSESSMENT

Patients undergoing thoracic surgery require pre-operative assessment of the risks of surgery along with education on the expected post-operative course and rehabilitation (National Lung Cancer

Forum for Nurses [NLCFN], 2013). Assessment prior to admission is important to:

- Identify medical issues which need further investigation, allowing for timely referral and preventing delays to the patient's pathway.
- Begin patient education prior to admission, as verbal patient information along with the provision of good quality written patient information allows patients time to learn about the procedure they will undergo.
- Have individual discussions with the patient and their family/carers which give them time to make appropriate arrangements for their admission and arrange support for their discharge (NHS Institute for Innovation and Improvement, 2008).

Research has demonstrated that pre-operative education can decrease length of stay, improve patient satisfaction and reduce the amount of analgesia required by patients (Garretson, 2004). Good quality written information combined with verbal information should be provided to all patients pre-operatively (NLCFN, 2014).

SMOKING CESSATION

Evidence demonstrates that the risk of in-hospital death and pulmonary complications after thoracic surgery is significantly higher for smokers than non-smokers (Mason et al., 2009). Smoking has many physiological effects including hypersecretion of mucus in the airways, along with airway narrowing and a reduced ability to clear airway secretions (Ambrose and Barua, 2004; Møller and Tønnesen, 2006). All current smokers who are being considered for thoracic surgical intervention should be encouraged to stop smoking as soon as possible prior to surgery (Nakagawa et al., 2001; Barrera et al., 2005; Mason et al., 2009). A range of smoking cessation interventions may be needed to help patients to stop smoking successfully and are explained in more detail in Chapter 18 (Huber and Mahajan, 2008).

PAIN MANAGEMENT

Thoracic surgery is painful, both thoracotomy and VATS incisions can cause severe pain. Intercostal

drains are also painful. Up to 50% of post-operative patients will complain of chronic pain after thoracic surgery with up to half of this group suffering from neuropathic pain, which is pain related to nerve damage (Steegers et al., 2008; Searle et al., 2009). Mobilisation and exercise are essential to recovery after surgery but these activities cause pain. Side effects from analgesics are common in thoracic surgery patients: common side effects are constipation, nausea and psychological disturbances (Joint Formulary Committee [JFC], 2014).

TYPES OF ANALGESIA

THORACIC EPIDURAL ANALGESIA

A thoracic epidural is inserted pre-operatively by the anaesthetist. The aim of a thoracic epidural is to selectively block pain from the site of surgery by infusion of a combination of local anaesthetic and opioid analgesia (McLeod and Cumming, 2004). Patients with thoracic epidural analgesia require regular monitoring of their vital signs, pain level and degree of motor and sensory block. Complications of thoracic epidural analgesia include hypotension, urinary retention, nausea and vomiting, respiratory depression, central nervous system toxicity, dislodgement of the epidural catheter and infection of the catheter site (Sawhney, 2012). Local guidelines for the management of epidural infusions should be followed when caring for a patient with a thoracic epidural infusion.

When discontinuing thoracic epidural analgesia care should be taken to ensure the patient receives adequate oral or intravenous step-down analgesia. Where possible, advice from a specialist pain team should be taken to ensure the patient continues to receive adequate pain relief.

THORACIC PARA-VERTEBRAL BLOCK

A thoracic para-vertebral block is an injection or infusion of local anaesthetic in the para-vertebral space which contains the thoracic spinal nerves and sympathetic trunk. When used in the thoracic surgery setting a para-vertebral block can be inserted by the anaesthetist prior to the start of surgery or by the surgeon during surgery under direct visualisation (Iyer and Yadav, 2013). They are usually used in a multimodal approach to pain relief along with opioid infusion or oral analgesia.

Table 14.2 Post-operative analgesia

Drug	Indication	Side effects
Strong opioid analgesics:		
Morphine	Severe acute pain	Sedation
		Respiratory depression
		Constipation
		Nausea and vomiting
		Itching
		Tolerance and dependence
		Euphoria
Oxycodone	Severe acute pain where morphine is not tolerated	Same as morphine but patients often tolerate oxycodone better
Weak opioid analgesics:		
Tramadol	Moderate to severe acute pain	Dizziness
		Convulsions
Codeine	Moderate to severe acute pain	Constipation
Other analgesic medication:		
Paracetamol	Mild to moderate pain, use in combination with weak opioid analgesics for a synergistic effect	Occasional allergic skin reactions
		Liver damage with overdose
Ibuprofen	Mild to moderate pain	Gastrointestinal disturbances
		Hypersensitivity reactions
Gabapentin	Neuropathic pain	Sedation
		Gastrointestinal disturbances

Source: Adapted from Joint Formulary Committee (JFC), *British National Formulary (BNF)* (68th ed.), BMJ Group and RPS Publishing, London, 2014; Rang, H. et al. *Rang and Dale's Pharmacology* (7th ed.), Elsevier Churchill Livingstone, Edinburgh, 2011.

The infusion of local anaesthetic via a paravertebral catheter will spread into the epidural space, giving some epidural analgesia effect. However, the incidence of side effects (hypotension, urinary retention, nausea and vomiting) are lower than in thoracic epidural analgesia (Piraccini et al., 2011). Other rare complications associated with para-vertebral blocks are pneumothorax, pleural puncture and vascular puncture. Studies have demonstrated that thoracic para-vertebral blocks offer similar pain relief and a superior safety profile to thoracic epidural analgesia (Daly and Myles, 2009; Piraccini et al., 2011).

As thoracic para-vertebral blocks are usually used in a multimodal approach to pain management they can be discontinued when appropriate and the oral or intravenous analgesia used alongside the block continued or increased to give adequate step-down analgesia.

PATIENT-CONTROLLED ANALGESIA

Patient-controlled analgesia (PCA) may be used alone or as part of a combined approach to pain relief in conjunction with a para-vertebral block. Strong opioid analgesics such as morphine or oxycodone are the most common drugs used in PCA pumps. PCA should be used in accordance with local guidelines and the patient closely monitored for the side effects of strong opioid analgesia such as respiratory depression, nausea and vomiting, pruritus, constipation, hallucinations and nightmares (Rang et al., 2011). It is important to monitor the patient's pain using a recognised pain score and to control side effects such as nausea and vomiting and constipation if the patient is to continue to use the PCA pump successfully (Chumbley and Mountford, 2010).

ORAL ANALGESIA

Oral analgesia is important for the management of post-operative pain once epidural or PCA pumps have been discontinued. It can be used in conjunction with a para-vertebral block. A standard analgesia prescription for an in-patient might include regular administration of a weak opioid analgesia plus a non-steroidal anti-inflammatory drug (NSAID) and paracetamol with a strong opioid prescribed on a PRN basis for breakthrough pain. See Table 14.2 for drugs commonly used for post-operative pain relief along with their side effects.

The effectiveness of the prescribed analgesia should be regularly monitored and advice sought from the specialist pain team if required. It is important that patients receive education about post-operative pain relief both prior to their surgery and during the post-operative period. Patients should be discharged with the same analgesia regime as they have received in hospital along with advice on how to continue to manage their pain at home and how to slowly step-down their analgesia once their pain starts to reduce. Pain levels should continue to be monitored on subsequent follow-up and treated aggressively if not controlled (Gottschalk et al., 2006).

PSYCHOLOGICAL CARE

Patients undergoing thoracic surgery can be under a great deal of psychological stress at the time of their surgery. In addition to stress related to undergoing surgery with its associated risks many patients have recently been diagnosed with cancer or are aware that they may have cancer. Studies have demonstrated that up to half of patients diagnosed with cancer report psychological distress (Vachon, 2006). Nurses play an important role in supporting patients at this difficult time. Legg (2011) cites good communication which provides an empathetic approach, and the provision of good quality information that is understood by the patient as important in supporting cancer patients. It is also important to be aware of the specialist resources available to patients locally, such as provision of specialist cancer nursing services and patient support groups.

Patients having surgery for non-malignant pathology may also suffer from anxiety and psychological distress. The same empathetic approach with provision of information should be used and their anxieties treated with the same importance as those with malignant disease.

CHEST DRAIN MANAGEMENT

Refer to Chapter 8 for information on the indications for and management of chest drains.

The clinical need for chest drainage arises any time the negative pressure in the pleural cavity is disrupted by the presence of air and/or fluid, resulting in pulmonary compromise. Small injuries to the lung parenchyma and visceral pleural during the normal course of thoracic surgery can lead to air leaks into the pleural space. There will also be some blood and fluid loss from the operative site. The purpose of chest drainage is to evacuate the air and/or fluid from the chest cavity to help re-establish normal intrathoracic pressure. This facilitates the re-expansion of the lung to restore normal breathing dynamics. Most post-operative air leaks will resolve with the apposition of the pleural surfaces; however, a number of patients will have a prolonged air leak, defined as an air leak persisting for more than 5 days post-operatively (Mueller and Marzluf, 2013). The numbers of patients developing a prolonged air leak after surgery varies, with studies reporting rates of 8% to 26% (Lee et al., 2011; Rivera et al., 2011; Mueller and Marzluf, 2013; Burt and Shrager, 2014). The risk factors for developing a prolonged air leak are older age, low FEV_1, poor nutritional status and use of steroids (Singhal et al., 2010). Additionally, prolonged air leaks are more common with segmental resections, in redo surgery, with the use of mechanical ventilation and where there is incomplete lung expansion (Deslauriers and Mehran, 2005). Persistent air spaces in the pleural cavity occur when there is failure of one of the normal mechanisms that obliterate pleural spaces. These are the shift of adjacent dynamic structures such as the mediastinum and diaphragm, hyperinflation of the residual lung and accumulation of blood and pleural fluid in the space. Patients who have bi-lobectomy, underlying pulmonary fibrosis or a persistent air leak are more likely to have a post-resection space (Deslauriers and Mehran, 2005).

The application of suction to chest drain post thoracic surgery is a controversial subject with a number of studies finding no benefits from the practice (Sanni et al., 2006), whereas others have advocated its use (Brunelli et al., 2004; Zardo et al., 2015). The recent introduction of electronic chest drainage systems that provide regulated suction in a unit that can be carried by the patient has allowed patients who need thoracic suction via their chest drains to mobilise freely. These electronic chest drains also provide a digital assessment of the air leak measured in millilitres/minute, giving a more accurate measure of the air leak (Cerfolio and Bryant, 2008; Rathinam et al., 2011).

DISCHARGE WITH CHEST DRAINS

Patients who require continued chest drainage and are otherwise fit for discharge home may be considered for discharge home with a chest drain *in situ* (Mueller and Marzluf, 2013; Burt and Shrager, 2014). The most common reasons for discharge with a chest drain are prolonged air leak and continued drainage after surgical treatment of empyema. A number of ambulatory drains are available for this purpose (Carroll, 2003; Joshi, 2009). Ambulatory drains contain a one-way valve and are able to be worn on the body. Patients discharged home with a chest drain should be reviewed regularly in an appropriate clinic setting and the drain removed when clinically appropriate (Mueller and Marzluf, 2013). Nurse-led clinics for review of patients discharged home with chest drains are a successful tool for managing this group of patients (Williams et al., 2012).

MOBILISATION AND EXERCISE

Mobilisation and deep breathing exercises are essential after thoracic surgery as they aid the expectoration of secretions from the airways and promote lung expansion (Iyer and Yadav, 2013). Thoracic surgery is performed on a deflated lung. Post-operatively the lung needs to fully re-expand and secretions that have accumulated in the airways need to be cleared. Impairment of the mechanisms of coughing due to surgery are common and anatomical rearrangement due to surgery is also thought to play a part in decreasing the clearance of mucus (Deslauriers and Mehran,

2005). Patients undergoing thoracic surgery should be seen by a physiotherapist post-operatively. Common interventions include breathing and coughing exercises and promotion of mobilisation (Varela et al., 2011; Agostini et al., 2013). Patients who are current or recent ex-smokers will need increased physiotherapy input post-operatively due to the increase in bronchial secretions associated with smoking.

ENHANCED RECOVERY IN THORACIC SURGERY

Enhanced recovery is an approach to the pre-operative, intra-operative and post-operative care of patients undergoing surgery that aims to ensure that patients are in the best possible condition for surgery, have the best possible management during and after their operation, and experience the best post-operative rehabilitation (NLCFN, 2014).

There are four founding principles of all enhanced recovery programmes:

1. All patients should be on a pathway to enhance their recovery. This enables patients to recover from surgery, treatment, illness and leave hospital sooner by minimising the physical and psychological stress responses.
2. Patient preparation ensures the patient is in the best possible condition, identifies the risks and commences rehabilitation prior to admission or as soon as possible.
3. Pro-active patient management components of enhanced recovery are embedded across the entire pathway; pre, during and after operation/ treatment.
4. Patients have an active role and take responsibility for enhancing their recovery (NHS Improvement, 2012).

An underlying principle within enhanced recovery programmes is to empower patients to actively contribute to their own recovery (Driver, 2011). Enhanced recovery programmes advocate a number of interventions:

- Utilisation of innovative technologies
- Early resumption of oral intake
- Early mobilisation
- Pain management

- Reduction of surgical stress
- Utilisation of advanced techniques in anaesthesia

These measures ensure that patients are in optimal condition for their operation and post-operative rehabilitation. There have been a number of studies and trials demonstrating that implementing at least four of the elements of enhanced recovery can lead to a reduction in the length of stay in hospital and a reduction in morbidity and complication rates (Arumainayagam et al., 2008; Govas et al., 2009; Husted et al., 2010; Lemanu et al., 2013). Some studies report an improvement in patient experience with patients on an enhanced recovery pathway feeling happier and less anxious (Polle et al., 2007).

CASE STUDY

Mr Taylor is a 63-year-old gentleman who visited his GP complaining of pain in his right shoulder and arm that initially started at the front of his chest and had subsequently moved to the area around his scapula. The pain was waking him at night. He was a smoker of 10–15 cigarettes per day from age 14 and was otherwise fit and well with an active job as a school caretaker. His chest was clear on examination and there was no tenderness in the painful area so his GP arranged a chest X-ray.

The chest X-ray demonstrated opacification at the right apex suspicious for a tumour. The GP explained the result to Mr Taylor and made a 2-week wait referral to the lung cancer team.

Mr Taylor underwent investigations including a chest computerised tomography (CT) scan, molecular resonance imaging (MRI) of his brachial plexus, positron emission tomography-CT (PET-CT), CT-guided biopsy of the tumour and pulmonary function testing. These investigations demonstrated a tumour in keeping with a right apical bronchogenic carcinoma, which was extremely avid (metabolically active, dense area) on positron emission tomography (PET-CT). No (PET-CT) avid disease was demonstrated elsewhere. The tumour involved the right first and second ribs and adjacent soft tissues. It extended up to but did not involve the T1 vertebra. Pathology was in keeping with a primary non-small cell lung cancer (Pancoast tumour). It was staged by the radiologists as cT3/4N0M0. Mr Taylor's FEV_1 was 86% predicted and his WHO performance status was 0 (see Chapter 11 for more information on diagnostic tests and measures used to assess patients with lung cancer).

Following discussion at the lung cancer multidisciplinary team meeting (MDT), Mr Taylor was referred for consideration of surgery. The surgeon was prepared to proceed with lung and chest wall resection, he advised Mr Taylor to stop smoking prior to his surgery to reduce the risk of post-operative respiratory complication. Unfortunately, owing to the stress of the diagnosis of lung cancer and impending surgery Mr Taylor was not able to stop smoking in the 4 weeks between his out-patient appointment and his surgery.

Mr Taylor underwent a right thoracotomy, upper lobectomy, chest wall resection with en bloc resection of the first to third ribs and chest wall reconstruction with a porcine biomaterial patch. Systematic lymph node dissection of station 4R, 7, 10 and 11 was performed. Two drains were inserted and placed on −3kPa suction. An epidural was placed by the anaesthetist.

On the first post-operative day Mr Taylor was in an acceptable condition, his pain was well controlled by his epidural, his observations were satisfactory and he had good air entry bilaterally. Mr Taylor had a very small air leak via his chest drains initially, which had resolved by mid-morning, and drainage of less than 20 millilitres per hour. His drains were taken off suction. A chest X-ray was performed and demonstrated fully expanded lungs with a raised right hemidiaphragm and no fluid collection. Mr Taylor sat out of bed and went for some short walks with assistance.

On the second post-operative day Mr Taylor had his basal drain and epidural removed and began to mobilise independently, carrying his chest drain. He required morphine sulphate slow release 20 mg twice daily plus morphine sulphate liquid 10 mg as required to control his pain. His chest X-ray remained satisfactory. Mr Taylor continued to make good progress on day 3 and his remaining chest drain was removed. His post-drain removal chest X-ray demonstrated atelectasis on the right side, as Mr Taylor was asymptomatic a plan was made for regular physiotherapy, continued mobilisation and regular review. By day 5 Mr Taylor's oxygen saturations were dropping to 91% on air and his chest X-ray demonstrated complete collapse on the right side, he continued to mobilise around the ward and was asymptomatic. He returned to theatre for a rigid and flexible bronchoscopy. This demonstrated copious endobronchial secretions in the right sided airways, which were cleared. Over the following 12 days Mr Taylor continued to receive regular physiotherapy to assist him in clearing secretions and mobilise around the ward but required a further four rigid and flexible bronchoscopies for total collapse on the right side. Each bronchoscopy demonstrated copious secretions. Microbiology specimens sent from each procedure were all negative. Following the last bronchoscopy Mr Taylor was able to expectorate his secretions more effectively and was discharged home 22 days after surgery.

On follow-up 4 weeks later Mr Taylor was increasing his activity levels and was independent in activities of daily living. He complained of numbness on his chest wall and decreased function in his right hand. Pathology from his surgery demonstrated squamous cell carcinoma of the lung which was fully excised and staged as pT3N0M0. The plan from the lung MDT was that he should follow a lung cancer follow-up pathway. At six months post-operatively Mr Taylor had returned to work as a school caretaker. He still had some issues with decreased function in his right hand and although he still had some chest wall numbness he did not find this particularly troublesome. Mr Taylor had not started smoking again.

CASE STUDY DISCUSSION

Mr Taylor's pathway to surgery demonstrates the steps needed to assess a patient as suitable for radical therapy. Surgery is the main recognised curative treatment for lung cancer so it is important to ensure that all patients who will benefit from a curative resection are offered surgery (Health and Social Care Information Centre, 2014). Mr Taylor's post-operative course was prolonged by his respiratory problems. He had an operation that involved resection of the chest wall, which decreased his ability to breathe deeply and cough. This combined with the early effects of smoking cessation to prolong his recovery from surgery and delay his discharge home.

A Pancoast tumour is a lung cancer situated at the apex of the lung (Spaggiari et al., 2007). It is often associated with invasion of the structures of the thoracic inlet including the ribs, brachial plexus, subclavian blood vessels and vertebra (Parissis and Young, 2010). Shoulder and chest pain is the most common presenting symptom of this type of tumour (Foroulis et al., 2013). The aim of surgery is to remove the entire tumour including the upper lobe of the lung and any invaded structures. The best outcomes are obtained when the tumour is completely removed with no cancer cells present at the margins of the resected area (Parissis and Young, 2010). At surgery Mr Taylor's tumour was adherent to the chest wall at the first and second ribs. A chest wall resection including ribs 1–3 to give at least 3 cm of clear margin from the tumour was performed. The defect in the chest wall was closed with a porcine biomaterial patch to prevent chest deformity. Examination of the resected specimen by the pathologist demonstrated invasion of the chest wall fat and early invasion of the ribs, and there were clear margins around the specimen. Ongoing symptoms of pain and muscle weakness in the hand are common side effects of surgery for Pancoast tumours, due to damage to the structures of the thoracic outlet (Foroulis et al., 2013).

Mr Taylor's recovery from his surgery was prolonged due to hypersecretion of mucus in his airways, which he had difficulty clearing without assistance. Hypersecretion of mucus in the airways is associated with smoking and can increase in the period immediately after cessation of smoking as the airway cilia regenerate (Ambrose and Barua, 2004; Møller and Tønnesen, 2006). This combined with changes in the airway anatomy and impaired respiratory function led to build up of secretions in his airways, which he was unable to clear without further intervention. Prompt action to clear these secretions is important in preventing chest infection (Iyer and Yadav, 2013). In addition to regular bronchoscopy to clear the accumulated secretions in his airways Mr Taylor required intensive physiotherapy to help him to clear secretions from his chest and to promote mobilisation, which aids lung expansion. Mr Taylor had been asked to stop smoking at all of his out-patient consultations with the chest physician and the thoracic surgeon prior to his surgery. He was referred to his local smoking cessation service at the time of his pre-operative assessment where he was offered nicotine replacement therapy and support from a smoking cessation counsellor. He was unwilling to use the nicotine replacement and was not receptive to the counselling offered, stating that the stress of his diagnosis of lung cancer and the prospect of major surgery meant that he did not feel he could stop smoking.

Pain control was an important part of Mr Taylor's post-operative care. In addition to the pain from his surgery and drain sites he was being asked to cough regularly and clear secretions. As it was known that the lung and chest wall resection would cause considerable pain Mr Taylor had an epidural inserted prior to his surgery. This provided good pain relief in the initial post-operative period and was removed on the second day after his surgery. He was assessed by the hospital pain team who recommended oral morphine sulphate, which was effective in controlling his pain so that he was able to undertake his physiotherapy. Mr Taylor gradually reduced his oral analgesia dose after discharge home and had stopped all analgesia medication by 6 weeks after discharge.

While Mr Taylor had a prolonged and complicated recovery immediately after his surgery, in the longer term his recovery was very good and he was able to return to his normal daily activities with minimal effects from his surgery.

SUMMARY

Thoracic surgery is undertaken to treat many conditions affecting the chest. The most common reason for undergoing thoracic surgery is to treat lung cancer, but patients with a wide range of other malignant and non-malignant disease also have surgery (SCTS, 2011). Patients with diseases affecting the chest often have other health issues and careful assessment is needed to ensure patients are fit to undergo surgery and can cope with the reduction in respiratory capacity from resection of lung tissue.

Patients need specialist care after their surgery with emphasis placed on controlling pain and preventing complications, particularly pulmonary complications which are common in this group of patients (Agostini et al., 2010). Most patients will have chest drains and these should be monitored and managed to ensure air and fluid are effectively drained from the pleural cavity.

This chapter has discussed the common operations for respiratory conditions. There are many specialist thoracic surgery resources available to readers interested in researching other aspects of thoracic surgery not covered in this text, for example thoracic trauma, pectus deformity correction and thymectomy for myasthenia gravis.

REFERENCES

Agostini, P., Cieslik, H., Rathinam, H., Bishay, F., Kalkat, M., Rajesh, P., Steyn, R., Singh, S. and Naidu, B. 2010. Postoperative pulmonary complications following thoracic surgery: Are there any modifiable risk factors? *Thorax* 65 (9): 815–818.

Agostini, P., Reeve, J., Dromard, S., Singh, S., Steyn, R.S. and Naidu, B. 2013. A survey of physiotherapeutic provision for patients undergoing thoracic surgery in the U.K. *Physiotherapy* 99 (1): 56–62.

Ambrose, J.A. and Barua, R.S. 2004. The pathophysiology of cigarette smoking and cardiovascular disease: An update. *Journal of the American College of Cardiology* 43 (10): 1731–1737.

Andreetti, C., Menna, C., Ibrahim, M., Ciccone, A.M., D'Andrilli, A., Venuta, F. and Rendina E.A. 2014. Postoperative pain control: Videothoracoscopic versus conservative mini-thoracotomic approach. *European Journal of Cardio-Thoracic Surgery* 46 (5): 907–912.

Arumainayagam, N., McGrath, J., Jefferson, K. and Gillat, D. 2008. Introduction of an enhanced recovery protocol for radical cyctectomy. *British Journal of Urology International* 101 (6): 689–701.

Aziz, K.A.A., Oey, I.F., Waller, D.A., Morgan, M.D., Steiner, M.C. and Singh, S.J. 2010. P141 Lung volume reduction surgery – The first 200 operations in a UK centre: The benefits of a multidisciplinary strategy and minimally invasive approach. *Thorax* 65 (Suppl 4): A137–A138.

Barrera, R., Shi, W., Amar, D., Thaler, H.T., Gabovich, N., Bains, M.S. and White, D.A. 2005. Smoking and timing of cessation: Impact on pulmonary complications after thoracotomy. *Chest* 127 (6): 1977–1983.

Begum, S., Hansen, H.J. and Papagiannopoulos, K. 2014. VATS anatomic lung resections-The European experience. *Journal of Thoracic Disease* 6 (Suppl 2): S203–S210.

Brunelli, A., Charloux, A., Bolliger, C.T., Rocco, G., Sculier, J.P., Varela, G., Licker, M. et al. 2009. ERS/ESTS clinical guidelines on fitness for radical therapy in lung cancer patients (surgery and chemo-radiotherapy). *The European Respiratory Journal* 34 (1): 17–41.

Brunelli, A., Monteverde, M., Borri, A., Salati, M., Marasco, R.D., Al Refai, M. and Fianchini, A. 2004. Comparison of water seal and suction after pulmonary lobectomy: A prospective, randomized trial. *The Annals of Thoracic Surgery* 77 (6): 1932–1937.

Burt, B.M. and Shrager, J.B. 2014. Prevention and management of postoperative air leaks. *Annals of Cardiothoracic Surgery* 3 (2): 216–218.

Carroll, P. 2003. Ask the experts…Atrium dry suction chest drainage system. *Critical Care Nurse* 23 (4): 73–74.

Cerfolio, R.J. and Bryant, A.S. 2008. The benefits of continuous and digital air leak assessment after elective pulmonary resection: A prospective study. *The Annals of Thoracic Surgery* 86 (2): 396–401.

Chambers, A., Routledge, T., Dunning, J. and Scarci, M. 2010. Is video-assisted thoracoscopic surgical decortication superior to open surgery in the management of adults with primary empyema? *Interactive Cardiovascular and Thoracic Surgery* 11 (2): 171–177.

Chumbley, G. and Mountford, L. 2010. Patient-controlled analgesia infusion pumps for adults. *Nursing Standard* 25 (8): 35–40.

Clark, S.J., Zoumot, Z., Bamsey, O., Polkey, M.I., Dusmet, M., Lim, E., Jordan, S. and Hopkinson, N.S. 2014. Surgical approaches for lung volume reduction in emphysema. *Clinical Medicine* 14 (2): 122–127.

Daly, D.J. and Myles, P.S. 2009. Update on the role of paravertebral blocks for thoracic surgery: Are they worth it? *Current Opinion in Anaesthesiology* 22 (1): 38–43.

Davies, H.E., Davies, R.J.O and Davies, C.W.H. 2010. Management of pleural infection in adults: British thoracic society pleural disease guideline 2010. *Thorax* 65 (Suppl 2): ii41–ii53.

Demmy, T.L. and Curtis, J.J. 1999. Minimally invasive lobectomy directed toward frail and high-risk patients: A case-control study. *The Annals of Thoracic Surgery* 68 (1): 194–200.

Deslauriers, J. and Mehran, R. 2005. *Handbook of Perioperative Care in General Thoracic Surgery.* Elsevier Mosby, Philadelphia.

Driver, A. 2011. How enhanced recovery is transforming surgical care pathways. *Health Service Journal.* Available at: http://www.hsj.co.uk/resource-centre/best-practice/care-pathway-resources/how-enhanced-recovery-is-transforming-surgical-care-pathways/5033030.article

Du Rand, I.A., Barber, P.V., Goldring, J., Lewis, R.A., Mandal, S., Munavvar, M., Rintoul, R.C. et al. 2011. Summary of the British Thoracic Society guidelines for advanced diagnostic and therapeutic flexible bronchoscopy in adults. *Thorax* 66 (11): 1014–1015.

European Society of Thoracic Surgery Database Committee 2014. *European Society of Thoracic Surgeons Database Annual Report 2014 edition.* Dendrite Clinical Systems Ltd, Henley.

Falcoz, P.E., Conti, M., Brouchet, L., Chocron, S., Puyraveau, M., Mercier, M., Etievent, J.P. and Dahan, M. 2007. The Thoracic Surgery Scoring System (Thoracoscore): Risk model for in-hospital death in 15,183 patients requiring thoracic surgery. *The Journal of Thoracic and Cardiovascular Surgery* 133 (2): 325–332.

Fishman, A., Martinez, F., Naunheim, K., Piantadosi, S., Wise, R., Ries, A., Weinmann, G. and Wood, D.E. 2003. A randomized trial comparing lung-volume-reduction surgery with medical therapy for severe emphysema. *The New England Journal of Medicine* 348 (21): 2059–2073.

Fisseler-Eckhoff, A. and Demes, M. 2012. Neuroendocrine tumors of the lung. *Cancers* 4 (3): 777–798.

Foroulis, C.N., Zarogoulidis, P., Darwiche, K., Katsikogiannis, N., Machairiotis, N., Karapantzos, I., Tsakiridis, K., Huang, H. and Zarogoulidis, K. 2013. Superior sulcus (Pancoast) tumors: Current evidence on diagnosis and radical treatment. *Journal of Thoracic Disease* 5 (Suppl 4): S342–S358.

Garretson, S. 2004. Benefits of preoperative information programmes. *Nursing Standard* 18 (47): 33–37.

Gottschalk, A., Cohen, S.P., Yang, S. and Ochroch, A.E. 2006. Preventing and treating pain after thoracic surgery. *Anesthesiology* 104 (3): 594–600.

Govas, N., Tan, E., Windsor, A., Xynos, E. and
Tekkis, P. 2009. Fast-track vs standard care
in colorectal surgery: Meta-analysis update.
International Journal of Colorectal Disease 24 (10):
1119–1131.

Gridelli, C., Rossi, A., Airoma, G., Bianco, R.,
Costanzo, R., Daniele, B., Chiara, G. et al.
2013. Treatment of pulmonary neuroendocrine
tumours: State of the art and future developments. *Cancer Treatment Reviews* 39 (5):
466–472.

Health and Social Care Information Centre.
2014. *National Lung Cancer Audit Report 2014*.
Government Statistical Service, London.

Huber, G. and Mahajan, V. 2008. Successful smoking cessation. *Disease Management & Health
Outcomes* 16 (5): 335–343.

Husted, H., Hansen, H., Holm, G., Bach-Dal, C.,
Rud, K., Anderson, K. and Kehlet, H. 2010. What
determines length of stay after total hip and knee
arthroplasty? A nationwide study in Denmark.
Archives of Orthopaedic and Trauma Surgery 130
(2): 263–268.

Iyer, A. and Yadav, S. 2013. Postoperative care
and complications after thoracic surgery. In:
Firstenberg, M. (ed.) *Principles and Practice of
Cardiothoracic Surgery*. InTech, Rijeka.

Joint Formulary Committee (JFC). 2014. *British
National Formulary (BNF)* (68th ed.). BMJ Group
and RPS Publishing, London.

Joshi, J.M. 2009. Ambulatory chest drainage. *The
Indian Journal of Chest Diseases & Allied Sciences*
51 (4): 225–231.

Kaiser, L. 2006. Bronchoplastic procedures. In:
Kaiser, L. and Jamieson, G. (eds). *Operative
Thoracic Surgery* (5th ed.). Hodder Arnold,
London.

Kwon, Y.S. 2014. Pleural infection and empyema.
Tuberculosis and Respiratory Diseases 76 (4):
160–162.

Leao, L. 2006. Video-assisted thoracic surgery. In:
Kaiser, L. and Jamieson, G. (eds.). *Operative
Thoracic Surgery* (5th ed.). Hodder Arnold,
London.

Lee, L., Hanley, S.C., Robineau, C., Siroiss C.,
Mulder, D.S. and Ferri, L.E. 2011. Estimating
the risk of prolonged air leak after pulmonary

resection using a simple scoring system. *Journal
of the American College of Surgeons* 212 (6):
1027–1032.

Legg, M.J. 2011. What is psychosocial care and how
can nurses better provide it to adult oncology
patients. *Australian Journal of Advanced Nursing*
28 (3): 61–67.

Lemanu, D., Singh, P., Berridge, K., Burr, M.,
Birch, C., Babor, R., MacCormick, A., Arroll, B.
and Hill, A. 2013. Randomized clinical trial of
enhanced recovery versus standard care after
laparoscopic sleeve gastrectomy. *British Journal of
Surgery* 100 (4): 482–489.

Li, S., Feng, Z., Wu, L., Huang, Q., Pan, S., Tang, X.
and Ma, B. 2014. Analysis of 11 trials comparing
muscle-sparing with posterolateral thoracotomy.
The Thoracic and Cardiovascular Surgeon 62 (4):
344–352.

Light, R.W. 2003. Pleurodesis: What agent should be
used? *Jornal de Pneumologia* 29:53–54.

Lim, E., Baldwin, D., Beckles, M., Duffy, J., Entwisle
J., Faivre-Finn, C., Kerr, K. et al. 2010. Guidelines
on the radical management of patients with lung
cancer. *Thorax* 65 (Suppl 3): iii1–iii27.

Litzky, L.A. 2010. Pulmonary neuroendocrine
tumors. *Surgical Pathology Clinics* 3 (1): 27–59.

MacDuff, A., Arnold, A. and Harvey, J. 2010.
Management of spontaneous pneumothorax:
British thoracic society pleural disease guideline
2010. *Thorax* 65 (Suppl 2): ii18–ii31.

Marshall, M. 2006. Thoracic incisions. In: Kaiser,
L. and Jamieson, G. (eds.). *Operative Thoracic
Surgery* (5th ed.). Hodder Arnold, London.

Mason, D.P., Subramanian, S., Nowicki, E.R., Grab,
J.D., Murthy, S.C., Rice, T.W. and Blackstone, E.H.
2009. Impact of smoking cessation before resection of lung cancer: A Society of thoracic surgeons general thoracic surgery database study.
The Annals of Thoracic Surgery 88 (2): 362–370.

McLeod, G.A. and Cumming, C. 2004. Thoracic
epidural anaesthesia and analgesia. *Continuing
Education in Anaesthesia, Critical Care & Pain* 4 (1):
16–19.

Møller, A. and Tønnesen, H. 2006. Risk reduction: Perioperative smoking intervention. *Best
Practice & Research. Clinical Anaesthesiology* 20 (2):
237–248.

Molnar, T.F. 2007. Current surgical treatment of thoracic empyema in adults. *European Journal of Cardio-Thoracic Surgery* 32 (3): 422–430.

Mueller, M.R. and Marzluf, B.A. 2013. The anticipation and management of air leaks and residual spaces post lung resection. *Journal of Thoracic Disease* 6 (3): 271–284.

Nakagawa, M., Tanaka, H., Tsukuma, H. and Kishi, Y. 2001. Relationship between the duration of the preoperative smoke-free period and the incidence of postoperative pulmonary complications after pulmonary surgery. *Chest* 120 (3): 705–710.

National Health Service (NHS) Improvement. 2012. *Fulfilling the Potential: A Better Journey for Patients and a Better Deal for the NHS.* NHS Improvement, Leicester.

Nantional Health Service (NHS) Institute for Innovation and Improvement. 2008. Pre-operative Assessment and Planning. http://www.institute.nhs.uk/quality_and_service_improvement_tools/quality_and_service_improvement_tools/pre-operative_assessment_and_planning.html. Accessed 27 October 2015.

National Institute for Health and Care Excellence (NICE). 2005. *Lung Volume Reduction Surgery for Advanced Emphysema (IPG114).* NICE, London.

National Institute for Health and Care Excellence (NICE). 2011. *The Diagnosis and Treatment of Lung Cancer (CG 121).* NICE, London.

National Lung Cancer Forum for Nurses (NLCFN). 2013. *Guideline to Prepare and Support Patients Undergoing a Lung Resection.* http://www.nlcfn.org.uk. Accessed 27 October 2015.

National Lung Cancer Forum for Nurses. 2014. *Guideline for Patient Information on Enhanced Recovery in Thoracic Surgery.* http://www.nlcfn.org.uk. Accessed 27 October 2015.

Oberg, K., Hellman, P., Kwekkeboom, D. and Jelic, S. 2010. Neuroendocrine bronchial and thymic tumours: ESMO Clinical Practice Guidelines for diagnosis, treatment and follow-up. *Annals of Oncology: Official Journal of the European Society for Medical Oncology/ESMO* 21 (Suppl 5): v220–v222.

Parissis, H. and Young, V. 2010. Treatment of Pancoast tumors from the surgeons prospective: Re-appraisal of the anterior-manubrial sternal approach. *Journal of Cardiothoracic Surgery* 5: 102.

Piraccini, E., Pretto Jr, E.A., Corso, R.M. and Gambale, G. 2011. Analgesia for thoracic surgery: The role of paravertebral block. *HSR Proceedings in Intensive Care & Cardiovascular Anesthesia* 3 (3): 157–160.

Polle, S., Wind, J. and Fuhring, J. 2007. Implementation of a fast track perioperative care program: What are the difficulties? *Digestive Surgery* 24 (6): 441–449.

Pricopi, C., Mordant, P., Rivera, C., Arame, A., Foucault, C., Dujon, A., Le Pimpec Barthes, F. and Riquet, M. 2015. Postoperative morbidity and mortality after pneumonectomy: A 30-year experience of 2064 consecutive patients. *Interactive Cardiovascular and Thoracic Surgery* 20 (3): 16–321.

Rang, H., Dale, M., Ritter, J., Flower, R. and Henderson, G. 2011. *Rang and Dale's Pharmacology (7th ed.).* Elsevier Churchill Livingstone, Edinburgh.

Rathinam, S., Bradley, A., Cantlin, T. and Rajesh, P.B. 2011. Thopaz portable suction systems in thoracic surgery: An end user assessment and feedback in a tertiary unit. *Journal of Cardiothoracic Surgery* 6: 59.

Rena, O., Massera, F., Papalia, E., Della Pona, C., Robustellini, M. and Casadio, C. 2008. Surgical pleurodesis for Vanderschueren's stage III primary spontaneous pneumothorax. *The European Respiratory Journal* 31 (4): 837–841.

Rivera, C., Bernard, A., Falcoz, P-E., Thomas, P., Schmidt, A., Bénard, S., Vicaut, E. and Dahan, M. 2011. Characterization and prediction of prolonged air leak after pulmonary resection: A nationwide study setting up the index of prolonged air leak. *The Annals of Thoracic Surgery* 92 (3): 1062–1068.

Sanni, A., Critchley, A. and Dunning, J. 2006. Should chest drains be put on suction or not following pulmonary lobectomy? *Interactive Cardiovascular and Thoracic Surgery* 5 (3): 275–278.

Sawhney, M. 2012. Epidural analgesia: What nurses need to know. *Nursing* 42 (8): 36–41.

Sciurba, F.C., Ernst, A., Herth, F.J.F., Strange, C., Criner, G.J., Marquette, C.H., Kovitz, K.L., Chiacchierini, R.P., Goldin, J. and McLennan, G. 2010.

A randomized study of endobronchial valves for advanced emphysema. *The New England Journal of Medicine* 363 (13): 1233–1244.

Searle, R.D., Simpson, M.P., Simpson, K.H., Milton, R. and Bennett, M.I. 2009. Can chronic neuropathic pain following thoracic surgery be predicted during the postoperative period? *Interactive Cardiovascular and Thoracic Surgery* 9 (6): 999–1002.

Shaikhrezai, K., Thompson, A.I., Parkin, C., Stamenkovic, S. and Walker, W.S. 2011. Video-assisted thoracoscopic surgery management of spontaneous pneumothorax – long-term results. *European Journal of Cardio-Thoracic Surgery* 40 (1): 120–123.

Shapiro, M., Swanson, S.J., Wright, C.D., Chin, C., Cheng, S., Wisnivesky, J. and Weiser, T.S. 2010. Predictors of major morbidity and mortality after pneumonectomy utilizing the society for thoracic surgeons general thoracic surgery database. *The Annals of Thoracic Surgery* 90 (3) 927–934.

Singhal, S., Ferraris, V.A., Bridges, C.R., Clough, E.R., Mitchell, J.D., Fernando, H.C. and Shrager, J.B. 2010. Management of alveolar air leaks after pulmonary resection. *The Annals of Thoracic Surgery* 89 (4): 1327–1335.

Spaggiari, L., D'Aiuto, M., Veronesi, G., Leo, F., Solli, P., Elena Leon, M. et al. 2007. Anterior approach for Pancoast tumor resection. *Multimedia Manual of Cardio-Thoracic Surgery* 1018.

Steegers, M.A.H., Snik, D.M., Verhagen, A., van der Drift, M.A. and Wilder-Smith, O.H.G. 2008. Only half of the chronic pain after thoracic surgery shows a neuropathic component. *The Journal of Pain* 9 (10): 955–961.

Teh, E., Abah, U., Church, D., Saka, W., Talbot, D., Belcher, E. and Black, E. 2014. What is the extent of the advantage of video-assisted thoracoscopic surgical resection over thoracotomy in terms of delivery of adjuvant chemotherapy following non-small-cell lung cancer resection? *Interactive Cardiovascular and Thoracic Surgery* 19(4): 656–660.

The Society for Cardiothoracic Surgery in Great Britain and Ireland (SCTS). 2011. *Second National Thoracic Surgery Activity & Outcomes Report 2011 edition.* Dendrite Clinical Systems Ltd, Henley.

Travis, W.D., Giroux, D.J., Chansky, K., Crowley, J., Asamura, H., Brambilla, E., Jett, J. et al. 2008. The IASLC lung cancer staging project: Proposals for the inclusion of broncho-pulmonary carcinoid tumors in the forthcoming (seventh) edition of the TNM Classification for Lung Cancer. *Journal of Thoracic Oncology* 3 (11): 1213–1223.

Treasure, T., Internullo, E. and Utley, M. 2008. Resection of pulmonary metastases: A growth industry. *Cancer Imaging* 8:121–124.

Urschel, H. and Cooper, J. 1995. *Atlas of Thoracic Surgery.* Churchill Livingstone, New York.

Uzzaman, M.M., Robb, J.D., Mhandu, P.C.E., Khan, H., Baig, K., Chaubey, S. and Whitaker, D.C. 2014. A meta-analysis comparing muscle-sparing and posterolateral thoracotomy. *The Annals of Thoracic Surgery* 97 (3): 1093–1102.

Vachon, M. 2006. Psychosocial distress and coping after cancer treatment: How clinicians can assess distress and which interventions are appropriate – What we know and what we don't. *American Journal of Nursing* 106 (3 Suppl): 26–31.

Varela, G.N.M., Novoa, P., Agostini, P. and Ballesteros, E. 2011. Chest physiotherapy in lung resection patients: State of the art. *Seminars in Thoracic and Cardiovascular Surgery* 23 (4): 297–306.

Williams, S., Williams, J., Tcherveniakov, P. and Milton, R. 2012. Impact of a thoracic nurse-led chest drain clinic on patient satisfaction. *Interactive Cardiovascular and Thoracic Surgery* 14 (6): 729–733.

Younes, R.N., Gross, J.L., Taira, A., Martins, A.A.C. and Neves, G.S. 2009. Surgical resection of lung metastases: Results from 529 patients. *Clinics* 64 (6): 535–541.

Zardo, P., Busk, H. and Kutschka, I. 2015. Chest tube management: State of the art. *Current Opinion in Anaesthesiology* 28 (1): 45–49.

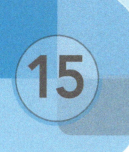

Tracheostomy care

15

DAVID WATERS AND LORRAINE MUTRIE

LEARNING OBJECTIVES

Upon completion of this chapter the reader should be able to:

- Describe the indications and contraindications associated with tracheostomy insertion
- Explain the component parts and types of tracheostomy tubes commonly utilised
- Understand the physiological and anatomical implications associated with an artificial airway
- Discuss the interventions and care considerations for a patient with a tracheostomy tube
- Describe the immediate actions required in tracheostomy-related emergency situations

INTRODUCTION

It is estimated that within the United Kingdom (UK) around 5000 surgical tracheostomies are performed during head or neck surgery. In addition, it is also speculated that around 10,000–15,000 percutaneous tracheostomies are inserted at the bedside, within critical care units (McGrath, 2014). Consequently, patients with tracheostomies are commonly located within critical care environments or specialist surgical wards, for example wards caring for patients following complex head or neck surgery. However, due to the rising numbers of patients receiving this intervention and pressures on critical care facilities, the patient with a tracheostomy may also be found in general or respiratory ward settings. This can pose unique patient safety challenges for the generalist

workforce, owing to the potential lack of specialist skills and knowledge required to care for this complex patient group (National Confidential Enquiry into Patient Outcome and Death [NCEPOD], 2014).

This chapter aims to explore the issue of tracheostomy care. Specifically, the types of tracheostomy will be defined; indications for their use discussed and the evidence base associated with tracheostomy care will be explored. Particular focus will be directed towards the role of the multidisciplinary team in delivering care to this patient population. Although not the focus of this chapter, a description of a laryngectomy will also be provided as tracheostomy and laryngectomy are closely interlinked and have particular issues regarding patient safety and resuscitation. In addition, this chapter will end with a tracheostomy case study, which aims to illustrate key patient considerations and associated interventions.

DEFINITION

A tracheostomy is a surgically created stoma through the anterior wall of the trachea, which is positioned just below the cricoid cartilage in percutaneous insertions, or between the first and second tracheal cartilage rings in surgical insertions (Tortora and Derrickson, 2011) (see Figure 15.1). A tracheostomy tube is commonly introduced through the tracheal stoma, forming an artificial airway and facilitating respiratory support interventions, such as airway protection, tracheal suction or mechanical ventilation.

Tracheostomy can be performed as an elective or emergency procedure and can be classified according to their insertion technique, i.e. surgical or percutaneous or with reference to their intended length of use, i.e. short term/temporary or long term/permanent.

SURGICAL TRACHEOSTOMY

A surgical tracheostomy is performed within the operating theatre setting, usually as part of a more complex surgical procedure of the head or neck, such as a neck dissection and flap formation for malignancy removal but can be performed instead of a

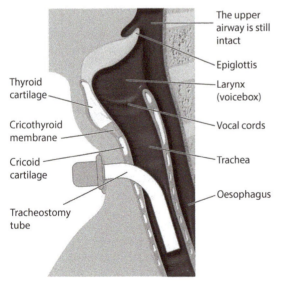

Figure 15.1 Anatomy of the neck and upper airways showing position of a tracheostomy. (From Shutterstock Image ID: 48386533. With permission.)

The upper airway is still intact

Epiglottis

Thyroid cartilage

Larynx (voicebox)

Cricothyroid membrane

Vocal cords

Cricoid cartilage

Trachea

Tracheostomy tube

Oesophagus

percutaneous procedure for patients that have anticipated complications, i.e. coagulation disorder or difficult anatomy. Although the procedure is commonly carried out under general anaesthesia, on occasions it can be undertaken with local anaesthesia.

Typically, a surgical incision is made through the anterior neck, with tissue being dissected down to the depth of the trachea. The trachea is then entered and a slit or window incision made through which the tracheostomy tube is inserted and secured in place.

PERCUTANEOUS TRACHEOSTOMY

Percutaneous tracheostomies are commonly performed within the critical care department at the patient's bedside. The procedure can be undertaken with sedation and local anaesthetic. This type of tracheostomy is commonly utilised for critically ill patients, who often are too clinically unstable for transfer to the operating theatre for a surgical tracheostomy, so a bedside percutaneous procedure offers a suitable solution for this patient group.

The percutaneous procedure commences with cannulation of the trachea by inserting a needle through the neck tissues into the tracheal cavity, followed by a guide-wire that is advanced through the needle. The needle is then removed and the tract made progressively bigger by inserting a series of dilators, each of increasing size until a stoma is formed that can accommodate the chosen tracheostomy tube. The tracheostomy tube is then inserted and secured in place.

TEMPORARY TRACHEOSTOMY

These are formed for patients who only require a tracheostomy for a short period of time, perhaps to facilitate airway protection, tracheal suction or mechanical ventilation. The intention is for this type of tube to be removed once the patient has recovered, or if their reason for tracheostomy has resolved.

PERMANENT TRACHEOSTOMY

This type of tracheostomy might be considered when the underlying condition/disease process is chronic or long term, i.e. following excision of a throat tumour, or for patients with a long-standing neurological condition.

LARYNGECTOMY

A laryngectomy refers to the complete or partial surgical removal of the larynx. This is a permanent procedure whereby the trachea is cut and then surgically attached to the front of the neck and forms the only mechanism through which the patient can breathe. A laryngectomy does not normally require a tracheostomy tube to be inserted but can require the use of some of the humidification and speech assistance valves discussed later in this chapter, sometimes making it difficult to immediately distinguish from a tracheostomy. Although this chapter focusses on tracheostomy, and many of the concepts are transferrable, it must be understood that in a laryngectomy the upper airway is no longer patent and therefore can no longer be used. This is essential for the emergency management of tracheostomies and will be covered later in this chapter (McGrath, 2014).

ALTERED PHYSIOLOGY

Insertion of a tracheostomy tube alters the patient's anatomy and will also influence a number of physiological processes, some of which are advantageous, whereas others present the patient and the healthcare team with additional challenges. These include:

- *Reduction in dead space.* Dead space refers to the volume of air that occupies the respiratory tract, which has no role within gas exchange (Tortora and Derrickson, 2011). A reduction in dead space is associated with a reduced work of breathing for the patient; this is achieved following insertion of a tracheostomy as the upper airway is bypassed. This can be likened to the effect of taking a breath through a hosepipe and then a drinks straw, with the drinks straw being associated with less effort and work of breathing, as less dead space is required to be displaced. In the context of a patient with respiratory insufficiency who requires weaning from mechanical ventilation within a critical care setting, the reduction in work of breathing

associated with a temporary tracheostomy can be beneficial and assist with the initial phase of weaning, but can be a barrier to overcome during the latter weaning process.

- *Loss of humidification.* In normal human physiology, the upper airway, namely the oropharynx and nasopharynx, play a vital role in warming, filtering and humidifying any inhaled breath (Tortora and Derrickson, 2011) (see Chapter 1). Following insertion of a tracheostomy, the upper airway is bypassed, with all respiratory effort passing through the tracheostomy, as opposed to the upper airway. Consequently, the warming, filtering and humidification processes that occur normally are lost following tracheostomy insertion; this can result in thick pulmonary secretions, sputum retention and potential tube blockage (Dawson, 2014). To avoid these complications, all patients with a tracheostomy must receive artificial humidification (see later in this chapter for more discussion regarding humidification strategies).
- *Taste and smell impaired.* Patients often report changes in their taste and smell senses following tracheostomy. The normal pathway of air during inhalation allows breath to pass over the olfactory (smelling) nerve endings that are located within the nasopharynx. As the upper airway is bypassed following tracheostomy, the airflow through the nasopharynx is impaired, resulting in a reduction in olfactory stimulation. The sensation of taste is closely associated with smell, with a large proportion deriving from the smell of food, rather than from taste stimuli. As taste relies heavily on the olfactory process, abnormal taste sensations due to the nasopharynx being bypassed is experienced following tracheostomy.
- *Compromised swallow mechanism.* Placement of the tracheostomy tube can cause some disruption to the normal swallowing mechanism and can make eating or drinking unsafe owing to potential aspiration. Inflation of a tracheostomy tube cuff when *in situ* can result in the posterior wall of the trachea being pushed towards the oesophagus, which could result in a physical obstruction to swallowing

(McGrath, 2014). In addition, the tracheostomy tube can restrict the movements of the larynx and other structures within the anterior neck, impairing the normal swallowing processes. Owing to these concerns, patients with a tracheostomy usually are fed via a nasogastric tube and only commenced on oral intake following consultation with a speech and language therapist; this will be discussed later in this chapter.

- *Inability to speak.* The normal vocalisation process involves exhaled breath being passed through the larynx and over the vocal cords. As the larynx and upper airway structures are being bypassed by a tracheostomy tube, patients will be unable to generate any vocal sounds. This can pose immense psychological distress and frustration for patients, so strategies that allow patients to communicate through other means should be considered, i.e. communication boards.

INDICATIONS FOR TRACHEOSTOMY

A tracheostomy may be required for a number of clinical reasons; these include:

- To assist in the weaning from mechanical ventilation, as tracheostomies are associated with increased patient comfort and reduced sedation requirements
- To enable the long-term mechanical ventilation of patients, due to chronic respiratory impairment
- To facilitate the removal of pulmonary secretions, for those patients with excessive secretions or who are unable to clear their secretions independently
- To maintain an airway, for example in upper airway obstruction or reduced levels of consciousness
- To provide airway protection in patients who are at high risk of aspiration, such as patients with head injuries or neuromuscular disorders

(Intensive Care Society [ICS], 2014; McGrath, 2014).

TYPES OF TUBE

A tracheostomy tube is a curved tube designed to sit within the trachea; the tip of the distal end of the tube sits above the carina. The tubes are made of either metal or plastic and are sized in millimetres according to their internal diameter (Dougherty and Lister, 2015). There are numerous types of tracheostomy tubes available; these can be classified according to the following criteria:

- Presence or absence of a cuff at the distal end of the tracheostomy tube
- Presence or absence of a removable inner cannula within the tracheostomy tube
- Presence or absence of a fenestration or hole within the posterior wall of the tracheostomy tube
- Fixed or adjustable flange

The above categories of the tracheostomy tube will be discussed below in greater detail.

Cuffed and uncuffed tracheostomy tubes

A cuffed tracheostomy tube consists of an air-inflated or sponge balloon that is positioned at the distal end of the device (Dawson, 2014) (see Figure 15.2). The inflated cuff produces a seal within the trachea. This offers some protection from aspiration of oral secretions or gastric contents, while also facilitating positive pressure ventilation if required, and thus facilitating gas exchange (Myatt, 2015). However, it must be noted that this seal is not absolute and aspiration can occur. Cuffed tracheostomy tubes all have

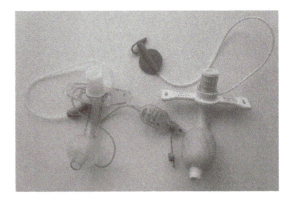

Figure 15.2 An example of cuffed tracheostomy tubes.

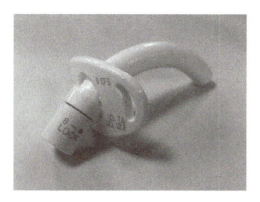

Figure 15.3 An example of an uncuffed tracheostomy tube.

a pilot balloon component, which allows the volume of gas within the cuff to be measured and titrated to ensure a sufficient seal is generated within the trachea. Further discussion concerning measuring cuff pressures will be included later in this chapter.

Uncuffed tracheostomy tubes lack the inflatable balloon that is present in conventional cuffed tracheostomy tubes (see Figure 15.3). Uncuffed tubes are commonly used for patients who require a long-term tracheostomy to assist with suctioning and secretion clearance. To be suitable for an uncuffed tube, the patient must be able to cough and have effective glottic function to prevent the risk of gastric aspiration.

A mini tracheostomy is a form of uncuffed tracheostomy tube with a smaller internal and external diameter that facilitates tracheal suction (see Figure 15.4). The patient does not breathe through the mini tracheostomy; the mechanism of breathing is through the normal passages of the upper airways. However, in an emergency situation oxygen can be applied to improve saturation or ventilation may be facilitated via a mini tracheostomy for a very short time.

Inner cannula

An inner cannula is a tube of smaller diameter, which is inserted and secured into the lumen of the tracheostomy (see Figure 15.5). This is a valuable safety feature, as regular monitoring and changing of the inner cannula can prevent tube occlusion due to encrustation or accumulation of pulmonary secretions. They are usually used in acutely unwell patients requiring tracheostomy but, although a common safety feature, some tracheostomy tubes might not include this component (ICS, 2014). Inner cannulas are available as re-useable or single use and use a variety of closure methods including hinge, snap lock and twist lock.

Fenestrations

A fenestration is a hole or a series of holes in the upper aspect of the tracheostomy tube and possibly also within the corresponding inner cannula (see Figure 15.5). A fenestrated tube facilitates air movement via the upper airway, in addition to through the actual tracheostomy tube. The movement of

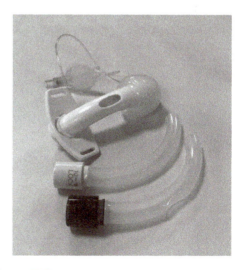

Figure 15.5 An example of a fenestrated tracheostomy tube, with unfenestrated and fenestrated inner cannula. Please note that fenestrated inner tubes are always coloured to alert staff to the fact that the inner tube has a fenestration and suctioning should not be performed until the inner tube has been changed to a non-fenestrated one.

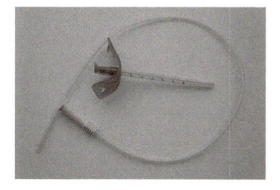

Figure 15.4 An example of a mini tracheostomy. Please note the diameter of the minitrach in comparison to a standard suction catheter.

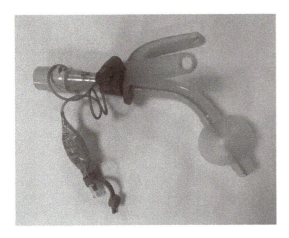

Figure 15.6 An example of a tracheostomy tube with an adjustable flange.

air through the upper airway allows the patient to vocalise. Typically, fenestrated tracheostomy tubes are used for long-term patients, or for those who have been weaned from a non-fenestrated tube but still require some degree of airway protection or assistance with secretion removal.

Fixed or adjustable flange

The flange (neck plate) of a standard tracheostomy tube is fixed. For patients that have a larger distance from their skin to their trachea (i.e. oedema or obesity), a tube with an adjustable neck flange may be required (McGrath, 2014) (see Figure 15.6). Care must be taken to ensure that the flange is securely fixed to prevent complications from movement or dislodgment.

CARE CONSIDERATIONS

HUMIDIFICATION

To avoid the complications associated with the loss of humidification, a number of methods of artificial humidification are available to patients. Both active and passive methods for providing humidification are available and the temperature of inhaled gas should be heated and humidified to the same level as in normal respiration (Wilkes, 2011).

Passive humidification uses the heat and moisture provided from exhalation to humidify inhaled gas using a heat moisture exchanger (HME) (Pierce, 2007). A HME is a device that contains a condenser material (foam or paper) that retains moisture and heat from exhaled gases to condition the inspired gas (Wilkes, 2011; McGrath, 2014). Commonly seen in practice is the 'Swedish nose' device, which attaches directly to the tracheostomy tube, and includes a port that allows supplemental oxygen to be incorporated if necessary. A 'Buchanan bib' is a stoma bib often used by patients with long-term stomas and consists of a foam-filled piece of material that sits discreetly over the stoma site. HMEs are small, easy-to-use devices that allow for portability and therefore ease of mobility for patients. They require regular checks for blockages from secretions, and device changes are recommended at least every 24 hours, or as necessary. HMEs should not be used on patients that are dehydrated or hypothermic as heat and moisture retention will not be effective (National Health Service Quality Improvement Scotland [NHS QIS], 2007; Pierce, 2007; St. George's Healthcare, 2012).

Active humidification is used in conjunction with oxygen therapy and consists of a heated water chamber that gases flow through or over prior to inspiration (Coombs et al., 2013). Complications of active humidification are the risks of overheating and the potential resistance to breathing caused by condensation within breathing circuit tubing. Bacterial colonisation is possible in all methods of artificial humidification, and therefore infection control principles must be considered (NHS QIS, 2007).

SECRETION MANAGEMENT AND SUCTION

Respiratory tract secretion management may be required for tracheostomised patients to prevent infection or tracheostomy tube blockage due to:

- The presence of an artificial airway preventing mucus travelling through the upper airways via the cilia cells
- Altered secretion consistency from inadequate humidification, leading to thicker secretions being more difficult to pass
- Impaired cough stimulation from incomplete closure of the epiglottis or decreased muscle tone due to clinical condition
- Increased mucus formation due to clinical condition

Cough exercises and secretion management techniques can be facilitated by physiotherapy referral; however, tracheal suction may still be required for some patients.

Suction can be performed using either a deep or shallow technique using an open or closed method (Coombs et al., 2013; McGrath, 2014). Shallow suction removes only secretions that are present within the tracheostomy tube and is the preferred method of suction (Dougherty and Lister, 2015). Deep suction advances the suction catheter beyond the end of the tracheostomy tube to facilitate secretion clearance lower down in the respiratory tract. Open suction requires a single-use flexible suction catheter to be passed through the tube using a sterile technique. Closed suction apparatus is available for patients that require regular suction or those that are being mechanically ventilated to prevent disconnection from the ventilator circuit.

Suction uses negative pressure to draw out secretions from the airway and as such, the vacuum effect can induce hypoxia, cause trauma and/or atelectasis, and patient discomfort; therefore, assessment of need should take place. Table 15.1 shows indications for tracheal suction. In an acute setting it has been suggested that suctioning every 8 hours is acceptable and that routine suctioning should be avoided (McGrath, 2014; Dougherty and Lister, 2015). There is a risk during suction of the catheter exiting through the hole of fenestrated tubes; this would result in ineffective suction as the catheter would not advance through to the lower trachea. This in turn could lead to mucosal damage of the upper trachea or larynx; therefore, suction should never be performed through a fenestrated tracheostomy tube unless a non-fenestrated inner cannula is *in situ*.

Table 15.1 Indications for tracheostomy insertion

Audible secretions
Respiratory distress
Decreased breath sounds
Decreased chest movement
Crackles
Decreased SaO_2
Reduced PaO_2
Increased $PaCO_2$
Change of ventilator pressures in mechanical ventilation

Other safety considerations during tracheal suction include:

- Selection of appropriately sized suction catheter to prevent complete airway occlusion
- Use of lowest pressure possible for suction to be effective. The National Tracheostomy Safety Project (McGrath, 2014) recommend a pressure of no greater than −150 mmHg (−20 kPa)
- Use of non-fenestrated inner cannula for fenestrated tracheostomy tubes
- The inability to pass a suction catheter could indicate a blocked tube and is considered a 'red flag' to an emergency (see Section 'Emergency Management')

HYGIENE AND STOMA SITE CARE

Tracheostomy tubes are at risk of dislodgement and should therefore have securing devices in place. It can take up to 7 days post insertion for an established stoma to form and sutures can be used in the initial post-operative period (NHS QIS, 2007; McGrath, 2014). However, the most common securing method is the use of tracheostomy ties. A tracheostomy tie is inserted through the eyelet hole on the flange of the tube, passed around the back of the patients' neck and secured through the other end of the flange. There should be one finger able to fit comfortably underneath the ties to ensure adequate security while minimising the risk of pressure damage from excess tightening (McGrath, 2014). The flange should sit neatly against the skin to prevent movement of the tube in and out of the trachea preventing mucosal damage from this action. A dressing can be placed between the flange and skin to absorb excess secretions and, although not essential for pressure damage prevention, they are often used in the acute setting for patient comfort. To prevent a moist environment for bacteria to multiply, both ties and dressings should be routinely changed at 24 hours or sooner if saturated in secretions (St. George's Healthcare, 2012).

The stoma site and outer tube should be cleaned with normal saline every 24 hours using a clean technique. Avoidance of cotton wool and gauze swabs is necessary owing to the risk of inhalation of fibre deposits (NHS QIS, 2007; St. George's Healthcare,

2012). Excoriated skin around the stoma can benefit from the application of a barrier film. If infection is suspected, a swab of the stoma should be sent for microscopy and for difficult stomas a specialist referral to tissue viability services may be required.

Inner cannulas should be inspected and changed regularly to maintain patency of the airway and potentially aid in the reduction of microbes present in an *in situ* cannula. A minimum of eight hourly changes are recommended and more regularly if tenacious secretions are present (ICS, 2014; McGrath, 2014). Re-usable inner cannula should be changed using the exchange technique (i.e. a spare inner tube available to replace the one *in situ*). Before any inner cannula is removed, attention must be paid to device connections to ensure quick replacement and securing, and to ensure any external equipment attachments remain compatible if the inner tube is removed and not replaced.

Many of the interventions required for stoma site care stimulate a patient cough, risking accidental decannulation; therefore, any manipulation of the stoma site should be carried out using a two-person technique: one to secure the airway and the other to carry out the procedure.

Stoma site care is often undertaken by nursing staff within the acute care setting, but for patients returning to the community with a tracheostomy early stoma site care education is required to promote independence, teach self-care and complication recognition (Dougherty and Lister, 2015; Harkin, 2015). Specialist nurses and district nurses play an active role in the education of patients and caregivers within the home and ongoing support is often necessary.

The benefits of good oral hygiene are well documented for all; in patients with a tracheostomy it is essential to prevent infection, ulceration and skin tears caused by secretions entering the mouth from the lower airway or from dry mucous membranes. In addition to twice-daily recommended tooth brushing, antiseptic agents can help to reduce the incidence of infection (Labeau et al., 2011).

CUFF MANAGEMENT

A cuffed tube provides a seal within the trachea to reduce the incidence of aspiration and facilitate positive pressure ventilation. Table 15.2 shows

Table 15.2 Complications of an over- or under-inflated tracheostomy tube cuff

Over inflation	Under inflation
Tracheal stenosis	Air leak
Tracheal dilation	Ineffective positive pressure ventilation
Necrosis	Aspiration (oral and gastric)
Fistula	Tube dislodgment/ movement friction
Weakened muscle and cartilage softening	

the complications that can arise from an over- and under-inflated cuff.

Modern tracheostomy tubes use high-volume, low-pressure cuffs that have a high surface area to prevent the complications that arise from over inflation, but cuff pressure must still be monitored. To achieve an adequate seal within the trachea, cuff pressure should be maintained at no more than $20–25\,cmH_2O$ and not exceed $35\,cmH_2O$ to reduce incidence of mucosal damage to the trachea from blood flow occlusion (ICS, 2014; McGrath, 2014).

The cuff should be inflated using the 'minimal occlusion volume (MOV)' technique (St. George's Healthcare, 2012) or the 'minimal leak technique (MLT)' (Pierce, 2007; Stacy, 2015) as described in local policy documents and measured using a manometer (Dawson, 2014) at least every 8 hours (McGrath, 2014) or every 4 hours for mechanically ventilated patients (Department of Health [DH], 2011). Increasing volumes needed to inflate the cuff indicate the presence of a leak, suggesting a defective cuff or incorrectly sized tube or flange.

Cuff deflation may be necessary for weaning, communication, nutrition or tube readjustment. Secretions can pool around the cuff; therefore, subglottic suction should be performed prior to cuff deflation. If cuff deflation is necessary, as with stoma site care, it should be a two-person technique.

COMMUNICATION

The loss of voice experienced in the presence of a cuffed tracheostomy tube can lead to communication difficulties for patients, giving rise to frustration and distress. Fenestrated tubes, as discussed earlier, allow for phonation and should be considered for use in patients that are not at risk of aspiration and are not mechanically ventilated. Similarly, the airflow present in an uncuffed tube allows for a degree of vocalisation.

Vocalisation with cuffed tracheotomy tubes is possible by using a one-way valve ('speaking valve') or the intermittent finger occlusion technique. Both methods force airflow up through the vocal cords and the larynx on expiration and can be used once the patient can tolerate the cuff being deflated (an inflated cuff causes complete occlusion of trachea, and therefore air cannot flow upwards). For patients that require mechanical ventilation a 'Passy-Muir' valve can be added to the breathing circuit for this purpose, with acknowledgement that pressures achieved will be altered owing to cuff deflation. Communication via this method can be tiring for acutely ill patients owing to the loss of positive pressure that a cuff allows for; therefore, gradual introduction and regular rest periods may be necessary.

When vocalisation is not tolerated, alternative communication techniques must be considered. Low-cost, non-verbal approaches to communication include lip reading, communication boards, picture/alphabet cards and hand/eye signals, whereas sophisticated methods include computers and handheld vibration devices (Dawson, 2014; Stacy, 2015).

Reassurance and explanation that voice loss is usually temporary for patients with a short-term tracheostomy, and that a weak voice is expected post decannulation, can allay fear for patients and their relatives. Concerning patients expected to have a long-term tracheostomy with permanent voice loss, pre procedure explanation and discussion of communication strategies can assist to facilitate their adjustment. Referral to a speech and language therapy service is recommended for all patients with a tracheostomy for ongoing advice and support.

SWALLOW AND NUTRITION

Owing to the altered swallow mechanism described previously, long-term nutritional care must be considered for all patients with a tracheostomy and for patients displaying signs of post decannulation dysphagia. Whereas for some that will mean long-term enteral support with the input of the dietetics service, many other patients can be supported and educated in oral intake.

A simple swallow test using water can be performed by trained staff to assess the safety and aspiration risk of a patient, advancing to a soft diet if deemed safe (ICS, 2014). This should be performed without the presence of an inflated cuff. In patients that demonstrate a problematic swallow, a speech and language therapy referral should be made for further assessment and ongoing support.

Any future evidence of swallow or speech difficulty in patients that have had a previous tracheostomy may require specialist follow up; therefore, notification of a temporary tracheostomy should be passed to the patient's GP.

TUBE CHANGE AND DECANNULATION

Tracheostomy performed for long-term management of an airway may require a change of tracheostomy tube. ICS (2014) recommend that the initial change of tracheostomy tube should be undertaken by a medical practitioner and that any subsequent change can be done by an experienced, trained healthcare professional.

The decannulation of a short-term tracheostomy should take place at the earliest, safe opportunity. Patients must be assessed to ensure that the reason for tracheostomy has been resolved, and that they have the ability to maintain and protect their own airway, with an effective cough and swallow. Respiratory preparation for decannulation could be considered in the form of cuff down trials to increase the work of breathing and allow the patient the opportunity to display their airway protection ability.

Downsizing the tracheostomy tube can be considered as a process for weaning (McGrath, 2014) with the aim of gradually reducing the size of the stoma. If secretion management remains a concern, downsizing to a mini tracheostomy could be considered.

An airtight dressing should be applied to the stoma site post decannulation and pressure applied to the site when coughing or speaking (McGrath, 2014). The need to recannulate a patient is greatest 4–24 hours post decannulation; therefore, close patient observation and availability of emergency equipment should be maintained during this period (Choate et al., 2009; St. George's Healthcare, 2012).

EMERGENCY MANAGEMENT

Emergency management of the airway could arise from a blocked or displaced tube, accidental decannulation or early or late bleeding. The National

Tracheostomy Safety Project (2012) has developed algorithms to assist in the management of an airway emergency in a patient with a tracheostomy (see Figure 15.7a) and a laryngectomy (See Figure 15.7b). The key difference for which algorithm to use is

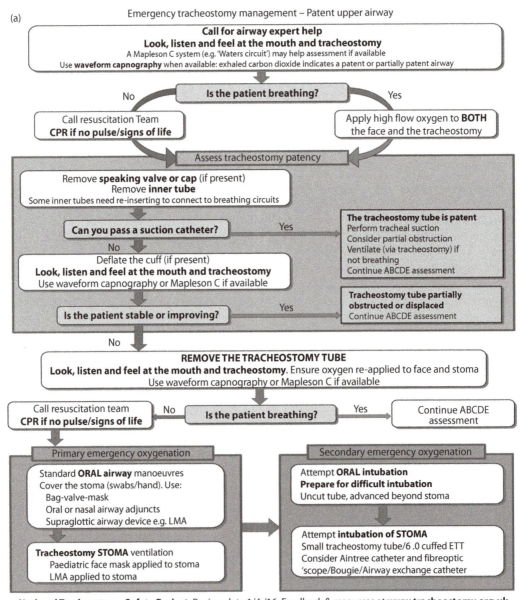

Figure 15.7 (a) Management of emergency airway algorithm. (Reproduced from McGrath, B.A. et al. 2012. *Anaesthesia*, 67 (9): 1025–1041. With permission from the Association of Anaesthetists of Great Britain & Ireland/ Blackwell Publishing Ltd.) *(Continued)*

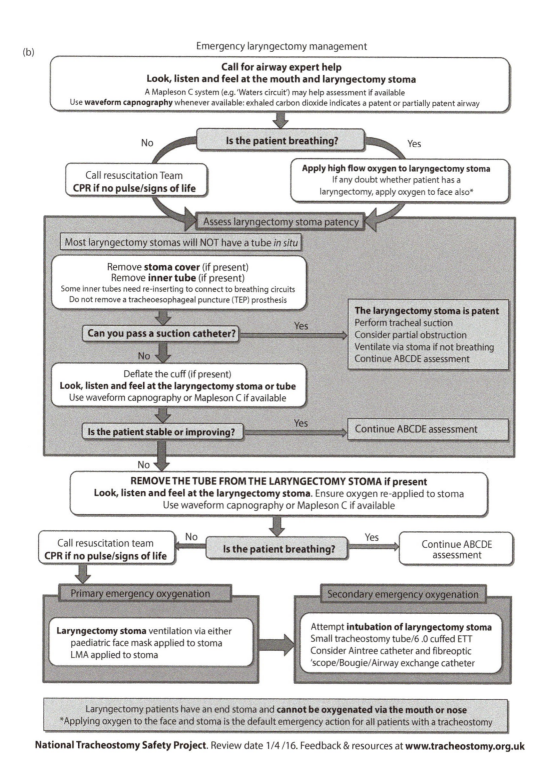

(b) Emergency laryngectomy management

Call for airway expert help
Look, listen and feel at the mouth and laryngectomy stoma
A Mapleson C system (e.g. 'Waters circuit') may help assessment if available
Use **waveform capnography** whenever available: exhaled carbon dioxide indicates a patent or partially patent airway

Is the patient breathing?

No → Call resuscitation Team **CPR if no pulse/signs of life**

Yes → **Apply high flow oxygen to laryngectomy stoma** If any doubt whether patient has a laryngectomy, apply oxygen to face also*

Assess laryngectomy stoma patency

Most laryngectomy stomas will NOT have a tube *in situ*

Remove **stoma cover** (if present)
Remove **inner tube** (if present)
Some inner tubes need re-inserting to connect to breathing circuits
Do not remove a tracheoesophageal puncture (TEP) prosthesis

Can you pass a suction catheter?

Yes → **The laryngectomy stoma is patent**
Perform tracheal suction
Consider partial obstruction
Ventilate via stoma if not breathing
Continue ABCDE assessment

No → Deflate the cuff (if present)
Look, listen and feel at the laryngectomy stoma or tube
Use waveform capnography or Mapleson C if available

Is the patient stable or improving?

Yes → Continue ABCDE assessment

No → **REMOVE THE TUBE FROM THE LARYNGECTOMY STOMA if present**
Look, listen and feel at the laryngectomy stoma. Ensure oxygen re-applied to stoma
Use waveform capnography or Mapleson C if available

Is the patient breathing?

No → Call resuscitation team **CPR if no pulse/signs of life**

Yes → Continue ABCDE assessment

Primary emergency oxygenation

Laryngectomy stoma ventilation via either
paediatric face mask applied to stoma
LMA applied to stoma

Secondary emergency oxygenation

Attempt **intubation of laryngectomy stoma**
Small tracheostomy tube/6 .0 cuffed ETT
Consider Aintree catheter and fibreoptic
'scope/Bougie/Airway exchange catheter

Laryngectomy patients have an end stoma and **cannot be oxygenated via the mouth or nose**
*Applying oxygen to the face and stoma is the default emergency action for all patients with a tracheostomy

National Tracheostomy Safety Project. Review date 1/4 /16. Feedback & resources at **www.tracheostomy.org.uk**

Figure 15.7 (Continued) (b) Emergency laryngectomy management. (Reproduced from McGrath, B.A. et al. 2012. *Anaesthesia*, 67 (9): 1025–1041. With permission from the Association of Anaesthetists of Great Britain & Ireland/ Blackwell Publishing Ltd.)

whether the patient has the presence of a functioning upper airway. The use of bedside information signs can be used to highlight the presence or absence of an upper airway, facilitating quick recognition of which algorithm to use (McGrath, 2014). With a laryngectomy, artificial ventilation including bag and mask must be performed via the tracheostomy tube or stoma.

CASE STUDY

Jack Woodburn is a 78-year-old gentleman who was admitted to hospital with community acquired pneumonia. He was diagnosed as having severe sepsis and required invasive mechanical ventilation owing to respiratory failure. After 8 days of ventilation via an endotracheal tube, Mr Woodburn underwent a percutaneous tracheostomy on the critical care unit to facilitate weaning from the ventilator. The use of a cuffed tracheostomy tube with an inner cannula was chosen. With input from a dietician, tailored nutritional support was already established and continued via an NG tube while Mr Woodburn remained sedated.

During the initial period after tracheostomy insertion Mr Woodburn appeared anxious and agitated as he tried to make his needs known to his family and staff. As Mr Woodburn's condition improved, vocal communication gradually took place using a one-way valve with the cuff down and Mr Woodburn was able to better communicate his needs and fears.

Pre-decannulation assessment took place and, on discussion between physiotherapist, nurse and doctor, a decision was made to step down to a mini tracheostomy before complete decannulation as excessive respiratory secretions were still present. A simple swallow assessment showed that Mr Woodburn was showing signs of difficulty when trying to swallow with the mini tracheostomy in place; therefore, a referral to speech and language therapy was made for swallow advice and support. A full assessment was made and a care plan devised to allow Mr Woodburn a Category C thick pureed diet.

Once the mini tracheostomy was removed, Mr Woodburn's wife informed nursing staff that her husband's voice did not sound the same as before he had had a tracheostomy. The nurse discussed this with Mr Woodburn and a further referral to speech and language therapy resulted in ongoing communication support for Mr Woodburn.

CASE STUDY DISCUSSION

This case study highlights some of the complexities of decision making in the care of a patient with a short-term tracheostomy in relation to the choice of tube and the time at which intervention should take place. There is currently no evidence indicating the optimum time for tracheostomy to take place for critically ill patients but as it was likely that Mr Woodburn was requiring sedative medication to tolerate the endotracheal tube, a tracheostomy would reduce the need for this and the resulting complications. The percutaneous method of insertion was used so that insertion could take place at the bedside, reducing the risk of transfer-related complications (ICS, 2014). A cuffed tube was used as the main purpose of the tracheostomy was to facilitate positive pressure ventilation; the cuff enables this by preventing any gas loss during ventilation (McGrath, 2014), and the inner cannula was chosen to prevent complication of blockage from excess secretions. NCEPOD (2014) recommend that professionals involved in tracheostomy must have knowledge of the variety of tubes available and select the one which is most appropriate. The ICS (2014), however, state that the tube most commonly used for an acutely unwell patient is a cuffed tube with inner cannula.

Stacy (2015) highlights impaired communication as a major cause of stress in patients with an artificial airway and this could have been compounded by the unexpected nature of the tracheostomy insertion (Harkin, 2015). Although the use of a speaking valve is recommended, careful observation of the patients' respiratory status is required as the valves can cause fatigue due to the increased respiratory effort required to overcome the airflow resistance and increase in dead space (ICS, 2014).

A multidisciplinary approach to all aspects of tracheostomy care is required if a patient is to receive safe and high quality care (NCEPOD, 2014). This case study demonstrates that without the input of specialist teams Mr Woodburn would have run the risk of unsafe decannulation owing to his inability to clear his own respiratory secretions and a high risk of gastric aspiration from an unsafe swallow, potentially resulting in the need to re-establish an artificial airway. It also draws attention to the positive impact that a multidisciplinary approach to care can have in fully addressing the needs of a complex patient. Although the case study does not address the care of a patient with a long-term tracheostomy, many of the approaches to care are the same, with early involvement pre-procedure referral to the MDT gold standard.

SUMMARY

The true number of tracheostomy insertions is still currently unknown, but it is likely that the numbers are rising and will continue to do so (ICS, 2014; NCEPOD, 2014). There are many considerations to make when caring for a patient with a tracheostomy, both practical and psychosocial. This chapter has presented a discussion on anatomy and physiology in relation to tracheostomy along with indications for, and explanation of, some of the devices available for use in practice.

The difficulties faced by a patient with a tracheostomy can arise whether the procedure is for short- or long-term management of a clinical condition, and some patients continue to have these difficulties indefinitely, as demonstrated by Mr Woodburn's ongoing need for communication support. Evidence from NCEPOD (2014) suggests that improvements must be made to knowledge and skills in relation to this patient group and as healthcare professionals it is imperative that we gain insight not only into the altered anatomy and physiology that a tracheostomy brings, but also understanding of some of the practical elements of care involved to adequately and effectively care for a patient with a tracheostomy. Special consideration must be given to airway management in an emergency situation for both tracheostomy and laryngectomy.

REFERENCES

Choate, K., Barbetti, J. and Currey, J. 2009. Tracheostomy decannulation failure rate following critical illness: A prospective descriptive study. *Australian Critical Care* 22 (1): 8–15.

Coombs, M., Dyos, J., Waters, D. and Nesbitt, I. 2013. Assessment, monitoring and interventions for the respiratory system. In: Mallett, J., Albarran, J.W. and Richardson, A. (eds.). *Critical Care Manual of Clinical Procedures and Competencies.* John Wiley and Sons, Chichester, 63–171.

Dawson, D. 2014. Essential principles: Tracheostomy care in the adult patient. *Nursing in Critical Care* 19 (2): 63–72.

Department of Health (DH). 2011. High Impact Intervention care bundle to reduce ventilation associated pneumonia. Available at: http://webarchive.nationalarchives.gov.uk/20120118164404/hcai.dh.gov.uk/files/2011/03/2011-03-14-HII-Ventilator-Associated-Pneumonia-FINAL.pdf. Accessed 11 November 2015.

Dougherty, L. and Lister, S. (ed.) 2015. *The Royal Marsden Manual of Clinical Nursing Procedures. Professional Edition* (9th ed.). John Wiley and Sons, West Sussex.

Harkin, H. 2015. Nursing patients with disorders of the ear, nose and throat. In: Brooker, C. and Nicol, M. (eds.). *Alexander's Nursing Practice* (4th ed.). Churchill Livingston, Edinburgh, 449–473.

Intensive Care Society (ICS). 2014. *Standards for the Care of Adult Patients with a Temporary Tracheostomy* [online]. Available at: http://www.ics.ac.uk/EasySiteWeb/GatewayLink.aspx?alId=2212. Accessed 4 February 2015.

Labeau, S.O., Van de Vyver, K., Brusselaers, N., Vogelaers, D. and Blot, S.I. 2011. Prevention of ventilator-associated pneumonia with oral antiseptics: A systematic review and meta-analysis. *Lancet Infectious Diseases* 11 (11): 845–854.

McGrath, B.A. 2014. *Comprehensive Tracheostomy Care. The National Tracheostomy Safety Project Manual.* John Wiley and Sons, Chichester.

McGrath, B.A., Bates, L., Atkinson, D. and Moore, J.A. 2012. Multidisciplinary guidelines for the management of tracheostomy and laryngectomy airway emergencies. *Anaesthesia* 67 (9): 1025–1041.

Myatt, R. 2015. Nursing care of patients with temporary tracheostomy. *Nursing Standard* 29 (26): 42–49.

National Confidential Enquiry into Patient Outcome and Death (NCEPOD). 2014. *On the Right Trach. A Review of the Care of Patients Who Underwent a Tracheostomy.* NCEPOD, London.

National Health Service Quality Improvement Scotland (NHS QIS). 2007. *Caring for the Patient with a Tracheostomy.* NHS QIS, Edinburgh.

National Tracheostomy Safety Project (NTSP). 2012. *Algorithm: Emergency tracheostomy management-patent upper airway.* Available at: http://tracheostomy.org.uk/Templates/Algorithms.html. Accessed 11 November 2015.

Pierce, L. 2007. *Management of the Mechanically Ventilated Patient* (2nd edn.). Saunders Elsevier, Missouri.

St. George's Healthcare NHS Trust. 2012. *Tracheostomy Guidelines.* Available at: https://www.stgeorges.nhs.uk/gps-and-clinicians/clinical-resources/tracheostomy-guidelines/. Accessed 12 November 2015.

Stacy, K. 2015. Pulmonary therapeutic management. In: Urden L., Stacy, K. and Lough, M. (eds.). *Priorities in Critical Care Nursing* (7th ed.). Elsevier Mosby, Missouri, 301–330.

Tortora, B. and Derrickson, G.J. 2011. *Principles of Anatomy and Physiology* (13th ed.). John Wiley and Sons, New Jersey.

Wilkes, A. 2011. Heat and moisture exchangers and breathing circuit filters: Their use in anaesthesia and intensive care. Part 1- history, principles and efficiency. *Anaesthesia* 66 (1): 31–39.

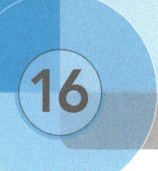

Oxygen therapy

16

ANDREW KERRY AND DAVID WATERS

LEARNING OBJECTIVES

Upon completion of this chapter the reader should be able to:

- Explain the physiological processes associated with oxygen therapy
- Describe the indications and contraindications associated with oxygen therapy
- Explain the various methods available to administer oxygen therapy
- Discuss the interventions and care considerations for a patient who is receiving oxygen therapy
- Discuss the use of home oxygen therapy

INTRODUCTION

It has been suggested that oxygen is the most commonly used drug globally, especially within the context of acutely unwell or deteriorating patients. Its use is often considered first line for many life-threatening or emergency clinical situations. The delivery of oxygen is not without risk, as its inappropriate use can be associated with an increased mortality and morbidity in some situations (National Patient Safety Agency, 2009). Consequently, healthcare professionals must possess the appropriate knowledge, skill and competence to safely administer oxygen therapy to patients under their care.

This chapter aims to explore the physiological responses to oxygen and the indications and contraindications associated with oxygen use. Attention will also be directed towards how oxygen is administered and the associated care considerations. The chapter will also include a patient case study, which aims to illustrate some key points related to oxygen therapy.

In 2008 the British Thoracic Society (BTS) published guidelines on the emergency administration of oxygen and this was followed in 2015 with guidelines on home oxygen therapy. It would be difficult to improve on the extensive evidence based approach the British Thoracic Society used to formulate the guidelines and so this chapter sets out to summarise the key points from the guidelines, supported with additional references. The reader is therefore encouraged to access the guidelines in full and to keep abreast of any future updates.

PHYSIOLOGY ASSOCIATED WITH OXYGEN THERAPY

At normal temperature and pressure, oxygen is a colourless, tasteless and odourless gas. In standardised conditions, two atoms of the element bind to form dioxygen, a diatomic molecule represented by the chemical formula O_2 (Marieb and Hoehn, 2010).

Oxygen is essential for normal cellular homeostasis and metabolism. Through the oxygen-dependent process of aerobic respiration, adenosine triphosphate (ATP) is produced by cellular mitochondria (Marieb and Hoehn, 2010). ATP is an energy-bearing molecule and in simplistic terms plays a role in 'fuelling' all cellular activities. A gross deficiency or absence of ATP will lead to cellular injury and eventually death (Wagstaff, 2014). Consequently, disease states that lead to insufficient oxygen levels can potentially have catastrophic effects on physiological function.

Atmospheric air consists of several gases in varying proportions. The chief constituent is nitrogen, which occupies 78% by volume followed by oxygen at 21%. The remaining 1% consists of a mixture of argon, carbon dioxide, neon, helium and methane. Healthy individuals with disease-free lungs are able to utilise this 21% of oxygen to fulfil all of their oxygen requirements. However, for those with lung disease (whose lungs are not functioning normally) and those who are critically ill (who may have increased oxygen demand) this 21% oxygen concentration may not be sufficient. Such individuals can become oxygen deprived, which leads to clinical manifestations such as hypoxemia (low levels of oxygen in the blood) and hypoxia (low levels of oxygen in the tissues). Oxygen therapy exposes the patient to air containing a higher percentage of oxygen, in which some of the other gases have been displaced in favour of oxygen. This may be a small percentage increase in the oxygen concentration, for instance to 24%, or it may, in severe circumstances, need to be increased to 100% where all of the inhaled gas the patient is breathing consists of oxygen, it having displaced all the other gases.

DEFINITION OF OXYGEN THERAPY

Oxygen therapy has been defined as delivery of oxygen at concentrations greater than those encountered in the ambient environment (O'Driscoll et al., 2008). Oxygen is usually administered to treat or prevent hypoxaemia, in turn reducing tissue hypoxia, which could lead to tissue injury or cellular death (O'Driscoll et al., 2008).

The indications for oxygen therapy include:

- All patients that are hypoxaemic (with oxygen saturations less than 94%) should receive supplementary oxygen therapy.
- Supplementary oxygen should also be given to all patients with life-threatening critical illness, such as shock states, major trauma or sepsis. This should be delivered initially through a high-concentration non-rebreather reservoir mark device; subsequently, the dose should later be weaned following further investigations or if the patient has stabilised.

(O'Driscoll et al., 2008).

OXYGEN ADMINISTRATION

In the self-ventilating patient, delivering of oxygen to the alveoli is usually achieved by increasing the environmental oxygen fraction (sometimes referred to as the FiO_2). This is usually achieved through the use of different types of face masks or nasal apparatus.

The actual FiO_2 that is delivered to the alveoli by the oxygen administration device can be influenced by a number of patient- or device-related factors (see Table 16.1); consequently, the amount of oxygen the patient actually receives is often unpredictable.

OXYGEN DELIVERY DEVICES

For patients that are self-ventilating there are a number of devices available to facilitate oxygen delivery.

Table 16.1 Factors that can influence the FiO$_2$ delivered to the patient's alveoli by oxygen delivery devices

Patient factors	Device factors
Size of patients inhaled breath (tidal volume)	Speed of oxygen delivery through device (flow rate)
Presence of an inspiratory pause during the respiratory cycle	Volume inside device mask
Speed of patient's inhaled breath (inspiratory flow rate)	Size of air vents in the device (if present)
	Tightness of device mask fit to patient's face

Source: Adapted from Wagstaff, A.J. 2014. *Oh's Intensive Care Manual* (7th ed.). Butterworth-Heinemann, Oxford, 327–340.

Although there is great variety in the appearance and operation of oxygen delivery devices, most delivery devices include several core components:

1. *Oxygen supply:* This can be from pressurised cylinders, plumbed in oxygen supplies, or if in the home setting an oxygen concentrator.
2. *Oxygen flow control:* A valve, which will include a flow meter facilitating adjustment of oxygen flow from the supply.
3. *Tubing:* A length of tubing that connects the oxygen flow control to the device.
4. *Reservoir:* All devices will utilise some form of oxygen reservoir, which aims to store oxygen ready for inhalation during the next inspiratory breath. With a nasal cannula, the nasopharynx acts as the reservoir; with a simple oxygen mask, the mask itself performs this function. A physical reservoir bag can also be observed attached to the mask of the non-rebreathing mask oxygen delivery device.
5. *Patient attachment:* This element provides the interface between the patient and the oxygen supply; this could be a mask or the prongs on a set of nasal cannulae.
6. *Expiratory gas facility:* To enable any exhaled gases to exit the oxygen administration

device and to prevent the 'rebreathing' of any expiratory breaths. This might take the form of physical holes in the side of a mask, which facilitate removal of exhaled gases, or a one-way-valve (such as seen in a non-rebreathe reservoir mask device), which promotes a unidirectional flow of gas, ensuring that exhaled gases are taken away from the patient.

(Wagstaff, 2014).

A great variety of delivery devices are available clinically; however, the most commonly utilised oxygen delivery devices will be explored below:

NON-REBREATHING RESERVOIR MASK (OR HIGH CONCENTRATION RESERVOIR MASK)

In addition to a face mask, this device includes an integrated reservoir bag, which facilitates administration of high-concentration oxygen to the patient (see Figure 16.1). Typically, this device will deliver an oxygen concentration of between 60%–90%, when used with oxygen supply flow rates of 10–15 L/minute (Marino, 2014). Owing to the high concentration of oxygen delivered through this device, its use is indicated for critically ill patients; for example, those who are acutely deteriorating.

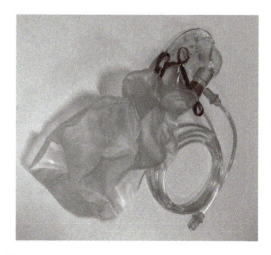

Figure 16.1 Non-rebreathing reservoir mask.

SIMPLE FACE MASK

This device consists of a face mask, which is attached via tubing to the oxygen supply (see Figure 16.2). The concentration of oxygen delivered is controlled by adjustment of the oxygen flow at its source. This oxygen flow is typically set between 5–10 L/minute, which equates to 40%–60% FiO_2. An oxygen flow of less than 5 L/minute is not recommended as this can lead to an increased resistance to breathing for the patient and a possible accumulation of exhaled carbon dioxide.

VENTURI MASK

A Venturi mask device consists of a simple face mask, a number of interchangeable Venturi valves (each with its own set oxygen concentration) and tubing which connects to the oxygen supply (see Figure 16.3). This device will provide the patient with an accurate and fixed concentration of oxygen, regardless of oxygen flow rate. The oxygen dosing is altered by changing the Venturi valve and by adjusting the oxygen flow rate. Venturi valves are available in the following oxygen concentrations: 24%, 28%, 35%, 40% and also 60%. Either 24% or 28% Venturi valves are recommended for patients who are at risk of carbon dioxide retention, i.e. patients who might have chronic obstructive pulmonary disease (COPD) (O'Driscoll et al., 2008).

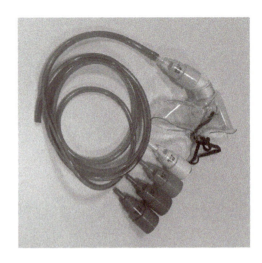

Figure 16.3 Venturi mask.

NASAL CANNULAE

This oxygen delivery device consists of a length of oxygen tubing, which originates at the oxygen supply source and ends with two small prongs that are inserted into the patient's nostrils (see Figure 16.4). The oxygen dose is altered by changing the oxygen flow rate, which can be set between 1–6 L/minute, which correlates to an FiO_2 of 24%–40% (Marino, 2014). Flow rates of 1–4 L/minute are more commonly used, as prolonged use of flow rates of 4–6 L/minute can be associated with patient discomfort and nasal dryness. Mouth breathing has been shown to have

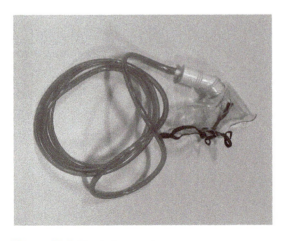

Figure 16.2 Simple face mask.

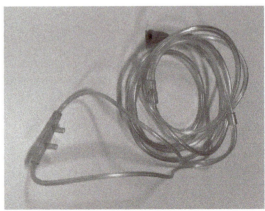

Figure 16.4 Nasal cannulae.

no negative effect on the inspired oxygen concentration delivered by nasal cannulae. Patients tend to tolerate nasal cannulae more than mask-based oxygen delivery devices; this is associated with greater comfort, the ability to eat and drink freely and reduced feelings of claustrophobia.

OTHER METHODS FOR OXYGEN DELIVERY

There are several other strategies that facilitate oxygen delivery. These include non-invasive ventilation, high-flow nasal oxygen and more invasive strategies such as extra-corporeal membrane oxygenation (ECMO); however, these are outside the remit of this chapter. Non-invasive ventilation (NIV) will be discussed in Chapter 17.

HUMIDIFICATION

In normal physiology, the upper airway will warm, filter and moisten each inspiratory breath (Marieb and Hoehn, 2010) (see Chapter 1). However, these normal processes may be impaired in critical illness or when the upper airway is bypassed, i.e. by an endotracheal tube, tracheostomy tube or following laryngectomy surgery (Galluccio and Bersten, 2014). In addition, oxygen therapy can have a drying effect on the respiratory tract owing to the fast moving flow of inhaled gas. Drying of the respiratory mucosa is associated with thickening of pulmonary secretions, airway mucosal damage, atelectasis and possible expectoration difficulties for the patient (Coombs et al., 2013; Galluccio and Bersten, 2014). Historically humidified oxygen therapy has been used to help resolve this issue and prevent any patient discomfort or symptoms associated with drying of the upper respiratory tract. The requirement for humidification for patients with bypassed airways is unquestioned (Galluccio and Bersten, 2014). However, there is little evidence to support routine humidification in the self-ventilating and non-intubated patient population (Dunk et al., 2013). Often there is sufficient moisture in atmospheric air and in the patient's own upper airway to provide effective humidification. Consequently,

the use of humidification in self-ventilating/non-intubated patients should be guided by patient comfort, i.e. if the patient complains of dry oral mucosa or experiences difficulty expectorating sputum. It is important to note that humidified oxygen can assist in the loosening of thick pulmonary secretions, so its use can be justified for those patients who may have excessive secretions or problems expectorating sputum, especially when combined with physiotherapy (O'Driscoll et al., 2008). Routine use of humidification should also be considered for those patients with a bypassed upper airway, i.e. patients with an endotracheal tube, tracheostomy tube or those following laryngectomy surgery (Coombs et al., 2013).

A typical humidified oxygen circuit for a self-ventilating, non-intubated patient will consist of a sterile water reservoir, a valve to regulate the percentage of oxygen delivered, a section of wide-diameter oxygen tubing (often referred to as elephant tubing) and usually a standard oxygen mask. Some circuits utilise cold humidification. However, most include a heater component that warms the oxygen before it is inspired.

Humidification equipment should be changed regularly following manufacturer's guidelines and local organisational policy. It is imperative that the pooling of water in the circuit is kept to a minimum as this provides opportunities for bacterial growth (Dunk et al., 2013). Oxygen tubing should be checked frequently for the presence of water, but also for kinks that may prevent oxygen being delivered to the patient. It is important that the tubing remains below the patient to prevent the movement of any pooled water towards the patient's face. For heated humidification systems, the correct temperature setting should also be monitored to ensure sufficient humidification levels and to prevent accidental burns or discomfort to the patient. Many of the circuits are noisy and can be quite disturbing to the patient. Explaining its purpose and educating the patient can help to alleviate some of this anxiety. Often patients complain that their face becomes damp and this can result in short-term discomfort and potential skin problems. Helping the patient to meet their personal hygiene needs and regularly reviewing facial skin integrity can help to prevent such issues.

IMPORTANT CONSIDERATIONS ASSOCIATED WITH OXYGEN THERAPY

OXYGEN PRESCRIPTION

Legally within the United Kingdom, medical oxygen is considered to be a medicinal product rather than a drug (O'Driscoll et al., 2008). However, for healthcare professionals the laws and regulations pertaining to the administration of medicines, in general, apply to oxygen in the same way, and therefore it is considered to be a drug. It is essential that all oxygen therapy is prescribed by a healthcare professional who is qualified to do so (O'Driscoll et al., 2008). For many years the prescribing of oxygen was not widely observed, but has become more commonplace in recent years, particularly as healthcare organisations have strengthened their prescribing practices and have introduced designated sections for oxygen prescribing into their drug administration documentation.

Healthcare professionals are often reminded that all medication should be accurately prescribed before it is dispensed and administered. The administration of non-prescribed medication or the taking of 'verbal orders' (the practice of taking a prescription order verbally from a prescriber, either directly or over the phone) is considered dangerous practice (Nursing and Midwifery Council [NMC], 2010). However, there are a very small number of exceptions where delaying administration of certain medications, in order to wait for a written prescription, could be detrimental to the patient; emergency oxygen administration is one of these exceptions. This does not, however, give the healthcare professional carte blanche to administer oxygen therapy, but does allow them to start oxygen therapy in an emergency situation without a prescription, providing they have been trained to do so (O'Driscoll et al., 2008). It is essential that a full oxygen therapy prescription is sought as soon as possible following the event. The very fact that a patient has commenced oxygen that is not prescribed should, in itself, be a trigger to refer the patient to a prescriber. Each healthcare organisation should have clear policies regarding the administration of unprescribed emergency oxygen therapy.

In the UK, it is commonplace for a drug administration chart to include a dedicated section for oxygen administration, which should include the following elements:

- Starting dose
- Method of delivery
- Target oxygen saturation levels
- Whether it is to be continuous or as required by the patient

(O'Driscoll et al., 2008).

The healthcare practitioner should review the patient regularly to ensure the oxygen therapy remains in place and that the patient's oxygen saturations are within the target ranges, taking appropriate action if required, in addition to signing the prescription whenever this review takes place (O'Driscoll et al., 2008).

INITIATING OXYGEN THERAPY

In emergency situations, it is justifiable to commence oxygen therapy immediately and then titrate the oxygen therapy to oxygen saturations (see below). It is important to stress that breathlessness alone, with no evidence of a hypoxemia (normal oxygen saturations and PaO_2 levels) is not a sufficient reason for initiating oxygen therapy. In the context of emergency oxygen therapy, blood gas analysis (arterial or an arterialised capillary earlobe sample) should be undertaken when available, as this can indicate the need for oxygen therapy or other respiratory support, such as NIV (O'Driscoll et al., 2008).

TARGET OXYGEN RANGES

In the context of a patient with a blood gas sample indicating a normal or low $PaCO_2$, with no risk factors for hypercapnic respiratory failure (e.g. COPD), it is recommended to aim for target SpO_2 levels within the normal range of 94%–98% (O'Driscoll et al., 2008). If a raised $PaCO_2$ is noted, especially when accompanied by a respiratory acidosis, a lower target SpO_2 is indicated (88%–92%). Patients with known COPD, or those at risk of hypercapnic respiratory failure, should also be managed with a target SpO_2 of 88%–92%. A target SpO_2 should be clearly documented within the patient's physiological observation chart and within their healthcare notes. Debate exists over the 'hypoxic drive' theory in relation to the delivery of high-concentration oxygen. Regardless of the underlying physiology it is important that patients with hypercapnia receive an adequate oxygen supply to maintain their saturation between 88% and 92%. Patients with COPD, who are critically unwell, should be managed initially like any other patient with a critical illness, but with emphasis on urgent and ongoing blood gas analysis to monitor carbon dioxide levels and tailoring oxygen therapy accordingly (O'Driscoll et al., 2008). These patients could suffer prolonged periods of hypoxaemia owing to the reluctance of clinical staff to provide adequate oxygenation for fear of reducing respiratory drive, despite the fact that the patient clearly has oxygen saturation levels well below the 88%–92% range.

MONITORING OXYGEN THERAPY

To evaluate the clinical effects of oxygen therapy and to detect possible complications, the patient should be monitored closely. Recording of physiological observations and use of 'track and trigger' systems such as the National Early Warning Score (NEWS) are recommended to facilitate this.

Once oxygen therapy has been initiated, detailed physiological monitoring should continue. Respiratory rate should be recorded, as tachypnoea can be a sensitive indicator of any emerging respiratory deterioration. The patient should have their SpO_2 levels checked for at least 5 minutes using a pulse oximeter (O'Driscoll et al., 2008). If the patient's target SpO_2 falls below their target level and they become unwell, urgent assistance should be sought. In situations when the patient is stable and their SpO_2 is above their target range, their oxygen dose should be reduced. For further guidance concerning the use of pulse oximetry see Chapter 4. In addition to SpO_2 monitoring, blood gas sampling (either arterial or arteriolised capillary) within 30–60 minutes of commencing oxygen therapy, is recommended for patients with the lower target SpO_2 of 88%–92% to detect possible hypercapnic respiratory failure (O'Driscoll et al., 2008).

WEANING OFF OXYGEN THERAPY

During episodes of acute or critical illness, patients may require oxygen therapy. As their symptoms improve, their oxygen requirements will most likely reduce, which in turn will allow their oxygen therapy to be weaned and hopefully later discontinued. The oxygen dose should be reduced if the patient's condition is stable and when their SpO_2 is consistently noted to be in the upper target range for a significant period of time, i.e. 4–8 hours (O'Driscoll et al., 2008). During the weaning of oxygen, the healthcare professional should closely monitor the patient's physiological observations for any signs of deterioration and to determine whether the patient is tolerating the reduction in oxygen dose. Specifically, the patient's SpO_2 should be monitored for 5 minutes following the reduction in oxygen dose, or rechecked 5 minutes following the change (O'Driscoll et al., 2008). Following the reduction in oxygen dose, if the patient remains clinically stable and their physiological observations remain within acceptable ranges, the weaning process can continue, with the eventual discontinuation of oxygen therapy.

HAZARDS OF OXYGEN THERAPY

Oxygen therapy is associated with a number of potential hazards, which healthcare professionals should be conscious of when caring for patients receiving this intervention. Oxygen from a piped supply or from a cylinder is highly compressed, with the gas being stored under significant pressure. Consequently, piped or cylinder oxygen poses an explosion risk, but also could cause barotrauma (pressure damage) to the airway or respiratory tract if the oxygen supply was not controlled by a pressure-limiting valve (Wagstaff, 2014). The combustion risk associated with oxygen should also be acknowledged; patients should be educated not to smoke while receiving oxygen therapy and situations where sparks might come into contact with oxygen should be avoided, such as ensuring oxygen is clear prior to defibrillation during a cardiac arrest (Resuscitation Council United Kingdom [RCUK], 2016).

CARDIAC, CEREBRAL AND RENAL IMPLICATIONS

Oxygen causes vasoconstriction in the vascular supply to the heart (coronary arteries), brain and kidneys (Marino, 2014). Consequently, although it may seem counterintuitive, the administration of oxygen therapy may reduce perfusion to these organs, by as much as 33% in the case of the brain and 29% in the coronary arteries. There is evidence to suggest that unnecessary administration of oxygen to people in the initial stages of a stroke or acute coronary syndrome may in fact make the situation worse by increasing existing ischaemia. This is yet another reason why oxygen therapy should only be commenced when there is a clear hypoxaemia present (Wagstaff, 2014).

DAMAGE TO LUNG TISSUE

Oxygen itself can have a direct damaging effect on the lung tissue, resulting in reduced lung compliance with interstitial oedema and fibrosis. The exact mechanism of this is unclear, but several factors have been implicated including an increase in production of oxygen-free radicals in the lungs and a reduction in surfactant (Marino, 2014; Wagstaff, 2014).

Other problems associated with oxygen therapy administration tend to be associated with how oxygen affects ventilation. Such problems are most commonly found in people who have pre-existing lung disease and those that have musculoskeletal conditions involving the thorax.

DENSITY OF OXYGEN

Oxygen is denser than air and more viscous and so at high concentrations it may become more difficult to breathe than air. In some people this may lead to a reduction in their forced expiration volume in 1 second (FEV_1) as they find the work of breathing harder (O'Driscoll et al., 2008).

VENTILATION/PERFUSION (V/Q) MISMATCH

Normally if there are poorly ventilated parts of the lung this leads to localised hypoxaemia in the capillaries of the alveoli and the flow of blood to such areas is reduced owing to the normal process of hypoxic pulmonary vasoconstriction (HPV). Pulmonary blood flows to the better ventilated parts of the lungs, but this is determined by the levels of hypoxaemia in the alveoli capillaries. If a patient receives oxygen at a high concentration, it will be absorbed into the alveoli capillaries and results in an increase of PaO_2 and therefore improved blood flow to that part of the lung. The problem is that, despite the increased blood flow, that part of the lung remains poorly ventilated and so there can be high levels of pulmonary $PaCO_2$. In a healthy individual an increase in ventilation compensates for this, but this may not be the case in those with respiratory disease and a systemic rise in $PaCO_2$ may therefore occur (O'Driscoll et al., 2008).

ABSORPTION ATELECTASIS

Air contains 78% nitrogen and it is not absorbed through the alveoli like oxygen. Its role in normal ventilation is to provide a residual volume of gas in the alveoli to maintain their patency during the breathing cycle. Oxygen therapy displaces some of that nitrogen and so there is less of it to maintain the patency of the alveoli. This can lead to collapse of the alveoli, particularly in people who have obstructed airways further up the respiratory tract (Wagstaff, 2014).

CO_2 BUFFERING (HALDANE EFFECT)

Oxygen therapy results in more haemoglobin being saturated with oxygen and so less will be available for carbon dioxide to bind to. This may result in an increase in partial pressure of carbon dioxide in the blood and an acidaemia (Wagstaff, 2014).

HOME OXYGEN THERAPY

Many patients require long-term oxygen therapy (LTOT) to be delivered at home. It can be valuable and in some situations essential for people with either respiratory or cardiac problems such as cystic fibrosis, COPD, severe asthma, pulmonary hypertension, obstructive sleep apnoea and heart failure.

INDICATIONS AND REFERRAL FOR LTOT

LTOT is indicated for the following patients:

- Those who have either stable COPD, cystic fibrosis, interstitial lung disease, advanced heart failure, with a resting $PaO_2 \leq 7.3$ kPa.
- Patients with stable COPD, cystic fibrosis, interstitial lung disease, with a resting $PaO_2 \leq 8.0$ kPa, who also exhibit more symptoms, such as: peripheral oedema, polycythaemia (with a haematocrit $\geq 55\%$) or pulmonary hypotension.
- For those with neuromuscular or chest wall conditions, receiving NIV, who require additional supplementary oxygen therapy to prevent hypoxaemia.

(Hardinge et al., 2015).

To instigate LTOT or home oxygen therapy, a referral should be made to a dedicated home oxygen service. A potential candidate for LTOT requires an in-depth assessment, which would include comprehensive review of their underlying respiratory or cardiac condition. The patient's SpO_2 or arterial blood gases will also assist the team in determining the need for LTOT and potential dosing. Detailed patient information is required at the point of referral. The National Institute of Health and Care Excellence (NICE, 2010) recommend the administration of LTOT for at least 15 hours/day (preferably longer).

NOCTURNAL OXYGEN THERAPY

A variant of LTOT is nocturnal oxygen therapy (NOT); this refers to the administration of oxygen only at night and is of benefit to patients who have moderate levels of hypoxia during sleep, but who have normal oxygen levels during waking/daytime hours. Reduction in nocturnal oxygen levels is thought to be associated with changes in V/Q associated with lying in the supine position and also owing to reduced respiratory drive during sleep (Hardinge et al., 2015).

AMBULATORY OXYGEN THERAPY

Ambulatory oxygen therapy (AOT) refers to the administration of supplementary oxygen during exercise or during everyday activities and utilises small mobile cylinders or oxygen concentrators. AOT is typically used for patients who are not sufficiently hypoxic to qualify for LTOT, but who become hypoxic during exercise or exertion. However, AOT can also be used alongside LTOT, to enable a patient who is established on home oxygen to mobilise more freely and to potentially leave the confines of their home and therefore improve quality of life.

METHODS OF LTOT DELIVERY

There are a variety of ways in which oxygen therapy can be delivered at home including oxygen cylinders, liquid oxygen and oxygen concentrators. Whichever method is used, home oxygen therapy in the UK can only be provided by a small number of authorised suppliers.

Oxygen concentrators are the most common device used for the delivery of the home oxygen therapy. These are static or portable electrical devices that filter out nitrogen from room air to supply a gas that is 85%–95% oxygen. Oxygen is typically delivered at flow rates of up to a maximum of 4 L/minute with incremental adjustments of 0.5 L/minute. If higher flow oxygen is required, then two concentrators can be joined together. Concentrators are recommended for patients who require significant amounts of oxygen throughout the day. The BTS guidelines suggest that patients needing more than 1.4 hours of oxygen a day would benefit from having a concentrator (Hardinge et al., 2015). Static oxygen concentrators often require long lengths of tubing around the house, which can be hazardous, and careful positioning of the tubing should be considered in order to reduce risk of tripping. Portable oxygen concentrators are lighter and run on a rechargeable battery, allowing the individual to take them outside their homes.

Oxygen cylinders contain pressurised compressed oxygen and are coloured either all white or black with a white collar. They come in a variety of sizes, including a small cylinder that fits into a backpack, allowing the person to use the oxygen outside of the home. The flow of oxygen is regulated with a flow meter that delivers flow in litres per minute. Although cylinders are useful for patients who do not require oxygen for long periods of time, they are often used as a backup should there be problems with other delivery devices such as oxygen concentrators that require an electrical power supply (Hardinge et al., 2015).

Liquid oxygen is a less common form of home oxygen therapy. To convert oxygen to a liquid it has to be cooled and stored below −183°C. Therefore, it is stored in insulated containers such as Dewar flasks. Liquid oxygen requires the patient to have significant understanding of the equipment as there are risks of gas leakage and cold burns (Hardinge et al., 2015). Liquid oxygen is limited to use on the ground floor of a home owing to health and safety reasons, which include the requirement for adequate ventilation, and also the movement of liquid oxygen flasks upstairs may be difficult (Hardinge et al., 2015).

Home oxygen therapy is perfectly safe, providing certain precautions are taken. Before commencing home oxygen therapy patients require a home-based risk assessment to be undertaken by the oxygen supplier, which is repeated every six months (Hardinge et al., 2015). Most of the precautions centre on the fact that oxygen is highly flammable. Patients should be advised that they should not smoke when using oxygen therapy, nor should they allow others to smoke near them. It is recommended that the oxygen supply should be kept a minimum of 6 feet (1.8 metres) away from naked flames (BOC Healthcare, 2012a). It is also important not to use flammable products when using oxygen therapy; this could include cleaning and home improvement products. It is also advisable that the patient has a fire extinguisher readily available in the house and that smoke detectors are fitted. Notifying the local fire and rescue service that oxygen therapy is being used in the home is also recommended, although not mandatory (BOC Healthcare, 2012a). Furthermore, if patients are using or transporting oxygen in their car, they should have an oxygen sticker clearly displayed (BOC Healthcare, 2012b).

CASE STUDY

Trevor Jones is a 68-year-old gentleman who was admitted 4 days ago with a left fractured neck of the femur. Following initial investigations, he underwent a total hip replacement, which was uneventful. He has no past medical history, but is a smoker of 52 years.

Mr Jones calls the nurse to say that he feels more unwell and it is clear that he is finding breathing difficult. The nurse assesses Mr Jones using the ABCDE assessment tool. The findings are as follows:

Airway: His airway is patent (noted by him being awake and being able to speak).

Breathing: Respiratory rate is 38 bpm, his chest rises equally and bilaterally. He appears to be using his accessary muscles. He is taking a breath between every word when speaking. Oxygen saturations are 81% on 4 L/minute oxygen via nasal cannula. He has been expectorating thick green sputum over the past few hours.

The current 4 L/minute oxygen therapy has been prescribed on the medication chart but there is no alternative therapy prescribed. The nurse immediately changes the oxygen therapy to a non-rebreathe mask at an oxygen flow rate of 15 L/minute and ensures Mr Jones is sitting upright. She keeps Mr Jones on continuous oxygen saturation monitoring.

Circulation: His blood pressure is 98/56 mmHg and heart rate is 124 bpm. He reports no chest pain. His capillary refill time is delayed at 4 seconds. Mr Jones's hands and feet feel cool and peripherally under-perfused.

Disability: He appears fully conscious (Alert on Alert Voice Pain Unconscious [AVPU Scale]) and is orientated. His pupils are equal and reactive to light. His blood glucose is 4.8 mmol/L.

Exposure: Hip wound dressing is intact, with no swelling or discharge noted. His temperature is 37.8°C.

Recording Mr Jones's observations on the early warning score chart, it is clear that he needs to be reviewed urgently. The nurse contacts the doctor to report the deterioration and asks for urgent review, as she suspects possible hospital-acquired pneumonia. She continues to monitor and reassess Mr Jones, ensuring the oxygen mask stays in place and is being used correctly. She records his observations, noting that with the increase in oxygen therapy his saturations have increased to 95%.

On review by the doctor, course crackles can be heard on chest auscultation and a portable chest X-ray confirms pneumonic changes, suggestive of hospital-acquired pneumonia. The doctor prescribes the oxygen therapy of 15L/minute via the non-rebreathe mask, a course of intravenous antibiotics and intravenous fluids.

Arterial blood gases show: pH 7.36, PaO_2 7.8 kPa, $PaCO_2$ 4.0 kPa, HCO_3 24 mmol/L.

After 24 hours, Mr Jones's condition appears to improve. His observations are subsequently:

Blood pressure 120/78 mmHg, heart rate 100 bpm, respiration rate 26 bpm, SpO_2 100% on 15 L/mom via non-rebreathe mask and temperature 36.8°C.

Noticing the improved respiratory rate and oxygen saturation, the nurse reduces the oxygen to 40% via a Venturi device after discussion with the doctor, who changes the oxygen prescription. Mr Jones's saturations are subsequently 97% on the 40% oxygen. Mr Jones's observations indicate further improvement: Blood pressure 124/79 mmHg, heart rate 90 bpm, respiration rate 18 bpm, SpO_2 98% on 40% oxygen and temperature 36.7°C. The nurse is later able to reduce the oxygen therapy to 2 L/minute via nasal cannula and Mr Jones's oxygen saturations remain at 98%.

CASE STUDY DISCUSSION

This case study highlights very good use of the BTS guidelines for the emergency administration of oxygen (O'Driscoll et al., 2008) and illustrates many points discussed in this chapter.

- A rapid ABCDE assessment highlights, amongst other issues, Mr Jones's increased respiratory rate and reduced oxygen saturations. This demonstrates a clear hypoxia and not just shortness of breath and the nurse was therefore correct to increase oxygen therapy to 15 L/minute via a non-rebreathe mask despite there being no prescription for it.
- The patient's observations are recorded using an early warning score and so the situation is quickly escalated to the medical staff.
- The nurse continues to monitor and assess Mr Jones throughout the scenario, maintaining continuous oxygen saturation monitoring and ensuring the oxygen mask remains in place.
- Blood gas analysis is used as a further means of assessing the severity of the situation and a clear hypoxaemia is determined.
- The nurse weans the oxygen appropriately as Mr Jones' condition improves, meaning he does not receive an inappropriate oxygen dose.
- The nurse ensures that all oxygen therapy provided during the emergency is prescribed and signed for.
- There is no specific need to repeat the blood gas analysis as Mr Jones's condition clearly improves but it may be considered as an option.

SUMMARY

Oxygen therapy can be vital in the management of both the acutely ill and deteriorating patient as well as those with long-term respiratory conditions. It is essential for those involved in the administration of oxygen therapy to have a clear understanding of not only how it works and the variety of methods of administration, but to be clear when it should and should not be used. Oxygen therapy is not without its problems and patients need close supervision and monitoring, receiving sufficient oxygen dosing to ensure adequate oxygen saturations, with the weaning off of the oxygen being a primary goal as their condition improves. This chapter has set out the main principles involved in caring for patients receiving oxygen therapy and has relied heavily on the British Thoracic Society guidelines for the use of emergency oxygen and home oxygen therapy (O'Driscoll et al., 2008; Hardinge et al., 2015). As highlighted at the beginning of this chapter, the reader is encouraged to access these guidelines in full and to remain abreast of future updates.

REFERENCES

Coombs, M., Dyos, J., Waters, D. and Nesbitt, I. 2013. Assessment, monitoring and interventions for the respiratory system. In: Mallett, J., Albarran, J.W. and Richardson, A. (eds.). *Critical Care Manual of Clinical Procedures and Competencies*. Wiley Blackwell, Oxford, 64–171.

BOC Healthcare. 2012a. Home oxygen: A guide for professionals. BOC Healthcare, London. Available at: http://www.bochomeoxygen.co.uk/internet.lg.bocoxygenservice.gbr/en/images/406765_Healthcare_A_Guide_for_Professionals_Handbook_NHS_x3_RZ1109_176796.pdf. Accessed 14 September 2015.

BOC Healthcare. 2012b. The Home Oxygen Handbook. BOC Healthcare, London. Available at: http://www.bochealthcare.co.uk/internet.lh.lh.gbr/en/images/406900_Healthcare_Patient_Home_Oxygen_Handbook_NHS_A4_RZ409_66361.pdf. Accessed 14 September 2015.

Dunk, R., Whitson, E. and Allibone, L. 2013. *Oxygen Therapy Part 3: Humidification of Oxygen*. Available at: www.clinicalskills.net. Accessed 14 September 2015.

Galluccio, S.T. and Bersten, A.D. 2014. *Humidification and inhalation therapy*. In: Bersten, A.D. and Soni, N. (eds.). *Oh's Intensive Care Manual* (7th ed.). Butterworth-Heinemann, Oxford, 375–381.

Hardinge, M., Annandale, J., Bourne, S., Cooper, B., Evans, A., Freeman, D., Green, A. et al. 2015. British Thoracic Society guidelines for home oxygen use in adults. *Thorax* 70 (Suppl 1): i1–i43.

Marieb, E.N. and Hoehn, K. 2010. *Human Anatomy & Physiology* (8th ed.). Pearson Benjamin Cummings, San Francisco.

Marino, P.L. 2014. *Marino's The ICU Book* (4th ed.). Lippincott Williams and Wilkins, Philadelphia.

National Institute of Health and Care Excellence (NICE). 2010. *COPD Management of Chronic Obstructive Pulmonary Disease in Adults in Primary and Secondary Care. Clinical Guidelines 101*. NICE, London.

National Patient Safety Agency (NPSA). 2009. *National Reporting and Learning Service. Rapid Response Report NPSA/2009/RRR006: Oxygen Safety in Hospitals*. NPSA, London.

Nursing and Midwifery Council (NMC). 2010. *Standards for Medicines Management*. Nursing and Midwifery Council, London.

O'Driscoll, B.R., Howard, L.S. and Davison, A.G. 2008. British Thoracic Society guideline for emergency oxygen use in adult patients. *Thorax* 63 (Suppl 6): vi1–vi73.

Resuscitation Council United Kingdom (RCUK). 2016. *Advanced Life Support* (7th ed.). Resuscitation Council, London.

Wagstaff, A.J. 2014. Oxygen therapy. In: Bersten, A.D. and Soni, N. (eds.). *Oh's Intensive Care Manual* (7th ed.). Butterworth-Heinemann, Oxford, 327–340.

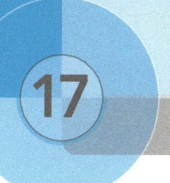

Non-invasive ventilation

17

CATHERINE PLOWRIGHT AND JANE KINDRED

LEARNING OBJECTIVES

Upon completion of the chapter the reader should be able to:

- Differentiate between Type 1 and Type 2 respiratory failure
- Understand the principles of non-invasive ventilation (NIV)
- Identify patients who may benefit from NIV
- Discuss the care required for people receiving NIV using an ABCDE approach

INTRODUCTION

This chapter will explain the principles of non-invasive ventilation (NIV), why it is used and the types of patients it should be considered for. NIV is an important treatment method in respiratory failure. It delivers intermittent positive airway pressure, which gives the patient ventilatory support using either a facemask or a nasal mask and may avoid intubation with an endotracheal tube and invasive ventilation (Halpin, 2003). In patients who have NIV started appropriately and timely there is less need for intubation and mortality rates are reduced (Halpin, 2003). The British Thoracic Society (BTS) published guidance in conjunction with the Intensive Care Society and the Royal College of Physicians (RCP) on the management of patients with Type 2

respiratory failure and these guidelines will provide readers with further information (Royal College of Physicians [RCP] et al., 2008). In 2016 the BTS and Intensive Care Society published guidelines for the ventilatory management of acute hypercapnic respiratory failure in adults (Davidson et al., 2016).

RESPIRATORY FAILURE

Respiratory failure can occur in many patients for a variety of reasons. Some of these reasons include pneumonia, pulmonary embolism, chronic obstructive pulmonary disease (COPD), conditions such as Guillain–Barre syndrome or muscular dystrophy, which affect nerves and muscle controlling breathing, drug or alcohol overdoses and chest trauma – please note this list is not exhaustive (Hughes and Black, 2011).

Respiratory failure occurs when there is inadequate gas exchange by the respiratory system and levels of arterial oxygen (PaO_2) and/or arterial carbon dioxide ($PaCO_2$) cannot be maintained within normal limits. Respiratory failure is diagnosed after obtaining an arterial blood gas (ABG) sample and analysing the results (Woodrow, 2012) (see Chapter 4 for a detailed explanation on arterial blood gases).

Respiratory failure is categorised into Type 1 and Type 2 respiratory failure. In Type 1 failure the level of oxygen is low (PaO_2 is less than 8 kPa) and the $PaCO_2$ is normal or low (BTS, 2002; Woodrow, 2012). Type 1 respiratory failure is also known as hypoxic respiratory failure. In Type 2 respiratory failure (also known as hypercapnic respiratory failure) the PaO_2 is less than 8 kPa and the $PaCO_2$ is greater than 6 kPa (BTS, 2002; Woodrow 2012).

In Type 1 respiratory failure there is damage to the lung tissue, which then prevents adequate oxygenation; but, as carbon dioxide diffusion requires less functioning lung tissue than that needed for oxygen diffusion, the lung tissue remaining is sufficient to excrete carbon dioxide. This results in the PaO_2 less than 8 kPa and the $PaCO_2$ normal or low. If the cause of the Type 1 respiratory failure is as a result of lack of oxygen alone, then treatment is supplementary oxygen for the patient (Higgins and Guest, 2008) (see Chapter 16).

In Type 2 respiratory failure, ventilation in the alveoli is insufficient to excrete the carbon dioxide and results in $PaCO_2$ greater than 6 kPa, and PaO_2 less than 8 KPa. The BTS (2002) further defined respiratory failure as acute, acute on chronic and chronic:

- *Acute type 2 respiratory failure:* Pre-existing respiratory disease will probably not have been present and arterial blood gases will show a low pH, high $PaCO_2$, and normal bicarbonate
- *Acute on chronic type 2 respiratory failure:* The patient has a history of Type 2 respiratory failure and experiences a sudden and acute deterioration. Arterial blood gases will show low pH, high $PaCO_2$ and a high bicarbonate
- *Chronic type 2 respiratory failure:* The patient has evidence of chronic respiratory disease. Arterial blood gases will show normal pH, high $PaCO_2$, and high bicarbonate

Table 17.1 summarises the differences between acute, acute on chronic and chronic.

Table 17.1 Differences between acute, acute on chronic and chronic Type 2 respiratory failure

	pH	$PaCO_2$	Bicarbonate
Acute Type 2 respiratory failure	Low	High	Normal
Acute on chronic Type 2 respiratory failure	Low	High	High
Chronic Type 2 respiratory failure	Normal	High	High

Type 2 respiratory failure is fatal if not treated as it causes hypoxia, which damages vital organs. Type 2 respiratory failure also results in central nervous system depression due to increasing carbon dioxide levels and respiratory acidosis as carbon dioxide is retained. NIV in the management of acute Type 2 respiratory failure has been a significant advance in respiratory care over the last 15 years (RCP et al., 2008). Most hospitals now use bi-level positive airway pressure (BiPAP), although there are other forms of NIV available (RCP et al., 2008). Prior to commencement of NIV, the medical staff should decide on alternative treatment plans if NIV should not achieve satisfactory improvements (RCP et al., 2008). Some patients who have Type 2 respiratory failure may be considered for invasive ventilation at first presentation or diagnosis, especially if they do not meet the inclusion and exclusion criteria for NIV. This is a decision that will be made in conjunction with the critical care and the referring team.

NON-INVASIVE VENTILATION

NIV is a way to provide support to patients who are having respiratory problems. The National Institute for Health and Care Excellence (2010) recommended that NIV should be available in all hospitals that admit patients with COPD. There are two main modes of providing NIV (RCP et al., 2008):

1. Continuous positive airway pressure – CPAP
2. Bi-level positive airways pressure – BiPAP

CPAP is indicated in patients who have Type 1 respiratory failure where there is acute hypoxemia without hypercapnia (RCP et al., 2008). It is also used when patients have sleep apnoea, pulmonary oedema and in post-operative respiratory problems. It is contraindicated for the following types of patients: those with facial injuries, surgery or burns, in those patients who cannot maintain an airway, recent gastrointestinal surgery, copious secretions, and in those patients who are haemodynamically unstable (RCP et al., 2008). A valve in the CPAP circuit provides the positive pressure in the circuit to create a resistance during expiration and this assists in keeping the alveoli open at the end of expiration for gas exchange.

BiPAP is a type of NIV that delivers gases at different pressures: inspiratory positive airway pressure (IPAP) and expiratory positive airway pressure (EPAP). On inspiration by the patient the BiPAP machine detects a drop in pressure and delivers a flow of air into the patient's airways until the predetermined inspiration pressure (IPAP) is reached, and on expiration the predetermined pressure (EPAP) is maintained in the alveoli to splint them open and enable improved gas exchange (Coombs et al., 2013).

PATIENTS WHO WOULD BENEFIT FROM BiPAP NIV

Patients with acute exacerbations of COPD and Type 2 respiratory failure may benefit from BiPAP. Patients should initially receive standard medical therapy within the first hour of presentation (RCP et al., 2008) and if this fails to improve the patients' arterial blood gases then NIV should be considered. Standard medical therapy (RCP et al., 2008) includes:

- Controlled oxygen to maintain SaO_2 88%–92%
- Nebulised salbutamol 2.5–5 mg
- Nebulised ipratroprium 500 µg
- Prednisolone 30 mg
- Antibiotic agent (when indicated)

There are strict inclusion and exclusion criteria for patients potentially requiring NIV, which must be considered (see Table 17.2). It is vitally important to consider the patient's pre-morbid condition, the severity and reversibility of the condition and the previous perceptions that the patient has of their condition. The multidisciplinary team should all have a role to play in determining the need for NIV and considerations must be made about what should happen if NIV does not work for the patient. The

Table 17.2 Inclusion and exclusion criteria for NIV

Inclusion criteria	Exclusion criteria
• Primary diagnosis of COPD exacerbation (known diagnosis or history and examination consistent with diagnosis) • Respiratory acidosis persisting after a maximum of one hour of standard medical therapy (controlled oxygen, and nebuliser of salbutamol and ipratroprium) • pH between 7.26 and 7.35 • Able to protect airway independently • Conscious and cooperative • Potential for recovery to quality of life acceptable to the patient • Patient's wishes taken into consideration	• Life-threatening hypoxaemia • Severe co-morbidity • Confusion/agitation/severe cognitive impairment • Facial burns/trauma/recent facial or upper airway surgery • Vomiting • Fixed upper airway obstruction • Undrained pneumothorax • Upper gastrointestinal surgery • Inability to protect the airway • Copious respiratory secretions • Haemodynamically unstable requiring inotropes/vasopressors (unless in a critical care unit) • Patient moribund • Bowel obstruction

Source: Royal College of Physicians (RCP), British Thoracic Society (BTS) and Intensive Care Society (ICS). 2008. *Non-Invasive Ventilation in Chronic Obstructive Pulmonary Disease: Management of Acute Type 2 Respiratory Failure.* Royal College of Physicians, London.

RCP et al. (2008) have an example of a NIV prescription checklist that could be used. This covers issues such as patients' mental capacity to provide consent for NIV and what should happen if NIV fails and whether the patient is a suitable candidate for admission to a critical care unit.

Healthcare professionals need to remember that NIV is not the treatment of choice for patients whose primary diagnosis is heart failure or pneumonia, but may be used in COPD patients with these complications if escalation to intubation and ventilation is deemed inappropriate. NIV may be considered in unconscious patients if endotracheal intubation is deemed inappropriate or NIV is to be provided in a critical care setting. Diaz et al. (2005) demonstrated that the use of NIV in patients who were comatosed secondary to hypercapnia respond rapidly to NIV.

If, after an hour of receiving maximum standard medical treatment, patients still have a respiratory acidosis ($PaCO_2 > 6$ kPa, pH <7.35 ≥7.26), then NIV must be considered. It should be noted that there is a higher rate of failed NIV in patients who are more acidotic (Conti et al., 2002). The reasons for considering NIV will vary dependent on the patient, the severity of condition and associated complicating factors (Davidson et al 2016). Table 17.3 summaries these.

ESTABLISHING NIV

A competent healthcare professional or specialist trainee doctor level 2 or above (RCP, 2015) must make the decision regarding whether NIV is the treatment of choice and a competent practitioner must commence the therapy (RCP et al., 2008). Patients requiring NIV must be cared for in the right clinical environment. Some hospitals may limit NIV to specialised areas such as emergency departments, critical care units or respiratory wards. This is more likely to enable staff to maintain their competence associated with NIV. If patients require NIV in other clinical areas then specialist advice must be sought, either from respiratory teams, critical care outreach or critical care teams. A patient requiring NIV must be safely managed in the optimisation, maintenance and weaning phases of non-invasive ventilation.

The ABCDE approach is a good clinical tool and it will be utilised to describe the care that patients requiring NIV need (Thim et al., 2012). Readers are directed towards the Thim et al. (2012) article for further detail concerning the ABCDE patient assessment approach.

AIRWAY AND BREATHING

It is vital to ensure that airway and breathing are assessed, maintained and monitored. Patient cooperation and compliance are important at the initiation of NIV and it should be remembered that many patients will be frightened and anxious at this stage due to their dyspnoea and abnormal gas exchange. Furthermore, many patients will experience claustrophobia associated with mask placement. The healthcare professional commencing the NIV should calmly explain the procedure to the patient, to ensure they fully understand the underlying rationale for the intervention. If possible, two staff should be with the patient at the initiation of treatment; one member of the staff can position the mask and adjust the NIV settings, while the other person spends time reassuring the patient, explaining to them what is happening.

MASK SIZE

An appropriately fitted and sized face mark will be better tolerated by the patient and will promote better therapeutic benefit, so time should be taken to ensure that the correct mask shape and size is obtained for the patient. There are numerous different masks available to purchase and most hospitals will have the product that they consider to be the most suitable for the majority of their patients. Healthcare professionals should be trained on how to choose and fit masks to patients, as products may have different fitting procedures. The full-face mask is usually used in the first 24 hours of therapy as it is thought to be more comfortable and better for patients who are mouth breathers (Hess, 2004) (see Figure 17.1). If masks are the correct size and in the correct position, then a good seal will be achieved and this will prevent some of the problems associated with NIV (Brill, 2014). Some of the problems associated with poorly fitting masks include corneal irritations due to leakages onto eyes, pressure ulcerations on the bridge of nose, as well as nasal and buccal mucosal irritations and dryness particularly when there is mask leakage.

The healthcare professional must assess the patient for use of accessory muscles, co-ordination of

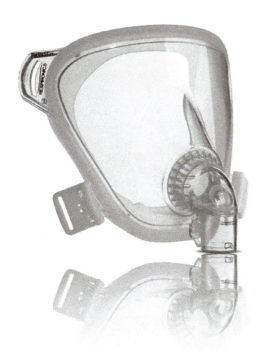

Figure 17.1 Shows an example of full face NIV mask. The mask pictured is the PerforMax mask. (Reproduced with permission from Philips Respironics.)

respiratory effort with the NIV machine and bilateral chest wall movement. Respiratory rates and oxygen saturations must be recorded and documented at least every 15 minutes in the first hour, every 30 minutes up to 4 hours and then at least hourly up to 12 hours (Lane et al., 2007; RCP et al., 2008). If the patient's condition should deteriorate, then the frequency of observations must be increased and appropriate action taken. Pulse oximetry should be continuous. These respiratory observations should be recorded on the National Early Warning Score (NEWS) system (RCP, 2012) along with the other physiological parameters. Some hospitals may utilise a locally adapted NEWS system.

INITIATION OF NIV

For a more detailed exploration of the required steps associated with the initiation of NIV therapy, the reader is encouraged to consult the flow chart diagram contained within RCP et al. (2008). The 2016 guidelines (Davidson et al., 2016) also suggest steps

to follow in initiating NIV – see Figure 17.2. Before commencing NIV the patient should be sitting or in a semi-recumbent position, and they should be as calm as possible.

The starting pressures (RCP et al., 2008) on the NIV BiPAP are recommended as follows:

- Inspiratory pressure (IPAP) of 10 cmH$_2$O
- Expiratory pressure (EPAP) of 4–5 cmH$_2$O

The new guidance (Davidson et al., 2016) suggests different starting pressures as follows (Figure 17.2):

- Inspiratory pressure (IPAP) of 15 cmH$_2$O
- Expiratory pressure (EPAP) of 3 cmH$_2$O

and hospitals should ensure that their policies are adjusted accordingly.

The majority of patients can tolerate these initial settings. IPAP can be increased gradually in 2 to 5 cmH$_2$O increments over about 20 minutes up to a maximum 20 cmH$_2$O in order to achieve a therapeutic response (RCP et al., 2008). If patients are unable to tolerate the maximum level, then the level they are most comfortable at should be maintained. EPAP may also be increased to a maximum of 6 cmH$_2$O in 1 cmH$_2$O increments (RCP et al., 2008). The new guidance (Davidson et al., 2016) suggests that IPAP should not exceed 30 and EPAP 8 without seeking expert opinion. Oxygen, if needed, can be entrained into the circuit and adjusted to maintain saturations usually between 88% and 92% in patients with COPD (RCP et al., 2008).

Arterial blood gases (ABGs) should be performed one hour after NIV has started and one hour after changes in IPAP or EPAP settings. The results of the ABGs will determine the further management plan regarding NIV for the patient. If a decision is made that the patient may require an indwelling arterial line for frequent ABG sampling, then the patient will need to be moved to a critical care unit. Some hospitals may use capillary blood samples to measure blood gases; however, the gold standard method is arterial blood samples (Higgins, 2008). Capillary blood samples are considered acceptable if pH and pCO$_2$ are the parameters of main interest; if pO$_2$ levels are important then it is recommended that an arterial blood gas should be obtained (Higgins, 2008).

If bronchodilators are prescribed, then they must be administered. They should preferably be

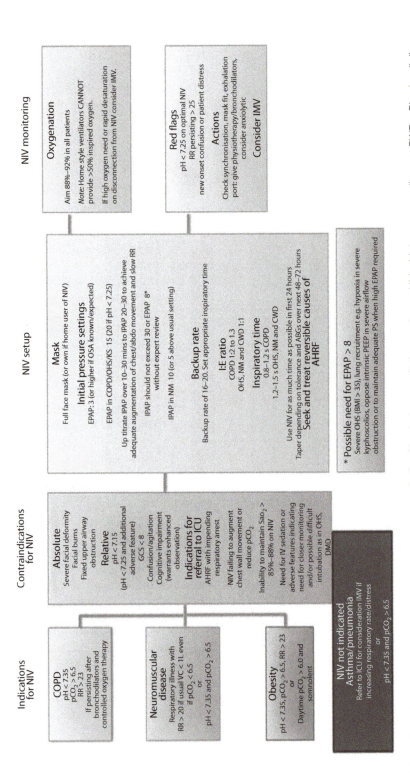

Figure 17.2 Brief summary for providing NIV in acute cases. OHS – Obesity hypoventilation syndrome, NM – Motor-neurone disease, CWD – Chest wall disease. (Adapted from Davidson, A.C., Banham, S., Elliott, M. et al. 2016. *Thorax* 71: ii1–ii35.)

administered with the NIV system off but if necessary can be given with the NIV in progress (Calvert et al., 2006; RCP et al., 2008).

DURATION OF TREATMENT

Patients who benefit and improve in the first few hours of NIV treatment should continue for as long as possible to achieve a pH ≥ 7.35 (Davidson et al., 2016; RCP et al., 2008). Once this is achieved and maintained and all underlying causes are treated then weaning should be considered (RCP et al., 2008).

ESCALATION

A decision should be made by the medical staff prior to commencement of NIV on what the management plan will be should NIV fail (RCP et al., 2008). Ideally the patient and their family should be involved in this decision-making process. This must include whether NIV is the ceiling of treatment, what the patient's resuscitation status is, and whether they are ready for admission to a critical care unit should escalation of treatment be required. A decision to proceed to intubation and ventilation ought to be made within the first few hours of treatment (RCP et al., 2008). If the patient is considered suitable for invasive ventilation should NIV fail, then the critical care team should be involved early (RCP et al., 2008). Treatment alternatives may need to be considered if NIV is deemed inappropriate; this may include palliative care.

WEANING

RCP et al. (2008) suggest that weaning should take place over a 4-day period, although for some patients weaning can be achieved in 2 to 3 days. Furthermore, on day 2 of weaning, NIV should continue for 16 hours, including 6 to 8 hours overnight; on day 3 NIV should continue for 12 hours, including 6 to 8 hours overnight; NIV may be discontinued on day 4 unless continuation is clinically indicated, for example, two hours in the morning, two hours in the afternoon and six hours or more overnight. The 2016 guidance (Davidson et al., 2016) suggests that NIV can be discontinued when there has been

a sustained normal pH and pCO_2 and a general improvement in the patient's condition. Like the 2008 guidance (RCP, 2008) it is still suggested that the time on NIV should be maximised in the first 24 hours depending on patient tolerance and/or complications. Davidson et al. (2016) suggest that NIV use during the day can be tapered in the following 2–3 days, depending on pCO_2 before being discontinued overnight.

RECORD KEEPING

A record of all NIV settings and whether the patient is receiving oxygen or not should be maintained. An example of an 'NIV prescription and changes to settings chart' can be found within RCP et al. (2008) guidelines. Respiratory improvements are often seen in the first few hours of NIV and are usually accompanied by improvements in neurological status. Therefore, a full clinical review and an ABG review should be made after 1–2 hours of treatment. A decision should then be made as to whether NIV is being effective.

While patients are receiving NIV, it is essential that good records are maintained, as this will enable healthcare staff to monitor the patient's progress with the therapy.

CARDIOVASCULAR

Patients must have cardiovascular observations performed at least every 15 minutes in the first hour, every 30 minutes up to 4 hours and then at least hourly up to 12 hours. These observations must include blood pressure, pulse rate and cardiac rhythm. If at any time the patient's condition deteriorates or the NEWS score increases, then the frequency of observations must be increased and acted upon, including escalation to an appropriate healthcare professional, e.g. senior doctor or critical care outreach team. Staff should be looking for reductions in blood pressure, as well as any increases in pulse rate.

There is some evidence that the effects of the positive pressure used in NIV can result in reductions in blood pressure. As pressure increases inside the lungs from the positive pressure, which is generated or supplied by the ventilator, this increases the pressure on the heart, which reduces venous return and causes a reduction in filling of the heart chambers. This in turn will reduce cardiac output and ultimately results in a fall in blood pressure. In a randomised control trial, Duran-Cantolla et al. (2010) reviewed patients with newly diagnosed hypertension and with sleep apnoea. They randomised the patients into two groups: one group received CPAP and one group placebo CPAP. Results found that those patients receiving CPAP produced a statistically significant reduction in blood pressure in patients with systemic hypertension and obstructive sleep apnoea. In patients who are invasively ventilated, the positive pressure and positive end expiratory pressure (PEEP) used have been found to decrease cardiac output and therefore blood pressure (Michard, 2005). A recent meta-analysis by Hu et al. (2015) also showed that CPAP does provide immediate improvements in patients who are hypertensive by lowering the blood pressure. The same effect is often seen in patients when NIV is first commenced – thus the importance of doing physiological observations at the frequency described. Particular care must be taken if the patient is hypotensive prior to commencing the NIV, as the patient may experience a further reduction in blood pressure when the NIV is initiated. There may be a medical discussion to administer intravenous fluids to some patients who are hypotensive.

DISABILITY

The conscious level of patients must be monitored using the Alert, Voice, Pain, Unresponsive (AVPU) method recorded on the NEWS system. Frequency of these observations must be at least every 15 minutes in the first hour, then every 30 minutes up to 4 hours and then at least hourly up to 12 hours. If AVPU alters, then a Glasgow Coma Score (GCS) must be performed. If there are any variations from 'A' or a deteriorating GCS, it is essential to repeat an ABG to check for a rise in carbon dioxide level. The blood glucose levels in all patients who have an altered AVPU or GCS score must be checked, even if the patient is not known to be diabetic, as a low blood glucose level can be easily corrected and will improve conscious level (Thim et al. 2012).

EXPOSURE/ENVIRONMENT

Staff must ensure that the patients have care to eyes and mouth. Eye care is essential as corneal irritations can occur owing to leakages onto eyes from the mask. Both eyes should be visually checked and the patients asked about any dryness or irritation in the eyes. It may be necessary to consider the use of eye lubricants, although repositioning and re-fitting of the mask may reduce the problem. For further information on eye assessment and care please see Woodrow et al. (2013). The oral cavity must be assessed each time the mouth is cleaned, which should be ideally twice a day (Woodrow et al., 2013). Patients should be encouraged and assisted to brush their teeth; the aim of mouth care is to ensure that the mouth is clean, moist and intact, that the lips are clean, soft, moist and intact, and that there is no pain or discomfort (Dougherty and Lister, 2008). Patients should be encouraged to maintain oral fluids and nutrition intake, and ideally the break from NIV should be minimal. It is considered good practice to plan NIV breaks to enable the patients to have meals, fluids, physiotherapy and oral medications within the same time period. Patients should have fluid balance carefully monitored. While patients are off NIV, oxygen therapy must be maintained.

Pressure ulceration is considered one of the more serious mask-related complications and usually develops on the nasal bridge (Sleilati et al., 2008; Gay, 2009). Healthcare professionals must assess the skin around the nose and back of ears at an appropriate frequency for the patient and if necessary take preventative measures using suitable dermal application materials. Weng (2008) showed that preventative measures could be taken to reduce pressure ulcers during NIV. If pressure ulcers develop, they have to be reported via the organisation's local incident reporting systems and in extreme cases the patient may ultimately require a skin graft (Sleilati et al., 2008; Gay 2009).

The safety of the patient is important and all information related to the NIV must be recorded. There is an example from the RCP et al. (2008) guidelines on how to document IPAP/EPAP recordings and ABGs in relation to these changes. The RCP et al. (2008) guidelines also provide a guide to trouble shooting and a method of audit NIV practices which are extremely useful.

CASE STUDY

Joe Ross is a 65-year-old gentleman who was diagnosed with COPD 6 years ago and had had one previous admission for his COPD. His latest spirometry demonstrated an FEV_1 of 28%, which represents a severe obstruction. He had stopped smoking two years ago. Joe's activity was limited and he could only walk 50 metres on the flat.

He presented to the Emergency Department (ED) with a one-week history of increasing shortness of breath and green sputum. He had commenced his rescue pack of steroids and antibiotics at home, but his wife was concerned that he was no better, and that he appeared a little confused and he was sleeping more than usual.

When the ambulance arrived at Joe's house his saturations were 85% on air. On arrival in ED, Joe was on 28% oxygen therapy via a Venturi mask which maintained oxygen saturation at 92%. Joe was not on long-term oxygen therapy at home. Routine physiological observations were taken using the NEWS system and an ABG was performed which showed an acute Type 2 respiratory failure:

- pH 7.28
- $PaCO_2$ 9.6 kPa
- PaO_2 7.3 kPa
- HCO_3 24.6 mmol/L

Joe lives with his wife in a bungalow. He stopped smoking two years ago, as did his wife. They have two children and four grandchildren. One of Joe's brothers also has COPD. Joe's mother is still alive but she suffers from hypertension and slight dementia. Joe's medications on admission were:

Triotropium 18 mcg of seretide 500 one puff twice a day salbutamol via a spacer as and when required.

The ED team prescribed nebulised bronchodilators, oral steroids, oral antibiotics and requested that 28% oxygen be continued, and they would review him after 30 minutes. After 30 minutes the nursing staff reported that Joe appeared to be drowsier, and a repeat ABG showed:

- pH 7.26
- $PaCO_2$ 10 kPa
- PaO_2 7.0 kPa
- HCO_3 24 mmol/L

As the acute Type 2 respiratory failure was not improving, the team assessing Joe requested that NIV be commenced and contacted the respiratory nurse.

It was policy at the hospital that Joe was admitted to that a full-face mask be used, as this had been found to reduce the prevalence of pressure area breakdown. Joe was measured for the correct size, fitted and commenced onto NIV with a starting IPAP of 15 cmH_2O and an EPAP of 3 cmH_2O.

Physiological observation monitoring using NEWS was increased to every 15 minutes to observe for a potential drop in blood pressure. Inspiratory and expiratory pressures were increased over the next 20 minutes; Joe was able to tolerate an IPAP of 26 (above the usual target pressure) and an EPAP of 8 (above the usual target pressure). This gave an estimated tidal volume of 600 mL, oxygen was entrained at 30% and he tolerated the NIV well. His blood pressure did drop slightly to 98/70 mmHg and intravenous fluids were commenced, and BP improved to 110/70 mmHg.

Joe was reassured throughout the whole of the initiation of NIV. After 60 minutes on the above pressures a repeat ABG was taken which showed:

- pH 7.30
- $PaCO_2$ 8.6 kPa
- PaO_2 9.7 kPa
- HCO_3 24.6 mmol/L

The medical team were satisfied with his progress and did not wish for further increase in NIV pressures. The respiratory consultant reviewed Joe and a management plan was devised. Joe had previously stated to his family that he did not wish to be resuscitated, as he felt that his overall quality of life was poor. A decision was made in conjunction with Joe that his care would be on a respiratory ward, and he was transferred.

On arrival to the respiratory ward Joe was allowed off the ventilator for a 10-minute break; therefore, he was able to drink, take medication and ensure that the nursing staff could review his pressure areas. These were found to be intact, hourly monitoring of his physiological observations continued and the ventilator check chart was maintained.

Joe was to remain on NIV for as long as he was able to tolerate, he felt he could manage if he was still able to have the 10-minute breaks, and began to clock watch. These 10-minute breaks were negotiated with Joe, as the aim of NIV is for it to continue as long as possible, uninterrupted. Joe remained on NIV for 4 days and he was discharged home after a further 4 days.

CASE STUDY DISCUSSION

Patients with acute exacerbations of COPD and Type 2 respiratory failure may benefit from BiPAP (RCP et al., 2008). Joe was initially treated with standard medical therapy but, as can happen, his condition deteriorated. The staff closely observed him and they became aware of an increasing drowsiness. It is important to closely monitor and observe all patients with Type 2 respiratory failure as changes will be observed before ABG confirm worsening results (RCP et al., 2008).

When the BiPAP was commenced and increased, the levels Joe tolerated were an IPAP of 26 and an EPAP of 8. This was higher than the RCP et al. (2008) recommendations, but as Joe, in conjunction with medical staff, had decided he did not want to be resuscitated, BiPAP was the ceiling of his treatment, so staff increased pressures to obtain the desired outcome.

Joe did experience a drop in blood pressure as the IPAP and EPAP were increased. This was only observed by staff because they were performing physiological observations using NEWS (RCP, 2012) every 15 minutes in the first hour, then every 30 minutes up to 4 hours and then at least hourly up to 12 hours (RCP et al., 2008). The staff ensured that Joe was adequately hydrated so his blood pressure was maintained. It is important to consider using intravenous fluids if patients on BiPAP are unable to maintain an adequate oral intake. Subcutaneous fluids could also be given if necessary.

This case study demonstrates how BiPAP was effectively used to treat a man with COPD and acute Type 2 respiratory failure.

SUMMARY

The RCP et al. (2008) guidelines make a number of recommendations about NIV. These include that NIV services should be managed by named clinical leads as well as having experienced staff available to support the service 24 hours a day, 7 days a week. Healthcare professionals should have the appropriate competencies, experience and skills to care for respiratory patients and staff who use NIV should attend annual courses. Staff should understand the criteria for commencing NIV in patients with COPD and be aware that those patients with predictors for further deterioration should be admitted to environments where early intubation can be performed. Patients should be selected appropriately for NIV by a specialist trainee doctor (RCP, 2015) or by a competent designated healthcare professional (RCP et al., 2008).

Good care for these patients is essential to ensure that all activities of living are managed and there should be a staffing ratio of one nurse to two patients receiving NIV for at least the first 24 hours of NIV. Duration of NIV will be dependent on the individual patients and throughout therapy they must continue to be monitored using the NEWS system. NIV is a vital therapy in the treatment of patients with respiratory failure.

REFERENCES

Brill, A. 2014. How to avoid interface problems in acute non-invasive ventilation. *Breathe* 10 (3): 231–241.

British Thoracic Society Standards of Care Committee. 2002. BTS Guideline: Non-invasive ventilation in acute respiratory failure. *Thorax* 57 (3): 192–211.

Calvert, L.D., Jackson, J.M., White, J.A., Barry, P.W., Kinnear, W.J. and O'Callaghan, C. 2006. Enhanced delivery of nebulised salbutamol during non-invasive ventilation. *Journal of Pharmacy and Pharmacology* 58 (11): 1553–1557.

Conti, G., Antonelli, M., Navalesi, P., Rocco, M., Bufi, M., Spadetta, G. and Meduri, G.U. 2002. Noninvasive vs. conventional mechanical ventilation in patients with chronic obstructive pulmonary disease after failure of medical treatment in the ward: A randomized trial. *Intensive Care Medicine* 28 (12): 1701–1707.

Coombs, M., Dyos, J., Waters, D. and Nesbitt, I. 2013. Assessment, monitoring and interventions for the respiratory system. In: Mallet, J., Albarran, J.W. and Richardson, A. 2013. *Critical Care Manual of Clinical Procedures and Competencies*. Wiley Blackwell, Oxford.

Davidson, A.C., Banham, S., Elliott, M. et al. 2016. BTS/ICS guideline for the ventilatory management of acute hypercapnic respiratory failure in adults. *Thorax* 71: ii1–ii35.

Diaz, G.G., Alcaraz, A.C., Talavera, J.C., Pérez, P.J., Rodriguez, A.E., Cordoba, F.G. and Hill, N.S. 2005. Noninvasive positive-pressure ventilation to treat hypercapnic coma secondary to respiratory failure. *Chest* 127 (3): 952–60.

Dougherty, L. and Lister, S. 2008. *The Royal Marsden Hospital Manual of Clinical Nursing Procedures Student Edition* (7th ed.). Wiley Blackwell, Oxford.

Duran-Cantolla, J., Aizpure, F., Montserrat, J.M. et al. 2010. Continuous positive airway pressure as treatment for systemic hypertension in people with obstructive sleep apnoea: Randomised controlled trial. *British Medical Journal* 341 (7783): 1142.

Gay, P.C. 2009. Complications of noninvasive ventilation in acute care. *Respiratory Care* 54 (2): 246–258.

Halpin, D.M.G. 2003. *Your Questions Answered COPD*. Churchill Livingstone, London.

Hess, D.R. 2004. The evidence for non-invasive positive pressure ventilation in the care of patients in acute respiratory failure: A systematic review of the literature. *Respiratory Care* 49 (7): 810–829.

Higgins, C. 2008. Capillary-blood gases: To arterialize or not. *Medical Laboratory Observer.* November: 42–47.

Higgins, D. and Guest, J. 2008. Acute respiratory failure 2: Nursing management. *Nursing Times* 104 (37): 22–23.

Hu, X., Fan, J., Chen, S., Yin, Y. and Zrenner, B. 2015. The role of continuous positive airway pressure in blood pressure control for patients with obstructive sleep apnea and hypertension. A meta-analysis of randomized controlled trials. *The Journal of Clinical Hypertension* 17 (3): 215–222.

Hughes, M. and Black, R. 2011. *Advanced Respiratory Critical Care.* Oxford University Press, Oxford.

Lane, A., Wood, M., Murray, P. and Boot, J. 2007. The use of a noninvasive ventilation (NIV) proforma improves successful weaning from NIV on a respiratory ward. *Thorax* 62 (Supp iii) A91–A92.

Michard, F. 2005. Changes in arterial pressure during mechanical ventilation. *Anesthesiology* 103 (2): 419–428.

National Institute for Health and Care Excellence (NICE). 2010. *Chronic Obstructive Pulmonary Disease: Management of Chronic Obstructive Pulmonary Disease in Adults in Primary and Secondary Care (partial update).* NICE, London.

Royal College of Physicians (RCP). 2012. *National Early Warning Score (NEWS): Standardising the Assessment of Acute-Illness Severity in the NHS.* Royal College of Physicians, London.

Royal College of Physicians (RCP). 2015. *Core and Speciality Trainees.* Available at: https://www.rcplondon.ac.uk/medical-careers/core-and-specialty-trainees Accessed 17 February 2015.

Royal College of Physicians (RCP), British Thoracic Society (BTS) and Intensive Care Society (ICS). 2008. *Non-Invasive Ventilation in Chronic*

Obstructive Pulmonary Disease: Management of Acute Type 2 Respiratory Failure. Royal College of Physicians, London.

Sleilati, F.H., Stephan, H.A., Nasr, M.W. and Riachy, M.A. 2008. An unusual pressure sore of the nasal bridge. *British Journal of Oral and Maxillofacial Surgery* 46 (5): 411–412.

Thim, T., Krarup, N.H.V., Grove, E.L., Rohde, C.V. and Løfgren, B. 2012. Initial assessment and treatment with the Airway, Breathing, Circulation, Disability, Exposure (ABCDE) approach. *International Journal of General Medicine* 5: 117–121.

Weng, M-H. 2008. The effect of protective treatment in reducing pressure ulcers for non-invasive ventilation patients. *Intensive and Critical Care Nursing* 24 (5): 295–299.

Woodrow, P. 2012. *Intensive Care Nursing: A Framework for Practice*. (3rd ed.) Routledge, London.

Woodrow, P., Elliot, J. and Beldon, P. 2013. Assessment and care of tissue viability, and mouth and eye hygiene needs. In: Mallet, J., Albarran, J.W. and Richardson, A. 2013. *Critical Care Manual of Clinical Procedures and Competencies*. Wiley Blackwell, Oxford.

Smoking cessation

18

BARBARA FOGGO

LEARNING OBJECTIVES

Upon completion of this chapter the reader should be able to:

- Describe the addictive effects of nicotine
- Identify the major health consequences of smoking
- Discuss the economic burden of smoking
- Identify current interventions available for smoking cessation

INTRODUCTION

The burden of smoking remains exponential in both financial and societal costs. Smoking remains the most preventable cause of chronic long-term conditions, premature death and generic ill health. In spite of the numerous campaigns and health warnings the prevalence of smoking remains a concern. One in five adults over the age of 16 continue to smoke; as a direct result over 200,000 men and women die each year due to smoking-related issues (Health and Social Care Information Centre [HSCIC], 2014a).

This chapter will discuss the harmful effects of smoking on the respiratory system and the addictive properties of nicotine. The major health consequences of smoking will be identified and discussed. Cancer will be referred to, but for a fuller discussion of lung cancer please refer to Chapter 11. Current interventions and therapies to aid smoking cessation will be identified and discussed.

SMOKING PREVALENCE

The October 2007 report of the Tobacco Advisory Group of the Royal College of Physicians (RCP) acknowledged that smoking is the single most important public health problem in Britain (RCP, 2007). It continues to be a high priority as currently there are approximately 10 million adults (age 18 or over) who smoke (Action on Smoking and Health [ASH], 2015). If 11–15 years old were included this number would increase by 200,000.

In 1971, 51% of the male population smoked and in comparison 42% of smokers were women (Forey et al., 2012). A growing concern with regards to health and healthy lifestyle along with the increased awareness of the dangers of smoking can also account for a decrease in the percentage of smokers. The current statistics demonstrate this reduction with 21% of all men who smoke and 19% of all women (HSCIC, 2014a). The recent data, although reassuring, highlight the comparable figures of men and women: the gap between the sexes is minimal and the consequence of this is the rise in lung cancer rates in women (HSCIC, 2015).

Twenty per cent of the United Kingdom (UK) population continues to smoke; the levels vary for men and women. The North East has the greatest percentage of female smokers at 25% and in the region of Yorkshire and Humber it is estimated that 24% of males currently smoke (HSCIC, 2014a). UK smoking rates peaked between the 1940s and 1960s, but fell steadily during the 1970s and 1980s (General Lifestyle Survey, 2011). However, by the mid-1990s this decline had levelled out, and in 1996 smoking rates rose for the first time in more than 20 years and 1998 rates were similar (HSCIC, 2014a). People in the age group 20–24 years are more likely to smoke than those in any other age group, reflecting the fact that the majority of smokers start smoking as teenagers (General Lifestyle Survey, 2011).

There are wide variations in smoking prevalence by socio-economic group. There is a large variation in smoking rates for professionals compared to manual workers, and this is duplicated across the sexes. Only 14% of managerial workers compared with 33% of routine and manual workers persist in smoking. The National Institute for Health and Care Excellence (NICE) have advised that smoking cession services target the socially disadvantaged and the minority ethnic populations within the community (NICE, 2008, 2013).

PATHOPHYSIOLOGY

Cigarette smoke contains over 4000 chemicals of which over 50 are carcinogenic, and many are poisonous. The chemicals include pesticides, paint stripper, lighter fuel, insecticides, industrial solvent and tar (Dalmandis, 2009). Some of the chemicals are found naturally in the tobacco plant and others are formed when the tobacco is processed or burnt. When inhaling, a cigarette burns at 700°C at the tip and around 60°C in the core. The heat breaks down the tobacco to produce various toxins.

Yellow staining on the fingers and teeth of smokers is a result of tar from the cigarette smoke: tar is the particulate sticky matter that is deposited within the lungs. Cells line the respiratory system and have fine hair-like projections called cilia, which protect the lungs by moving in a wave-like motion, transferring deposits up towards the throat to be coughed up or swallowed. When irritants such as smoke are inhaled, the cilia become paralysed and do not move the mucus and deposits, the smaller airways become inflamed, narrow and block as a result of the inflammation. This leads to the smoker coughing in an attempt to remove the mucus.

Nicotine is a potent alkaloid derived from the leaves of tobacco plants (*Nicotiana tabacum* and *Nicotiana rustica*), which are part of the nightshade family of plants and is the primary addictive agent in tobacco products. Nicotine is rapidly absorbed in the bloodstream via cigarette smoke inhalation, with arterial levels peaking 20 seconds after each inhalation (Rose et al., 1999).

There are two pathways in the brain that are important in nicotine addiction: the 'reward' pathway consisting of a network of dopaminergic neurons in the mesolimbic system; and the 'withdrawal' pathway, which involves noradrenergic neurons in the locus coeruleus.

REWARD PATHWAY

Like other addictive drugs, nicotine activates the mesolimbic system, resulting in a promotion of the release of dopamine in the nucleus accumbens. This dopamine surge induces feelings of pleasure or elation that become essential for the reinforcing effects of nicotine (Benowitz, 2010). The rapid action of inhaled nicotine on these pathways provides immediate positive reinforcement. Although the transfer of nicotine to the brain is not fully comprehended, it is estimated that it takes approximately 10 seconds to reach the brain, making it quicker than intravenous drug administration (Rose et al., 1999). The smoker is then motivated to repeat the behaviour, leading to compulsive use of the drug.

Chronic nicotine administration produces tolerance so that smokers need to smoke more to achieve the same effect.

WITHDRAWAL PATHWAY

A second factor involved in the development of nicotine addiction is the occurrence of withdrawal symptoms on deprivation of nicotine. These are believed to develop as a result of adaptive changes in the brain during chronic nicotine use and to be mediated by noradrenergic activity in the locus coeruleus. In February 2000, the Royal College of Physicians published a report on nicotine addiction which concluded that cigarettes are very effective nicotine-delivery devices and are as addictive as drugs such as heroin or cocaine (RCP, 2000). When a regular smoker abstains from smoking (either on stopping completely or enduring a long break between cigarettes), a state of nicotine deprivation ensues, resulting in altered levels of dopamine, noradrenaline and other neurotransmitters and altered activity in the associated neurons. These alterations support the cravings and withdrawal symptoms which follow that create the vicious cycle that is very difficult to break.

THE EFFECTS OF SMOKING ON HEALTH

Compared with most other countries in the European Union (EU), the UK has a worse mortality rate from smoking-related disease. Smoking is responsible for the death of 100,000 people in the UK per year and from the total deaths in the UK almost half will die of smoking-related diseases (Aveyard and West, 2007). In 2011, cigarette smoking accounted for almost 80,000 deaths (HSCIC, 2014a). Smoking is therefore responsible for about one in every five deaths in the UK each year. This translates into about 1500 people killed by smoking every week, and over 200 people per day. The World Health Organisation (WHO) estimate that tobacco kills around 6 million people each year (WHO, 2016). Relative mortality due to smoking is greater in younger age groups. Half of life-long smokers will die prematurely and

lose approximately 10 years of their life expectancy (ASH, 2014a).

The major effects of smoking on health include:

- *Cancer:* Smoking is a major cause of cancer and is responsible for a quarter of all cancer deaths (ASH, 2015), but also causes leukaemia and cancers of the kidney, stomach and liver. Smokers have twice the risk of death from cancer as non-smokers, and heavy smokers are four times at risk. See Chapter 11 for more detailed discussion of lung cancer.
- *Chronic obstructive pulmonary disease (COPD):* Smoking is the main cause of COPD (Decramer et al., 2012), accounting for 25,000 deaths from the disease per year (Health and Safety Executive [HSE], 2014). Smokers have at least 10 times the risk of dying from COPD compared with non-smokers. According to the WHO (2008), COPD is currently the fourth biggest cause of death, with this increasing to the third leading cause by 2030. Smoking accounts for a third of the respiratory deaths in the UK (ASH, 2015). See Chapter 5 for a more detailed discussion of COPD.
- *Coronary heart disease:* Up to 50% of cases of coronary heart disease are attributed to smoking. Under the age of 65 years, smokers are almost twice as likely to die from coronary heart disease than non-smokers, and heavy smokers (defined as those who smoke more than 20 per day by HSCIC [2014a]) are even more at risk. ASH (2015) estimate 14% of deaths as a result of cardiovascular disease are related to smoking.
- *Cerebrovascular disease:* Smokers are at a greater risk of having a stroke; a smoker is three times more likely to have a stroke compared to a non-smoker (Wannamethee et al., 1995). Around a fifth of all cases of stroke and 11% of deaths due to stroke are estimated to be caused by smoking. The HSCIC (2014a) report the largest number of hospital admissions, in excess of 711,000, were attributable to circulatory disease.

Many of the chemicals associated with smoking can pass across the placental barrier. The percentage of pregnant women smoking varies across the UK, from 5.1% in London to 20.6% in Durham and Darlington (HSCIC, 2014b). The complications of pregnancy and birth such as miscarriage, premature labour, low-birthweight baby and stillbirth occur more frequently with smokers than non-smokers (RCP, 2010). If a woman stops smoking before or in the early months of pregnancy, this reduces the risk of having a low-birthweight baby to that of a woman who has never smoked (McCowan et al., 2009).

There are various other health consequences associated with smoking, including worsening of existing disease, e.g. asthma (British Medical Association [BMA], 2002), ulcers, Crohn's disease and osteoporosis. The reproductive system is also affected, causing male impotence, sperm abnormalities and early menopause. The development and deterioration of current conditions can cause years of debilitating illness and other non-life-threatening problems.

Aside from the more serious effects imposed on health, smoking can impact cosmetically, causing facial wrinkles, discolouring skin, gingivitis, and impacting on wound healing (Metelitsa and Lauzon, 2010). Furthermore, smoking not only affects the individual but also their family and friends, potentially being exposed to passive or second-hand smoking, which can impact the non-smoker. The exposure to second-hand smoke can exacerbate asthma or other respiratory conditions, and long-term exposure can increase the risk of lung cancer, heart disease and stroke. Relatives and friends may also have to learn to live with a sick relative and/or come to terms with a premature death.

THE ECONOMIC BURDEN OF SMOKING

Smoking is associated with substantial healthcare and social costs. The annual cost to the NHS for treating diseases caused as a result of smoking according to ASH (2014a) is approximately £2 billion per year, equating to 5.5% of total healthcare costs (Alexander et al., 2009). The costs increase phenomenally if the associated social security payments for disability and widows' pension are added.

The annual cost of prescriptions for smoking cessation items in 2012/13 was over £58.1 million (HSCIC, 2014a). Diseases associated with smoking account for 1.6 million NHS hospital admissions for adults over the age of 35, which equates to 4300 admissions to hospital per day (HSCIC, 2014a). There are approximately 95,000 hospital admissions of children with illnesses caused by passive smoking (Department of Health [DoH], 2013). Millet et al. (2013) found that the number of hospital admissions with exacerbations of asthma decreased following smoke-free legislation in England. Treatment of passive smoking-related illnesses for children is estimated to cost the NHS £23.3 million annually (RCP, 2010).

In addition to direct medical costs, the economic burden of smoking extends to indirect costs. Smoking breaks and smoking-related sick leave are estimated to cost UK businesses £8.7 billion in lost productivity every year (Centre for Economics and Business Research, 2014).

Within the home, the fires caused by materials associated with smoking are estimated to cost approximately £391 million. Other costs include the payment of sickness or invalidity benefits to those suffering from disease caused by smoking and the payment of widow(er)s' pension and other social security benefits to the dependants of those who die as a result of smoking (ASH, 2014a).

It has been estimated that if these societal costs are taken into account, the total annual cost of smoking to the UK exceeds the £12.9 billion annual revenue collected in tobacco taxation (Tobacco Manufacturers Association, 2014).

LEGISLATION

The government in the UK had previously set Commissioning for Quality and Innovation (CQUIN) targets looking at referral rates and number of quitters; however, there are no current national targets associated with smoking cessation.

The Tobacco Control Policy (DOH, 2011) include the following strategies:

- Reduce smoking prevalence among adults to 18.5% or less by 2015.

- The end of all tobacco promotion in 2014.
  In April 2012 the government banned the display of tobacco products within shops and supermarkets.
  - Smoke-free public places – the introduction of the smoke-free policy in July 2007 resulted in an increase in the uptake of sought advice for smoking cessation (Bauld, 2011).

In October 2015 it became illegal to smoke in a car in England and Wales with passengers under the age of 18. The ban already existed in Scotland.

Although advertising of cigarettes is now illegal in the UK, previous to the Tobacco Advertising & Promotion Act 2002, advertising was promoted on many platforms including sponsorship particularly of sporting events. This advertising was not limited to male sporting events: industry efforts to target women saw campaigns associated with emancipation, independence, feminism, success and sophistication (Amos and Haglund, 2000). Advertising in this way impacted on the smoking rates of women (Shafey et al., 2004). In the UK, 27% of girls aged 16–19 years smoked compared to only 19% of the boys (HSCIC, 2014a). Since the introduction of Virginia Slims in 1968, there was an explosion of female-only brands linking smoking with weight control. Incentives ranged from free introductory samples to the sponsoring of women's tennis. In the Third World, where restrictions are laxer, the tobacco industry sponsors raves and discos in which people (often young girls) are employed to hand out free cigarettes to girls and young women (Hammond, 2000).

SMOKING CESSATION

The majority of surveys find smokers would like to give up: 70% of smokers in the UK say they want to stop, but only half make an attempt to quit (NICE, 2008). Nearly 80% have attempted to stop at least once, with about 30% actively trying each year. Of the current 13 million adult smokers in the UK, about 9 million want to stop and about 4 million will actually try each year, with only about 300,000 succeeding in giving up for good (HSCIC, 2014b). Cessation rates increase with age, starting at about 2% per year among smokers in their 20s and 30s, rising to about 4% per year among smokers in their late 40s and 50s. Overall, 2% to 3% of all smokers manage to stop permanently each year.

Even people with potentially life-threatening smoking-related diseases continue to smoke: 40% of those who have had a laryngectomy try smoking again soon afterwards; nearly 50% of lung cancer patients resume smoking within a year of surgery; and 38% of smokers who suffer a heart attack return to smoking while still hospitalised.

People who manage to stop smoking live longer and healthier lives than those who continue to smoke. The benefits, while greatest for younger smokers, also extend to those who stop at older ages. The benefits apply to people with and without smoking-related diseases and include improvements in fitness, general health status, teeth, skin and nails.

The risk of morbidity and death continues to drop as the abstinence period lengthens. Although the damage caused to the lungs by smoking is permanent, stopping smoking prevents further deterioration. Smoking cessation slows the progression of COPD, slowing the age-related decline in lung function to that of a non-smoker within a few months (Fletcher and Peto, 1977). Ten years after stopping, an ex-smoker's risk of lung cancer is reduced to become a third to a half of that for a continuing smoker. The risk continues to decline with abstinence.

The risk of coronary heart disease declines rapidly after smoking cessation. After just one year, the risk of coronary heart disease is halved compared with someone who continues to smoke. The risk continues to decline over time and after 10 to 15 years it is similar to that for a person who has never smoked.

TREATMENT, INTERVENTIONS AND THERAPY

Working within the context of a healthcare environment, it is a fundamental role of healthcare professionals of all grades to promote health and give health promotion advice at all opportunities and with every patient encounter (NICE, 2006, 2013). Advice given from a physician increases the rate of quitting from 1% to 3% (Stead et al., 2008). It is estimated by the Office for National Statistics (2012) that two thirds of current smokers want to quit. Self-help materials are a useful source of information, but a Cochrane review concluded that the benefit from these materials is small (Hartmann-Boyce et al., 2014).

There are many different approaches to stopping smoking and they vary in their effectiveness. Strategies may be used alone or several may be combined simultaneously. The use of a pharmacological treatment in combination with some form of motivational support provides better cessation rates than either component alone and appears to be the most effective way of helping smokers to stop (NICE, 2013). Interventions and therapies include:

NICOTINE REPLACEMENT THERAPY (NRT)

NRT is available on prescription and on general sale within the UK. There is an abundance of products available to smokers, and there has been an increase in the number of healthcare professionals trained to provide smoking cessation service, and many more are able to give brief advice. The variety and availability of locations to seek and attend smoking cessation services has improved to meet the needs of the population (NICE, 2008, 2013).

During 2012/2013 there were 1.3 million prescriptions written for NRT (HSCIC, 2014a). Nevertheless, one treatment does not suit all smokers and the development and enhancement of NRT products continues. The amount of nicotine provided from NRT does not equate to the high level of nicotine and the speed of delivery received by a cigarette. Ensuring that information is passed to the service user is essential for the acceptance of the product and the expectations of the service user. The NRT is a treatment to assist with the nicotine withdrawal by weaning the patient off nicotine through a reduction in dose and frequency, thereby reducing the nicotine dependence and the associated symptoms. It does not remove the urge to smoke and strategies for behaviour and changing habits should be discussed.

There are a number of NRT methods which are available for the delivery of NRT. The choice of which form is chosen should reflect individual patient's needs, tolerability and cost considerations.

Patches: The patches are available in 16-hour and 24-hour format, and come in three strengths. This is to reduce the sleep disruption experienced by some

service users. This method is suitable to give a background level of nicotine.

Gum: Nicotine is released by chewing the gum and is absorbed through the lining of the mouth; once the taste becomes strong the gum should be placed between the cheek and the gums of the mouth. This should be repeated as the taste starts to fade.

Lozenges: 2–4 mg lozenge which is slowly dissolved in the mouth every 1–2 hours for the first few weeks and should gradually be reduced.

Microtab: This is placed under the tongue, no chewing or swallowing required, the nicotine is absorbed through the lining of the mouth.

Nasal spray: Is the fastest method of NRT delivery and is beneficial for heavy smokers. This method can cause runny nose and watering eyes, but this should resolve or ease in a few days.

Mouth spray: This is a fine spray delivered directly into the mouth, working quickly to provide relief from withdrawal.

Inhalators: This is a popular method of NRT delivery as it replaces the hand to mouth action, inhaling the nicotine without the additional tobacco chemicals.

BUPROPRION (ZYBAN®)

Buproprion was originally designed as an antidepressant, but it was also found to aid smoking cessation. It can reduce the cravings and symptoms of withdrawal. The reason behind its ability to reduce cravings is unclear, but it is thought to have an effect on the part of the brain that deals with addictive behaviour. Buproprion is usually commenced one to two weeks prior to quitting and the course lasts for at least 8 weeks (NICE, 2013). This treatment is not appropriate for smokers who are susceptible to seizures as there is an increased risk (Hughes et al., 2014). This product is available on prescription.

VARENICLINE (CHAMPIX®)

Varenicline is a partial antagonist on the nicotine receptors. It works by binding the receptors that accept nicotine, thereby reducing the sensation of rewarding and relieving the nicotine withdrawal symptoms. Varenicline is taken as a 12-week course to give the maximum support to cease smoking.

When Varenicline was first introduced as a method of smoking cessation there was a significant amount of concern linking commencement of Varenicline with depression and suicide. Thomas et al. (2013) explored a prospective cohort study of 349 general practices and of almost 120,000 men and women using smoking cessation products in the UK they found that there was no increased risk of suicide with Varenicline or Buproprion compared with other prescribed NRT. Smoking is often utilised as a method of stress and anxiety relief, and discussing alternative methods of stress relief and current levels of anxiety and depression may also assist compliance. Nicotine withdrawal can cause raised levels of anxiety, agitation, restlessness and irritation.

E-CIGARETTES

Electronic nicotine delivery devices, more commonly known as e-cigarettes, have grown in popularity since 2000 as a method of quitting smoking and 2.1 million people use them (ASH, 2014b). They are available to purchase in a variety of locations and there is little regulation regarding the sale of e-cigarettes in the UK. E-cigarettes consist of a rechargeable battery, nicotine liquid cartridge and heating element that converts the liquid into a vapour which can be inhaled and seen. They are available in a variety of different sizes and devices, some imitating a cigarette.

An ASH (2010) online survey found that one out of five users of e-cigarettes had quit smoking. The other users were using e-cigarettes as a replacement in areas where cigarettes are prohibited. Cahna and Siegelb (2011) determined that they were a safer option than tobacco cigarettes based on the safety data available. The U.S. Food and Drug Administration found that e-cigarettes contained toxic chemicals and carcinogens; they also found a lack of quality control with regards to dosage and labelling (Westenberger, 2009). Trading Standards in the UK have concerns with electrical safety, child-resistant packaging and appropriate labelling (Trading Standards Institute, 2010).

Until e-cigarettes are licenced the advice to patients will be to use a regulated and licensed nicotine replacement product in addition to behavioural support (NICE, 2012, 2013). If patients decline this advice, they need to be made aware of the lack of safety data available. Perhaps once regulated, the use of e-cigarettes may be an additional smoking cessation agent, but in the absence of robust safety and efficacy data their use should be with caution. The British Thoracic Society (BTS) (2014) have called for more research into e-cigarettes.

ADDITIONAL SUPPORT

Combining pharmacological therapy and stop smoking counselling increases the chances of quitting and prolonged abstinence compared to quit attempts without any assistance (Ferguson et al., 2005). The prevalence of social media offers another method of support to stop smoking. There are a variety of online approaches, including websites, mobile device apps and well-known social media platforms such as Twitter and Facebook. The most popular type of material are self help leaflets (33%) and approximately 15% of smokers ask advice from healthcare professionals to help them stop (HSCIC, 2014a).

Alternative therapies also assist with stopping smoking; nevertheless, there is a lack of evidence to support the effectiveness of these treatments. Healthcare practitioners need to be receptive and support smokers to quit, while providing them with the relevant information. This enables service users to choose the best method for them. Parrot et al. (1998) suggest that cold turkey is the least successful method of quitting. Other alternative therapies such as acupressure and acupuncture replicate placebo in their long-term abstinence rates.

COST INTERVENTIONS

Due to the major gains in health, smoking cessation is one of the most cost-effective healthcare interventions that can be made (West et al., 2000). Even the most intensive smoking cessation interventions offer remarkably good value for money compared with many other widely accepted healthcare interventions. The cost to a Health Authority of saving one year of life through helping a smoker to stop has been estimated at £174 for brief advice. For more intensive intervention, which includes advice, NRT and self-help materials, the cost is approximately £269 (Parrot et al., 1998). The BTS (2014) also support the fact that smoking cessation interventions are cost-effective, but many healthcare professionals are inadequately trained to deliver optimal smoking cessation interventions. As well as bringing health gains for relatively modest expenditure, smoking cessation is likely to reduce the healthcare costs associated with managing smoking-related illnesses, which are currently estimated to be at £2.8 billion per year (BTS, 2014) and, in the longer term, treatment costs may well be offset by the savings that result.

CASE STUDY

Tess Bates is a 62-year-old lady who has smoked since she was a teenager. She had thought about giving up smoking many times and had said to friends that she wished she could give up. Despite saying this, she was in two minds. On the one hand she liked smoking, while on the other she knew the risks of smoking. Smoking had got her through some challenging life situations. Tess was from a working-class background and became pregnant at 15. She married young and then had two further children. By the time Tess was 20 she had three small children, was living in a local authority flat and, although her husband was working, money was very tight. Tess worked in a series of part-time, low-paid jobs. Over the years Tess's husband was not faithful and their marriage was a difficult one. Tess had been prescribed anti-depressants many times by her GP.

When Tess began smoking in the 1960s, it was the thing to do. No one worried about the effects it might have on their health. However, Tess was now well aware of the danger to health posed by smoking but thought that, as that she had smoked for almost five decades, that it was pointless giving up now.

Tess had attended her GP practice regularly over the years and recently staff at the practice had taken the opportunity to briefly discuss smoking cessation. While Tess liked smoking, she thought that she should at least try to give up. However, she could not bear the thought of going to the surgery and being 'lectured' by the nurse. Tess therefore purchased her own nicotine patches. Tess stopped smoking and started using the patches, but felt ill almost straight away. Tess felt irritable and anxious, and she could not concentrate. When she went out of the house she was panicky, she hyperventilated and felt dizzy. Tess did not visit a healthcare professional to discuss her symptoms; instead, she stopped using the patches and started smoking again. She told her friends that the patches had made her ill.

CASE STUDY DISCUSSION

Tess's case highlights the complexity of smoking behaviours. In the twenty-first century the health effects of smoking are well documented, yet people smoke for many reasons (English and Spencer, 2007). Tess had smoked for almost five decades and was aware of the dangers, but did not realise the benefits of stopping smoking even after all of that time of being a smoker. If Tess had been prepared to go to a healthcare professional, she could have had more in-depth information given to her. However, she did not want to be 'lectured', which highlights the difficult task that healthcare professionals have in giving smoking cessation advice. Unfortunately, Tess was never very likely to succeed by trying to give up without support. The review by Stead and Lancaster (2012) demonstrates that combined behavioural support and medication are more successful at helping people quit smoking.

The symptoms that Tess displayed were as a result of abrupt nicotine withdrawal and not as a result of using the patches (McEwen and West, 2010). Blaming the patches was either a lack of understanding on Tess's part or, more likely, an excuse for starting smoking again. McEwen and West (2010) outline the PRIME model of stopping smoking where smokers move through four stages of smoking, planning to quit, attempting to quit and not smoking. What determines whether a smoker moves from one of the four states to another is their immediate desire at that moment. It is likely that Tess did not really want to give up smoking at that point in time. If she had consulted a healthcare professional, Tess could have been offered alternatives to nicotine patches or a combination of nicotine replacement, medications and support.

SUMMARY

Smoking cessation is a highly cost-effective healthcare intervention, comparing favourably with many other common healthcare interventions. To be successful, smoking cessation strategies need to address the overriding role of nicotine addiction in keeping smokers smoking, as well as the behavioural aspects of the disorder. For this reason, the more effective approaches to smoking cessation involve simultaneously targeting of both aspects, using pharmacological intervention combined with some form of motivational support and advice. It is well accepted that advice from a healthcare professional, even if brief, can increase smoking cessation rates (Stead and Lancaster, 2012). NRT can also help some smokers to stop smoking by reducing nicotine withdrawal symptoms through weaning schedules; however, there are some considerations to its use. The availability of new, effective and alternative pharmacological treatments for smoking cessation is clearly needed and will provide further impetus for healthcare professionals to help those smokers who are motivated to stop.

REFERENCES

Alexander, S., Balakrishnan, R., Scarborough, P., Webster, P. and Raynor, M. 2009. The burden of smoke-related ill health in the United Kingdom. *Tobacco Control* 18: 252–255.

Amos, A. and Haglund, M. 2000. From social taboo to "torch of freedom": The marketing of cigarettes to women. *Tobacco Control* 9: 3–8.

ASH. 2010. YouGov Survey. Sample size 10,000 adults. Fieldwork conducted between 27th February and 16th March 2012. www.ash.org.uk

ASH. 2014a. Smoking Statistics, Illness and Health, November 2014. www.ash.org.uk

ASH. 2014b. Use of Electronic Cigarettes in Great Britain. October 2014. www.ash.org.uk

ASH. 2015. Smoking Statistics January 2015. www.ash.org.uk

Aveyard, P. and West, R. 2007. Managing smoking cessation. *British Medical Journal* 7335 (7609): 37–41.

Bauld, L. 2011. The Impact of Smokefree Legislation in England: Evidence Review. Available at: https://www.gov.uk/government/uploads/system/uploads/attachment_data/file/216319/dh_124959.pdf. Accessed 5 July 2016.

Benowitz, N.L. 2010. Nicotine addiction. *New England Journal of Medicine* 362 (24): 2295–2303.

British Medical Association. 2002. *Towards Smoke Free Public Places*. British Medical Association, Board of Science and Education & Tobacco Control Resource Centre, London.

British Thoracic Society. 2014. *Position Statement: Tobacco*. BTS, London.

Cahna, Z. and Siegelb, M. 2011. Electronic cigarettes as a harm reduction strategy for tobacco control: A step forward or a repeat of past mistakes? *Journal of Public Health Policy* 32 (1): 16–31.

Centre for Economics and Business Research (CEBR). 2014. CEBR research for the British Heart Foundation outlines the costs of smoking to businesses in ahead of No Smoking Day on March 12th (2014) http://www.cebr.com/reports/smoking-costs-uk-businesses-8-7bn/. Accessed 29 April 2015.

Dalmandis, S. 2009. Tobacco contains over 4000 chemical compounds including tar, carbon monoxide, hydrogen, cyanide and arsenic. *Pharmacy News* 06/2009 23–26.

Decramer, M., Janssens, W. and Miravitlles, M. 2012. Chronic obstructive pulmonary disease. *The Lancet* 379 (9823): 1341–1351.

Department of Health. 2011. *Healthy Lives, Healthy People: A Tobacco Control Plan for England*. Department of Health, London.

Department of Health. 2013. Policy. Smoking. Available at: https://www.gov.uk/government/policies/reducing-smoking. Accessed 29 April 2015.

English, W.A. and Spencer, R. 2007. Effects of smoking on health. *Clinical Anaesthesia* 8 (3): 89–90.

Ferguson, J., Bauld, L., Chesterman, J. and Judge, K. 2005. The English smoking treatment services: One-year outcomes. *Addiction* 100 (S2): 59–69.

Fletcher, C. and Peto, R. 1977. The natural history of chronic airflow obstruction. *British Medical Journal* 1: 1645.

Forey, B., Hamling, J., Hamling, J., Thornton, A. and Lee, P. 2012. International Smoking Statistics Web Edition. A collection of worldwide historical data. United Kingdom. Available at: http://www.pnlee.co.uk/Downloads/ISS/ISS-United Kingdom_120111.pdf. Accessed 5 March 2015.

General Lifestyle Survey. 2011. (Released 07 March 2013). Available at: http://www.ons.gov.uk/ons/rel/ghs/general-lifestyle-survey/2011/index.html. Accessed 20 March 2015.

Hammond, R. 2000. *Tobacco Advertising & Promotion: The Need for a Coordinated Global Response*. World Health Organisation. Available at: www.who.int/tobacco/media/ROSS2000X.pdf. Accessed 27 April 2015.

Hartmann-Boyce, J., Lancaster, T. and Stead, L.F. 2014. *Print-Based Self-Help Interventions for Smoking Cessation*. The Cochrane Collaboration. John Wiley and Sons Ltd. Oxford, UK.

Health and Safety Executive. 2014. Chronic Obstructive Pulmonary Disease (COPD) in Great Britain in 2014. Available at: www.hse.gov.uk/statistics/causdis/copd/copd.pdf. Accessed 29 April 2015.

Health and Social Care Information Centre (HSCIC). 2014a. Statistics on Smoking: England, 2013. Available at: http://www.hscic.gov.uk/catalogue/PUB11454/smok-eng-2013-rep.pdf. Accessed 10 June 2016.

Health and Social Care Information Centre (HSCIC). 2014b. Statistics on NHS Stop Smoking Services, England – April 2013 to March 2014. Available at: http://www.hscic.gov.uk/catalogue/PUB14610. Accessed 27 April 2015.

Health and Social Care Information Centre (HSCIC). 2015. Statistics on Women's Smoking Status at Time of Delivery, England – Quarter 4, 2013–14. (Publication date June 2014.)

Hughes, J.R., Stead, L.F., Hartmann-Boyce, J., Cahill, K. and Lancaster, T. 2014. *Antidepressants for Smoking Cessation (Review)*. The Cochrane Collaboration. John Wiley and Sons Ltd. Oxford, UK.

McCowan, L.M., Dekker, G.A., Chan, E., Stewart, A., Chappell, L.C., Hunter, M., Moss-Morris, R. and North, R.A. 2009. Spontaneous preterm birth and small for gestational age infants in women who stop smoking early in pregnancy: Prospective cohort study. *British Medical Journal* 338 (7710): 1552–1558.

McEwen, A. and West, R. 2010. The PRIME approach to giving up smoking. *Practice Nursing* 21 (3): 149–153.

Metelitsa, A. and Lauzon, G.J. 2010. Tobacco and the skin. *Clinics in Dermatology* 28 (4): 384–390.

Millet, C., Tayu Lee, J., Laverty, A.A., Glantz, S.A. and Majeed, A. 2013. Hospital Admissions for Childhood Asthma after Smoke-Free Legislation in England. Available at: http://pediatrics.aappublications.org/content/131/2/e495.full.pdf+html. Accessed 29 April 2015.

National Institute for Health and Care Excellence. 2006. *Smoking: Brief Interventions and Referrals*. Public Health Guideline 1. NICE, London.

National Institute for Health and Care Excellence. 2008. *Smoking Cessation Services*. NICE Public Health Guideline 10. NICE, London.

National Institute for Health and Care Excellence. 2012. *Smoking Cessation Care*. NICE, London.

National Institute for Health and Care Excellence. 2013. *Smoking Cessation: Supporting People to Stop Smoking*. NICE Quality Standard 43. NICE, London.

Office for National Statistics. 2012. General Lifestyle Survey, 2010. Available at: http://www.ons.gov.uk/ons/rel/ghs/general-lifestyle-survey/2010/index.html. Accessed 27 April 2015.

Parrott, S., Godfrey, C., Raw, M., West, R. and McNeill, A. 1998. Guidance for commissioners on the cost effectiveness of smoking cessation interventions. Health Educational Authority. *Thorax* 53 (Suppl. 5 Pt 2): S1–S38.

Rose, J.E., Behm, F.M., Westman, E.C. and Coleman, R.E. 1999. Arterial nicotine kinetics during cigarette smoking and intravenous nicotine administration: Implications for addiction. *Drug Alcohol Depend* 56 (2): 99–107.

Royal College of Physicians. 2000. *Nicotine Addiction in Britain. A Report of the Tobacco Advisory Group of the Royal College of Physicians*. RCP, London.

Royal College of Physicians. 2007. Harm reduction in nicotine addiction. Helping people who can't quit. Available at: https://cdn.shopify.com/s/files/1/0924/4392/files/harm-reduction-nicotine-addiction.pdf?15599436013786148553. Accessed 5 July 2016.

Royal College of Physicians. 2010. *Passive Smoking and Children: A Report by the Tobacco Advisory Group of the Royal College of Physicians.* RCP, London.

Shafey, O., Fernandez, E., Thun, M., Schiaffino, A., Dolwick, S. and Cokkinides, V. 2004. Cigarette advertising and female smoking prevelance in Spain, 1982–1997. *Cancer* 100 (8): 1744–1749.

Stead, L.F., Bergson, G. and Lancaster, T. 2008. *Physician Advice for Smoking Cessation (Review).* The Cochrane Collaboration. John Wiley and Sons Ltd. Oxford, UK.

Stead, L.F. and Lancaster, T. 2012. *Combined Pharmacotherapy and Behavioural Interventions for Smoking Cessation. Review.* The Cochrane Collaboration. John Wiley and Sons Ltd. Oxford, UK.

Thomas, K.H., Martin, R.M., Davies, N.M., Metcalfe, C., Windmeijer, F. and Gunnell, D. 2013. Smoking cessation treatment and risk of depression, suicide, and self harm in the Clinical Practice Research Datalink: Prospective cohort study. *British Medical Journal* 347: f5704. Available at: http://www.bmj.com/content/347/bmj.f5704/rr/672291. Accessed 24 July 2015.

Tobacco Manufacturers Association. 2014. Taxation. Available at: http://www.the-tma.org.uk/policy-legislation/taxation/. Accessed 29 April 2015.

Trading Standards Institute. 2010. *Response of the Trading Standards Institute to MHRA Consultation on the Regulation of Nicotine Containing Products.* Trading Standards Institute, Basildon, Essex.

Wannamethee, S.G., Shaper, A.G., Whincup, P.H. and Walker, M. 1995. Smoking cessation and the risk of stroke in middle-aged men. *The Journal of the American Medical Association* 274 (2): 155–160.

West, R., McNeill, A. and Raw, M. 2000. Smoking cessation guidelines for health professionals: An update. *Thorax* 55 (12): 987–999.

Westenberger, B.J. 2009. *US Food and Drug Administration: Evaluation of E-Cigarettes.* US Food and Drug Administration, Centre for Drug Evaluation and Research, Division of Pharmaceutical Analysis, St Louis, MO.

World Health Organisation. 2008. World health statistics. Available at: http://www.who.int/whosis/whostat/EN_WHS08_Full.pdf. Accessed 20 March 2015.

World Health Organisation. 2016. Tobacco Fact Sheet N°339. Updated June 2016. Available at: http://www.who.int/mediacentre/factsheets/fs339/en/. Accessed 5 July 2016.

Pulmonary rehabilitation

19

EMMA TUCKER AND CATHERINE STOERMER

LEARNING OBJECTIVES

Upon completion of the chapter the reader should be able to:

- Recognise patients who would benefit from pulmonary rehabilitation
- Identify and discuss the evidence base for pulmonary rehabilitation
- Identify the elements of a pulmonary rehabilitation programme and discuss how it can be structured
- Debate evidence based outcome measures that can be used to assess exercise capacity and health-related quality of life
- Discuss how to appropriately prescribe exercise to an individual with chronic obstructive pulmonary disease

INTRODUCTION

Pulmonary rehabilitation (PR) is a recognised method of treatment for people with chronic obstructive pulmonary disease (COPD). The British Thoracic Society (BTS) Guidelines for PR, published in 2013, state that PR is an interdisciplinary programme of care for patients with chronic respiratory impairment (Bolton et al., 2013). This is predominantly COPD. However, research has demonstrated measured benefits in other respiratory diseases (Newall et al., 2005; Nishiyama et al., 2008; Holland et al., 2012).

The benefits of PR are well researched and documented with the main factors being significant increases in health-related quality of life (HRQoL), functional and maximal exercise capacity and a decrease in hospital days and hospitalisations (Griffiths et al., 2000; National Institute of Health and Care Excellence [NICE], 2010).

The focus of this chapter is to provide an overview of PR, its benefits, how PR programmes are structured and associated outcome measures.

In 2013 the BTS Guidelines on Pulmonary Rehabilitation in Adults were published and shortly after in 2014 the BTS also published 'Quality

Standards for Pulmonary Rehabilitation in Adults'. The purpose of these quality standards are to provide healthcare professionals, commissioners and patients with a clear guide to standards that should be met when delivering PR programmes, ensuring safe, effective and good practice. This chapter will refer to these guidelines as a reference point for best practice.

AIMS AND BENEFITS OF PULMONARY REHABILITATION

The two main aims of PR are to increase exercise capacity and HRQoL, by improving the symptoms associated with respiratory conditions (NICE, 2010; Bolton et al., 2013). The outcome measures used to assess these will be discussed later in the chapter. In order to achieve this, the proposed benefits of enrolling an individual on a PR programme are identified as:

- To reduce dyspnoea (see Figure 19.1)
- To manage the symptoms rather than the disease process
- To initiate physical training
- Increase exercise tolerance and promote efficient energy expenditure

- To maximise independence and decrease dependence
- Decrease anxiety and promote self-management
- Promote long-term adherence to health-enhancing behaviours (Spruit et al., 2013)

Dyspnoea (also referred to as breathlessness) can be a debilitating symptom associated with respiratory conditions in both its acute and chronic phases. The dyspnoea cycle describes the process that the symptoms of breathlessness can lead to.

When someone begins to become breathless they usually start to become less active; this subsequently leads to weaker and less efficient muscles. The quadriceps muscles in patients with COPD have been found to be significantly weaker even in those with mild disease, with 28% and 26% of patients with a Medical Research Council (MRC) dyspnoea score (see Table 19.1) level of 1 or 2 respectively and 43% of patients with a MRC of 4 or 5, demonstrating a reduction in quadriceps strength (Seymour et al., 2010). This weakness is largely due to muscle atrophy demonstrated by cross-sectional area and contributes to leg fatigue and exercise intolerance (Hamilton et al., 1995). It has also been found that the activity of oxidation enzymes is lower in people with COPD when compared to normal subjects. This

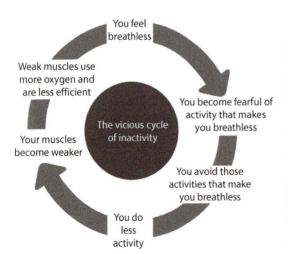

Figure 19.1 Dyspnoea cycle reproduced with permission of the British Lung Foundation www.blf.org.uk.

Table 19.1 Medical research council dyspnoea score

Grade	Degree of breathlessness related to activities
1	Not troubled by breathlessness except on strenuous exercise
2	Short of breath when hurrying or walking up a slight hill
3	Walks slower than contemporaries on level ground because of breathlessness, or has to stop for breath when walking at own pace
4	Stops for breath after walking about 100 metres or after a few minutes on level ground
5	Too breathless to leave the house, or breathless when dressing or undressing

Source: Adapted from Fletcher, C.M. 1960. *British Medical Journal* 2 (523): 1665.

results in premature lactic acid production during exercise (Maltais et al., 1996). This increase in lactic acid further drives ventilation, thereby increasing the respiratory rate and exacerbating any feeling of breathlessness experienced by the patient.

The muscle weakness and inactivity found in patients with COPD have been shown to be associated with more frequent hospital admissions and mortality (Garcia-Aymerich et al., 2006). It therefore follows that improving muscle strength and activity will reduce hospitalisation and mortality. It has been shown that muscle strength, endurance and how quickly someone tires all improve significantly following exercise training (Troosters et al., 2000; Mador et al., 2001). Exercise training can increase the cross-sectional area of muscle by at least 20% (Whittom et al., 1998), increase the oxidative capacity (Maltais et al., 1996) and reduce the lactic acid produced during exercise (Casaburi et al., 1991; Maltais et al., 1996). It has also been shown to improve exercise capacity and HRQoL (Lacasse et al., 1997).

Other exercise limitations that individuals with COPD encounter will be covered later in the chapter.

PATIENT SELECTION

A number of characteristics should be considered when selecting patients to be invited to participate in a PR programme.

MEDICAL RESEARCH COUNCIL DYSPNOEA SCALE

All patients with a clinical diagnosis of COPD (forced expiratory volume in 1 second [FEV_1]/forced vital capacity [FVC] <0.7) that are functionally limited by their breathlessness should be referred to PR (NICE, 2010). Predominantly this means patients with a MRC scale of dyspnoea score of 3–5 (see Table 19.1). However, recent research has also included a MRC score of 2. These are patients that are starting to become functionally limited by their shortness of breath (SOB) and complaining of symptoms.

In 2009, The London Respiratory Team produced the COPD 'Value' pyramid. This was then adopted by the BTS and the Improving and Integrating Respiratory Services (IMPRESS) Guide to the relative value of COPD interventions was produced (Williams et al., 2012). They investigated the cost-effectiveness of the most common interventions used in the treatment of COPD and promoted the use of PR at an early stage of diagnosis (i.e. MRC 2–3), prior to the introduction of some medical therapies. It was suggested that patients should be optimised on medical treatment prior to PR, not necessarily maximised. It was subsequently recommended by Bolton et al. (2013) that patients with COPD should be taking bronchodilator therapy, in line with the NICE (2010) COPD Guidelines, prior to referral to PR.

OTHER RESPIRATORY CONDITIONS

People with other respiratory conditions should also be considered for PR. Specifically there is evidence to support its use with individuals who have interstitial lung disease (ILD) and non-cystic fibrosis bronchiectasis (Newall et al., 2005; Nishiyama et al., 2008; Holland et al., 2012). It is important to remember that, when assessing these patients, the standard outcome measures used are validated in the COPD population and at present may not be transferrable to other respiratory diseases.

EXCLUSION CRITERIA

When selecting appropriate patients for PR it is important to refer to the exclusion criteria. There are four main reasons why a person would be excluded from PR. These are:

1. Unstable cardiovascular disease i.e. unstable angina or hypertension, or myocardial infarction within the last 6 weeks
2. Significant aortic stenosis >60 mmHg
3. Recent eye or abdominal surgery within last 3 months
4. Medical problems that severely restrict exercise or compliance with the programme.

It is also important when considering a patient for PR that they understand the level of motivation and commitment required as there is a high dropout rate within PR (Fischer et al., 2009).

POST-ACUTE EXACERBATION OF CHRONIC OBSTRUCTIVE PULMONARY DISEASE (AECOPD)

One of the most targeted areas for research over recent years has been the inclusion of patients recently discharged from hospital following an acute exacerbation of their COPD. Following an acute exacerbation of COPD there is an accelerated decline in an individual's lung function, reduced quality of life and an increased risk of death. In fact, the risk of readmission within 90 days of a hospital admission for COPD is increased by 33% in this population (Price et al., 2006). Therefore, if these patients can be enrolled in PR within 30 days of their admission following their exacerbation, subsequently this can reduce their short-term risk of readmission to hospital and improve their short-term HRQoL and exercise capacity (Puhan et al., 2011). Theories on why this is achieved include increasing patient strength and physical activity immediately post discharge from hospital and ensuring continuous contact with a healthcare professional. PR also teaches self-management strategies that may be utilised to prevent the risk of readmission.

SMOKERS/SMOKING CESSATION

Debate exists about whether or not smokers should be included in PR programmes. Studies have demonstrated that current smokers attend approximately two-thirds less sessions and had lower completion rates (Young et al., 1999; Sabit et al., 2008). However, there is also evidence to suggest that there are some smokers who do benefit from PR (Paone et al., 2008). PR can provide an opportunity to facilitate smoking cessation, through engagement with PR practitioners and peer support from fellow patients who have successfully ceased smoking. Smoking cessation should be addressed at assessment and referral made to appropriate services (Bolton et al., 2013). Authors have suggested that smoking cessation should ideally be addressed as a first-line treatment on the diagnosis of COPD prior to be being referred to PR (Williams et al., 2012) (see Chapter 18 for a detailed account of smoking cessation).

LOCATION OF PR DELIVERY

PR has predominately been run in a hospital-based setting, usually with the patients attending as outpatients. However, more and more courses are now being held in community venues, such as local leisure centres; this has been driven by trends to provide care closer to patients' homes and within their communities. With the government focus on increasing physical activity within all populations, this means that more and more healthcare can be carried out in local facilities. The recommendation of the NICE Guidelines for COPD states that PR sessions should be held at practical times, in conveniently located and accessible buildings, in order to increase concordance (NICE, 2010). Evidence suggests that PR is effective in all settings, including hospital in- and out-patient, in the community and the home (Morgan, 2001).

The most important aspects to consider when ensuring accessibility for the patient includes:

- Is the venue on a local bus route?
- Does the venue have adequate parking and adequate marked disabled bays?
- Is the gym area accessible and is there a lift if necessary?

DURATION OF PR PROGRAMMES

The recommended duration of PR programmes is between 6–12 weeks, with two supervised exercise sessions and one unsupervised session per week (Bolton et al., 2013). An example of a course may be constructed as follows:

Week 1: Pre-assessments (this should include medical assessment, exercise HRQoL outcome measures and specific, measurable, attainable, realistic and timely [SMART] goal setting).

Weeks 2–7: 2 × sessions per week of supervised exercise and education sessions (normally 2 hours in total).

Week 8: Post-assessments (re-assess exercise and HRQoL outcome measures and achievement of goals, plan for future exercise regime).

Evidence has shown that patients who attend the minimum of 12 supervised exercise sessions tend to have greater improvements in outcome measures (Lacasse et al., 2006). However, there is also well-documented research examining the causes of drop-out rates associated with courses and the percentage of patients who actually complete a whole course. Reasons for this are numerous and include: hospitalisations, social isolation, transport issues and exacerbations (Fischer et al., 2009).

How programmes are structured is dependent on local providers, commissioners, staffing, funding and venue availability. The development of PR services and programmes have changed dramatically across the UK in the last 5 years with the introduction of the Department of Health Service Specification for PR (2012): a document and tool designed to assist in setting up and commissioning PR services in local authorities, the most recent BTS PR Guidelines (2013) and the Quality Standards for PR in Adults (2014).

ELEMENTS OF A PR PROGRAMME

PR, as previously mentioned, is a structured programme consisting of both exercise and educational components. PR should be delivered by an interdisciplinary team (Bolton et al., 2013). This can include physiotherapists, therapy assistants, specialist respiratory nurses, occupational therapists, dieticians, respiratory consultants, general practitioners, members of local support groups and local exercise instructors.

EXERCISE COMPONENT

When exercising a group of individuals with varying levels of anxiety, perceptions and disease awareness, it is important to ensure that each patient is prescribed exercise at the correct intensity. This should always be done by a qualified healthcare professional with the relevant expertise. Various methods of training can be utilised within the exercise component of the session, but should always include a combination of resistance and aerobic exercise in order to increase exercise capacity and strength. Both continuous and interval training has shown to have equivalent benefits on endurance performance and so should be considered on an individual basis

when recommending and prescribing aerobic exercise (Zainuldin et al., 2011).

The Modified Borg Dyspnoea Scale is a very useful measure to guide and assess patients to ensure that they are exercising at the correct intensity to allow for exercise adaptations to occur. The Borg Scale (see Table 19.2) can be useful to assist in increasing and decreasing intensity of exercise, duration of aerobic exercise and a teaching tool for patents to understand how to exercise at a safe level within their breathlessness perceptions.

For ease of structuring exercise sessions for a group of patients, it is expected and recommended that there will be a generic training programme to follow. However, it is important to progress and prescribe exercises based on the individual's progression and physical performance at baseline testing. There should be large focus on individualised treatment within a group setting ensuring that PR needs to be individually tailored and designed to optimise each patient's physical and social performance and autonomy with all programmes comprising individualised programmes and education (Bolton et al., 2013).

When prescribing exercise, it is extremely important to recognise the exercise limitations that individuals encounter. A normal response to exercise is an increase in minute ventilation (VE) in order to meet metabolic demand. An increase in VE is achieved through increasing both the tidal volume (Vt) and the respiratory rate (RR), predominantly by increasing the Vt. Patients with COPD are unable to do this to

Table 19.2 Modified Borg dyspnoea scale

0	Nothing at all
0.5	Very, very slight (just noticeable)
1	Very slight
2	Slight
3	Moderate
4	Somewhat severe
5	Severe
6	
7	Very severe
8	
9	Very, very severe (almost maximal)
10	Maximal

Source: Adapted from Borg, G.A. 1982. *Medicine and Science in Sports and Exercise* 14 (5): 377–381.

the same extent due to the development of dynamic hyperinflation during exercise (O'Donnell et al., 2001). COPD results in expiratory flow limitation due to the obstructive nature of the disease so patients need a longer expiratory time to fully exhale. However, during exercise, when the RR is increased they do not have time to fully exhale, leading to an increase in end expiratory lung volume above the normal level. This is termed dynamic hyperinflation (DH). DH contributes to a lower oxygen consumption (VO_2) during exercise and a lower exercise tolerance and correlates better with patients' symptoms than spirometry (O'Donnell et al., 1999; O'Donnell and Webb 2008).

EDUCATION COMPONENT

The education element of the PR programme is comprehensive and it is recommended that specific elements should be delivered by the multidisciplinary team (Bolton et al., 2013). There are numerous suggested educational sessions that should be covered within the programme (Bolton et al., 2013). These include:

- Anatomy, physiology, pathology – in health and in chronic respiratory disease
- Medication (including oxygen therapy)
- Smoking cessation
- Dyspnoea/symptom management
- Chest-clearance techniques
- Energy conservation/pacing
- Patient support groups
- Nutritional advice
- Managing travel
- Benefits system and welfare rights
- Advance directives
- Anxiety management and relaxation
- Goal setting and rewards
- Relaxation
- Confidence, self-efficacy and self-management
- Identifying and changing beliefs about exercise and health-related behaviours

POST PULMONARY REHABILITATION COURSE

It is important that once a patient has completed a course of supervised exercise that they fully understand the benefits of continued exercise and are provided with the tools to enable this to happen. Research that looked at continued supervised exercise has shown that if patients continue to participate they can maintain their post-PR exercise capacity and prevent decline (Moullec et al., 2008; Ringbaek et al., 2010). Many options are available to patients on discharge from the PR course, although these are obviously dependent on local resources. Examples may include local walking groups, gym classes for the over-50s, leisure centre organised post-PR graduation classes, referral to GP exercise gym instructor, or patients may choose to purchase their own equipment and exercise at home.

USE OF SUPPLEMENTAL OXYGEN IN PULMONARY REHABILITATION

There are a percentage of patients that may require oxygen to exercise; these are usually those classified as having severe respiratory illness. Patients that are already prescribed long-term oxygen therapy (LTOT) are likely to require ambulatory oxygen in order to exercise safely and to the required intensity.

Evidence has shown that individuals that desaturate on exercise may benefit from the use of supplemental oxygen during the exercise component of the programme, with improvements in increased exercise capacity (Revill et al., 2000). It is important to ensure that these patients are assessed appropriately and by a member of staff with expertise in this field. Patients should be offered ambulatory oxygen therapy for use during exercise in a pulmonary rehabilitation programme following a formal assessment demonstrating improvement in exercise endurances (Hardinge et al., 2015) (see Chapter 16 for further detail on oxygen therapy).

OUTCOME MEASURES FOR PULMONARY REHABILITATION

The minimal standards for assessing the outcome of pulmonary rehabilitation should include the assessment of exercise capacity, dyspnoea and health status (Bolton et al., 2013; Bolton et al., 2014). These outcome measures demonstrate the aims of PR discussed earlier in the chapter. Methods for assessing outcomes should be used at the initial assessment and again at the final assessment so that any improvements as a result of PR can be identified and reported on. The minimal clinically important difference (MCID) is the minimal amount of improvement that should be seen in order to determine that the rehabilitation has been successful. The following section reviews some examples of outcome measures appropriate to PR.

EXERCISE CAPACITY

The definition of exercise capacity is the maximum amount of physical exertion that a patient can sustain (Walker et al., 1990) and is measured in a laboratory as VO_2 max. When working in the field, various walk tests have been developed as a measure of functional capacity that has been shown to correlate highly with a maximum VO_2 and therefore exercise capacity. The evaluation of exercise capacity can be used to both prescribe exercise and evaluate the response of a treatment. The main walk tests used in PR are the 6-minute walk test (6MWT), the incremental shuttle walk test (ISWT) and the endurance shuttle walk test (ESWT):

- The 6MWT (Butland et al., 1982) requires patients to walk on a level surface for 6 minutes at their own pace around a 30-metre course and the distance walked is measured. Results obtained from the 6MWT have been shown to correlate strongly with lung function tests, HRQoL, VO_2 max and mortality (Brown and Wise, 2007). For the 6MWT the MCID is 54–80 metres (Wise and Brown, 2005).
- The ISWT (Singh et al., 1992) is a progressive walk test over a 10-metre course which is set to a series of bleeps that increase in their frequency i.e. the patient needs to gradually increase their speed. The test finishes when the patient is too breathless to continue or is unable to keep up with the bleeps. The outcome measured is distance covered. During the ISWT there is a linear relationship between VO_2 max and speed. Therefore, VO_2 max can be estimated from the distance walked (Singh et al., 1994). The MCID for the ISWT is 47.5 metres, which is classified as being 'slightly better.' If an improvement of 78.7 metres is achieved, then a patient is 'better' (Singh et al., 2008).

- The ESWT (Revill et al., 1999) is similar to the ISWT. However, the bleeps are constant throughout. The outcome in this case is duration. While the ISWT measures maximal capacity, the ESWT measures the ability to use that capacity (Solway et al., 2001). As yet no MCID has been established for use in pulmonary rehabilitation (Pepin et al., 2011).

Due to a learning effect, it is important that two tests are done for both the 6MWT and the ISWT.

DYSPNOEA

Dyspnoea is often the main symptom that patients with chronic respiratory disease present with. However, it is subjective and the mechanism behind the sensation of dyspnoea is not fully understood. That being so, like pain, the sensation of dyspnoea should be whatever the patient says it to be. Ways of measuring dyspnoea include the MRC breathlessness scale (Fletcher et al., 1959) and the Borg scale (Borg, 1982). These have been discussed earlier in the chapter. For the Borg scale it has been suggested that a change of 1 point could be significant (Ries, 2005).

HEALTH STATUS

Symptoms of chronic respiratory disease do not always correlate with the clinical state of the airways. Therefore, pulmonary function testing does not necessarily give any information on how the disease is affecting the patient in day-to-day life; these data are obtained through health status questionnaires. Health status is 'the impact of health on a person's ability to perform and derive fulfilment from the activities of daily life' (Curtis and Patrick 2003, p. 36). It includes HRQoL and functional status. There are two types of health status questionnaires: disease specific or generic.

DISEASE SPECIFIC QUESTIONNAIRES FOR CHRONIC RESPIRATORY DISEASE

These questionnaires ask a variety of questions on how the patient is affected by their respiratory disease. These questions may refer to symptoms such as cough, wheeze, sputum and breathlessness, how the patient's function and activity is affected by the disease and how this affects them socially and psychologically. These are then given a score. Examples of disease-specific health status questionnaires are The St Georges Respiratory Questionnaire (SGRQ) (Jones et al., 1992), The Chronic Respiratory Questionnaire (CRQ) (Guyatt et al., 1987), the Clinical COPD Questionnaire (CCQ) (Van der Molen et al., 2003) and the COPD Assessment Test (CAT) (Jones et al., 2009). Both the CAT and CCQ are specific for COPD patients. The SGRQ has been shown to be a sensitive tool to look at quality of life in patients with interstitial lung disease (Chang et al., 1999).

GENERIC QUESTIONNAIRES FOR HEALTH STATUS

These questionnaires assess the psychological, physical and social aspects of a patient's quality of life. There are many examples of these questionnaires including the Medical Outcomes Study Short Form 36 (SF36), European Quality of Life Health Questionnaire (EQ5) and the Sickness Impact Profile.

The outcome measures discussed above are not an exhaustive list, but represent some of the more commonly used tools to assess the effectiveness of pulmonary rehabilitation. Measurement of lower limb muscle strength for example would seem to be an important outcome measure to assess due to the effect that a loss of quadriceps strength has on patients with chronic respiratory disease. The 30-second chair stand test has been shown to be a reasonably reliable and valid indicator of lower limb strength in older community living adults and is a quick and easy method that requires little equipment (Jones et al., 1999).

CASE STUDY

Mr Tait is a 72-year-old gentleman who was diagnosed with COPD 12 months ago. Since then he has suffered two exacerbations, one of which led to him being admitted to hospital. He is retired and used to enjoy playing golf, but is finding that he now needs to use a golf buggy to get around the course and feels that he is holding up his friends that he plays with. He gave up smoking when he was diagnosed with COPD, but has a history of 30-pack years. His GP referred him for pulmonary rehabilitation.

At his assessment for PR, Mr Tait had a productive sounding cough. He was not short of breath at rest or cyanosed. He looked generally well in himself and was motivated to take part in rehabilitation. At this stage Mr Tait had an FEV_1 of 55% of predicted value, his blood pressure was 138/88 mmHg and his SpO_2 was 95% on air. His MRC breathlessness score was 3 (walks slower than contemporaries on the level because of breathlessness or has to stop for breath when walking at own pace).

Mr Tait completed the COPD assessment test and scored 27 and on his walk test (the incremental shuttle walk test-ISWT) he managed 290 metres before he had to stop due to breathlessness. Mr Tait's modified Borg score prior to commencement of the ISWT is 0 (no breathlessness) and was 4 (somewhat severe) at the end. His SpO_2 dropped to 90% after the walk but recovered within a couple of minutes.

Mr Tait was taking the following medications: salbutamol, tiotropium, furosemide and ramipril and did not have any allergies.

Mr T started a 6-week course of PR attending twice a week. The programme included both exercise and education. At the end of the 6 weeks Mr Tait had another assessment. He completed the COPD assessment test again and this time scored 21. He also repeated the ISWT and managed to walk 370 metres (80 metres further than he did at the start of the programme), and his Borg scale after his walk was only a 2 (slight breathlessness). He stated that he feels less short of breath and is managing to walk a few holes on the golf course. He was given an 'exercise referral', which will get him a discount to continue to use the gym so that he can maintain the benefits that he has gained doing the programme. The results of his pre- and post-pulmonary rehabilitation questionnaires and walk test were sent back to his GP and he is discharged from the programme.

CASE STUDY DISCUSSION

Patients with an MRC score of 3–5 who are functionally limited by breathlessness should be referred to an outpatient PR programme (Bolton et al., 2013). This is what happened in the case of Mr Tait. The point of referral is a good time to explore the patient's understanding and motivation to attend a PR programme. Mr Tait had already given up smoking, but at referral smoking status should be addressed and the patient referred to smoking cessation if relevant as PR offers a good opportunity for patients to address lifestyle issues.

Mr Tait attended a 6-week course of PR with two supervised exercise sessions per week. This is the duration that is recommended by Bolton et al. (2013) and is based on randomised trials that show this duration offers the most significant benefits in terms of exercise, dyspnoea and health status. The programme included a combination of resistance and aerobic training to ensure maximal strength and endurance benefits. Each exercise session was followed by an education topic that aims to assist in self-management and understanding. Topics can include things such as lung pathology, medication, chest clearance techniques and energy conservation.

Mr Tait's post-programme tests showed that he gained a clinically significant improvement in his COPD assessment test, indicating an improvement in his symptoms and an improvement in his ISWT of 80 metres, which again is above the minimal clinically important difference indicating an improvement in his exercise capacity. Mr Tait was given an exercise referral at the end of his course to encourage the continuation of exercise beyond the duration of the course. Bolton et al. (2013) state that all patients completing PR should be encouraged to continue exercise beyond the programme.

SUMMARY

PR is a highly evidence-based, cost-effective treatment for individuals with COPD and other chronic respiratory disorders such as ILD and bronchiectasis. This wealth of evidence has led to guidelines and quality standards being published to help guide providers, commissioners and patients towards best practice for this area of healthcare. PR leads to improved self-management of a long-term condition and takes healthcare out of the hospital setting and back into the community.

REFERENCES

Bolton, C.E., Bevan-Smith, E.F., Blakey, J.D., Crowe, P., Elkin, S.L., Garrod, R., Greening, N.J. et al. 2013. British Thoracic Society pulmonary rehabilitation guideline group. Guideline on pulmonary rehabilitation in adults. *Thorax* 68 (suppl 2): i1–i30.

Bolton, C.E., Steiner, M., Bevan-Smith, E.F., Blakey, J.D., Crowe, P., Elkin, S.L., Goddard, S. et al. 2014. British Thoracic Society reports. In: *Quality Standards for Pulmonary Rehabilitation in Adults*. Vol. 6 (2), British Thoracic Society, London.

Borg, G.A. 1982. Psychological basis of perceived exertion. *Medicine and Science in Sports and Exercise* 14 (5): 377–381.

Brown, C.D. and Wise, R.A. 2007. Field tests of exercise in COPD: The six minute walk test and the shuttle walk test. *The Journal of Chronic Obstructive Pulmonary Disease* 4 (3): 217–223.

Butland, R.J.A., Pang, J. and Gross, E.R. 1982. Two, six and 12 minute walk tests in respiratory disease. *BMJ* 284 (6329): 1607–1608.

Casaburi, R., Patessio, A., Loli, F., Zanaboni, S., Donner, C. and Wasserman, K. 1991. Reductions in exercise lactic acidosis and ventilation as a result of exercise training in patients with obstructive lung disease. *American Journal of Respiratory Disease* 143 (1): 9–18.

Chang, J., Curtis, J., Patrick, D. and Raghu, G. 1999. Assessment of health related quality of life in patients with interstitial lung disease. *Chest* 116 (5): 1175–1182.

Curtis, J.R. and Patrick, D.L. 2003. The assessment of health status among patients with COPD. *European Respiratory Journal* 21 (suppl 41): 36s–45s.

Department of Health. 2012. *Service Specification: Pulmonary Rehabilitation Service*. Department of Health, London.

Fischer, M.J., Scharloo, M., Abbink, J.J., van't Hul, A.J., van Ranst, D., Rudolphus, A., Weinman, J., Rabe, K.F. and Kaptein, A.A. 2009. Drop-out and attendance in pulmonary rehabilitation: The role of the clinical and psychosocial variables. *Respiratory Medicine* 2009 (103): 1564–1571.

Fletcher, C.M. 1960. Standardised questionnaire on respiratory symptoms: A statement prepared and approved by the MRC Committee on the Aetiology of Chronic Bronchitis (MRC breathlessness score). *British Medical Journal* 2 (523): 1665.

Fletcher, C.M., Elmes, P.C. and Fairbairn, M.B. 1959. The significance of respiratory symptoms and the diagnosis of chronic bronchitis in a working population. *British Medical Journal* 2 (5147): 257–266.

Garcia-Aymerich, J., Lange, P., Benet, M., Schnohr, P. and Anto, J. 2006. Regular physical activity reduces hospital admission and mortality in chronic obstructive pulmonary disease: A population based cohort study. *Thorax* 61 (9): 772–778.

Griffiths, T.L., Lonescu, A.A., Thomas, J., Tunbridge, J., Burr, M.L., Campbell, I.A., Lewis-Jenkins, V. et al. 2000. Results at 1 year of outpatient multidisciplinary pulmonary rehabilitation: A randomised controlled trial. *Lancet* 355 (9201): 362–368.

Guyatt, G.H., Berman, L.B., Townsend, M., Pugsley, S. and Chambers, L. 1987. A measure of quality of life for clinical trials in chronic lung disease. *Thorax* 42 (10): 773–778.

Hamilton, A., Killian, K., Summers, E. and Jones, N. 1995. Muscle strength, symptom intensity, and exercise capacity in patients with cardiorespiratory disorders. *American Journal of Respiratory Critical Care Medicine* 152 (6 pt1): 2021–2031.

Hardinge, M., Annandale, J., Bourne, S., Cooper, B., Evans, A., Freeman, D., Green, A. et al. 2015. British Thoracic Society guidelines for home oxygen use in adults. *Thorax* 70 (suppl 1): i1–i43.

Holland, A.E., Hill, C.J., Glaspole, I., Goh, N. and McDonald, C.F. 2012. Predictors of benefit following pulmonary rehabilitation for interstitial lung disease. *Respiratory Medicine* 106 (3): 429–435.

Jones, C.J., Rikli, E. and Beam, W.C. 1999. A 30-s chair stand test as a measure of lower body strength in community-residing older adults. *Research Quarterly for Exercise and Sport* 70 (2): 113–119.

Jones, P.W., Harding, G., Berry, P., Wicklund, I., Chen, W.H. and Kline, L.N. 2009. Development and first validation of the COPD assessment test. *European Respiratory Journal* 34 (3): 648–54.

Jones, P.W., Quirk, F.H., Baveystock, C.M. and Littlejohns, P. 1992. A self complete measure of health status for chronic airflow limitation. The St Georges Respiratory Questionnaire. *American Review Respiratory Disease* 145 (6): 1321–1327.

Lacasse, Y., Goldstein, R., Lasserson, T.J. and Martin, S. 2006. Pulmonary Rehabilitation for chronic obstructive pulmonary disease. *Cochrane Database Systematic Reviews* 18 (4).

Lacasse, Y., Guyatt, G. and Goldstein, R. 1997. The components of a respiratory program: A sytematic overview. *Chest* 111 (4): 1077–88.

Mador, M., Kufel, T., Pineda, L., Steinwald, A., Aggarwal, A., Upadhyay, A. and Khan, M. 2001. Effect of pulmonary rehabilitation on quadriceps fatiguability during exercise. *American Journal of Critical Care Medicine* 163 (4): 930–935.

Maltais, F., LeBlanc, P., Simard, C., Jobin, J., Berube, C., Bruneau, J., Carrier, L. and Belleau, R. 1996. Skeletal muscle adaptation to endurance training in patients with chronic obstructive pulmonary disease. *American Journal of Respiratory Critical Care Medicine* 154: 442–447.

Morgan, M.D.L. 2001. British Thoracic Society standards of care subcommittee on pulmonary rehabilitation pulmonary rehabilitation. *Thorax* 56 (11): 827–834.

Moullec, G., Ninot, G., Varray, A., Desplan, J., Hayot, M. and Prefaut, C. 2008. An innovative maintenance follow-up program after a first inpatient pulmonary rehabilitation. *Respiratory Medicine* 102 (4): 556–566.

National Institute for Health and Care Excellence. 2010. *Chronic Obstructive Pulmonary Disease. Management of Chronic Obstructive Pulmonary Disease in Adults in Primary and Secondary Care.* NICE, London.

Newall, C., Stockley, R.A. and Hill, S.L. 2005. Exercise training and inspiratory muscle training in patients with bronchiectasis. *Thorax* 60 (11): 943–948.

Nishiyama, O., Kondoh, Y., Kimura, T., Kato, K., Kataoka, K. and Ogawa, T. 2008. Effects of pulmonary rehabilitation in patients with idiopathic pulmonary fibrosis. *Respirology* 13 (3): 394–399.

O'Donnell, D., Lam, M. and Webb, K. 1999. Spirometric correlates of improvement in exercise performance after anticholinergic therapy in chronic obstructive pulmonary disease. *American Journal of Respiratory Critical Care Medicine* 160 (2): 542–549.

O'Donnell, D., Revill, S. and Webb, K. 2001. Dynamic hyperinflation and exercise intolerance in chronic obstructive pulmonary disease. *American Journal Respiratory Critical Care Medicine* 164 (5): 770–777.

O'Donnell, D. and Webb, K. 2008. The major limitation to exercise performance in COPD is dynamic hyperinflation. *Journal of Applied Physiology* 105 (2): 753–755.

Paone, G., Serpilli, M., Girardi, E., Conti, V., Principe, R., Puglisi, G., De Marchis, L. and Schmid, G. 2008. The combination of a smoking cessation programme with rehabilitation increases stop-smoking rate. *Journal Rehabilitation Medicine* 40 (8): 672–677.

Pepin, V., Laviolette, L., Brouillard, C., Sewell, L., Singh, S.J., Revill, S.M., Lacasse, Y. and Maltais, F. 2011. Significance of changes in endurance shuttle walking performance. *Thorax* 66 (2): 115–120.

Price, L.C., Lowe, D., Hosker, H.R., Anstey, K., Pearson, M.G. and Roberts, C.M. On behalf of the British Thoracic Society and the Royal College of Physicians Clinical Effectiveness Evaluation Unit (CEEu) 2006. UK National COPD Audit 2003: Impact of hospital resources and organisation of care on patient outcome following admission for acute COPD exacerbation. *Thorax* 61 (10): 837–842.

Puhan, M.A., Gimeno-Santos, E., Scharplatz, M., Troosters, T., Walters, E.H. and Steurer, J. 2011. Pulmonary rehabilitation following exacerbations of chronic obstructive disease. *Cochrane Database Systematic Reviews* 5 (10).

Revill, S.M., Morgan, M.D.L., Singh, S.J., Williams, J. and Harman, A.E. 1999. The endurance shuttle walk: A new field test for the assessment of endurance capacity in chronic obstructive pulmonary disease. *Thorax* 54 (3): 213–222.

Revill, S.M., Singh, S.J. and Morgan, M.D. 2000. Randomized controlled trial of ambulatory oxygen and an ambulatory ventilator on endurance exercise in COPD. *Respiratory Medicine* 94 (8): 778–783.

Ries, A.L. 2005. Minimally clinically important difference for the UCSD shortness of breath questionnaire, Borg scale and visual analog scale. *Journal of Chronic Obstructive Pulmonary Disease* 2 (1): 105–110.

Ringbaek, T., Brondum, E., Martinez, G., Thogersen, J. and Lange, P. 2010. Long-term effects of 1-year maintenance training on physical functioning and health status in patients with COPD: A randomized controlled study. *Journal of Cardiopulmonary Rehabilitation and Prevention* 30 (6): 47–52.

Sabit, R., Griffiths, T.L., Watkins, A.J., Evans, W., Bolton, C.E., Shale, D.J. and Lewis, K.E. 2008. Predictors of poor attendance at an outpatient pulmonary rehabilitation programme. *Respiratory Medicine* 102 (6): 819–824.

Seymour, J., Spruit, M., Hopkinson, N., Natanek, S., Man, W., Jackson, A., Gosker, H. et al. 2010. The prevalence of quadriceps weakness in COPD and the relationship with disease severity. *European Respiratory Journal* 36: 81–88.

Singh, S.J., Jones, P.W., Evans, R. and Morgan, M.D.L. 2008. Minimum clinically important improvement for the incremental shuttle walk test. *Thorax* 63 (9): 775–777.

Singh, S.J., Morgan, M.D.L., Hardman, A.E., Rowe, C. and Bardsley, P.A. 1994. Comparison of oxygen uptake during a conventional treadmill test and the shuttle walk test in chronic airflow limitation. *European Respiratory Journal* 7: 2016–2020.

Singh, S.J., Morgan, M.D.L. and Scott, S. 1992. Development of a shuttle walking test of disability in patients with chronic airways obstruction *Thorax* 47 (12): 1019–1024.

Solway, S., Brooks, D., Lacasse, Y. and Thomas, S. 2001. A qualitative systematic overview of the measurement properties of functional walk tests used in the cardiorespiratory domain. *Chest* 119 (1): 256–270.

Spruit, M.A., Singh, S.J., Garvey, C., ZuWallack, R., Nici, L., Rochester, C., Hill, K. et al. 2013. American Thoracic Society/European Respiratory Society statement: Key concepts and advances in pulmonary rehabilitation. *American Journal Respiratory Critical Care Medicine* 188 (8): e13–64.

Troosters, T., Gosselink, R. and Decramer, M. 2000. Short and long term effects of outpatient rehabilitation in patients with chronic obstructive pulmonary disease: A randomised trial. *American Journal of Medicine* 109: 207–212.

Van der Molen, T., Willemse, B., Schokker, S., Ten Hacken, N., Postma, D. and Juniper, E. 2003. Development, validity and responsiveness of the clinical COPD questionnaire. *Health Quality Life Outcomes* 1 (1): 13.

Walker, H.K., Hall, W.D. and Hurst, J.W. 1990. *Clinical Methods: The History, Physical and Laboratory Examination* (3rd ed.). Butterworths, Boston.

Whittom, F., Jobin, J., Simard, P., LeBlanc, P., Simard, C., Bernard, S., Belleau, R. and Maltais, F. 1998. Histochemical and morphological characteristics of the vastus lateralis muscle in patients with chronic obstructive pulmonary disease. *Medicine and Science in Sports and Exercise* 30 (10): 1467–1474.

Williams, S., Baxter, N., Holmes, S., Restrick, L., Scullion, J. and Ward, M. 2012. British Thoracic Society reports. In: *British Thoracic Society and the Primary Care Respiratory Society IMPRESS Guide to the Relative Value of COPD Interventions*. Vol. 4 (2), British Thoracic Society, London.

Wise, R.A. and Brown, C.D. 2005. Minimally clinically important difference in the six minute walk test and the incremental shuttle walk test. *Journal of Chronic Obstructive Pulmonary Disease* 2 (1): 125–129.

Young, P., Dewse, M., Fergusson, W. and Kolbe, J. 1999. Respiratory rehabilitation in chronic obstructive pulmonary disease: Predictors of nonadherence. *European Respiratory Journal* 13: 855–859.

Zainuldin, R., Mackey, M.G. and Alison, J.A. 2011. Optimal intensity and type of leg exercise training for people with chronic obstructive pulmonary disease. *Cochrane Database Systematic Reviews* 11.

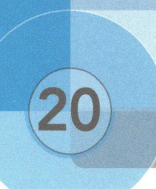

Cognitive behavioural therapy for respiratory conditions

20

KAREN HESLOP-MARSHALL

LEARNING OBJECTIVES

Upon completion of this chapter the reader should be able to:

- Discuss the psychological impact of respiratory disease on patients
- Identify ways to screen for anxiety and depression
- Understand the basic principles of cognitive behavioural therapy
- Describe how cognitive behavioural therapy can be used to help reduce symptoms of anxiety and depression for patients with respiratory disease

INTRODUCTION

In the United Kingdom (UK), life expectancy is increasing and continues to improve (Buck, 2014). People are living longer with health conditions such as chronic obstructive pulmonary disease (COPD). Many respiratory diseases are very disabling and lead to a gradual progression of disability over many years; as a consequence, day-to-day functioning can be very challenging and quality of life is often reduced (Ng et al., 2007; Department of Health [DH], 2011). Patients often focus on feeling unwell, their inability to perform everyday activities and on the emotional consequences of the disease (British Lung Foundation, 2006). A term used to describe ill-health or disease burden is 'disability-adjusted life years' (DALYs) (Buck, 2014). Research has ranked respiratory and cardiac diseases as the two most disabling disorders in terms of DALYs (Aydin and Ulusahin, 2001).

There is growing recognition that people with long-term physical health problems have an increased risk of developing symptoms of anxiety and depression and it is now widely accepted that anxiety and depression are extremely common co-morbidities in patients with COPD (Global Initiative for COPD [GOLD], 2015). Unfortunately, many healthcare professionals pay little attention to the psychological impact of respiratory diseases and do not screen for symptoms of anxiety and depression. This may be due to lack of understanding of the impact of such symptoms on patients' lives or lack of training in knowing how to treat symptoms of anxiety and depression.

This chapter aims to provide an overview of the use of cognitive behavioural therapy (CBT) for patients with respiratory problems such as COPD. The chapter includes a summary of anxiety and depression in COPD, methods of screening for symptoms of anxiety and depression, what CBT is and common CBT techniques that can help treat these symptoms. Finally, a case study will be presented which illustrates the impact of CBT for a patient with COPD who has very severe COPD and is experiencing symptoms of anxiety, panic attacks and low mood.

ANXIETY AND DEPRESSION

Maurer et al. (2008) argue that anxiety and depression are two of the most common co-morbidities associated with COPD. Prevalence estimates of anxiety and depression in COPD vary widely (Maurer et al., 2008). A systematic review and meta-analysis reported the prevalence of clinically significant symptoms of anxiety as 36% and 40% for depression in patients with COPD (Yohannes et al., 2006). However, symptoms of anxiety seem to be increasing and can be as high as 60%. In a large randomised controlled trial, 1518 patients were screened for symptoms of anxiety; more than half (60%) of patients screened had symptoms of anxiety based on a Hospital Anxiety and Depression Scale (HADS) of greater than seven (Heslop-Marshall and De Soyza, 2014). The impact of pulmonary disease on activities of daily life is adversely affected by anxiety and depression, even after controlling the effects of breathlessness (Weaver et al., 1997).

People with COPD are two to three times more likely to experience mental health problems than the general population (Naylor et al., 2012). Serious implications for people with COPD and mental health problems include poorer clinical outcomes, lower quality of life and reduced ability to manage physical symptoms effectively, and are associated with unhealthy behaviours such as smoking (Naylor et al., 2012). A number of variables have been associated with anxiety and depression in patients with COPD (Maurer et al., 2008). These can be found in Table 20.1.

ANXIETY

Anxiety is a common emotion experienced by us all. Anxiety can help people identify danger and respond appropriately (Pooler and Beech, 2014). However, the persistence of anxiety can leave people feeling

Table 20.1 Variables associated with depression and anxiety in patients with COPD

Physical disability
Long-term oxygen therapy
Low body mass index
Severe dyspnoea
Percentage of predicted FEV_1 <50%
Poor quality of life
Presence of co-morbidity
Living alone
Female gender
Current smoking
Low social class status

Source: Adapted from Maurer, J. et al. 2008. *Chest* 134 (4 Suppl): 43S–56S.

apprehensive and with a tendency to worry. When we perceive danger, the automatic fear response occurs faster than conscious thought. Surges of adrenaline are released; these subside quickly once the perceived or actual threat has passed. Anxiety causes a number of physical responses such as increased respiratory rate (David, 2006). These symptoms overlap with the symptoms of COPD (Giardino et al., 2010). In individuals who have normal lung function the physical symptoms of anxiety can be alarming. However, for people whose respiratory function is compromised, the symptoms of anxiety can lead to extreme fear and panic. Anxiety is reported across all ranges of COPD severity and is associated with lower levels of self-efficacy, impaired health status, poorer treatment outcomes and reduced survival (Ng et al., 2007). Anxiety is a significant predictor of the frequency of hospital admissions and re-admissions for acute exacerbations of COPD.

Panic disorder is a severe form of anxiety. Panic is up to ten times more prevalent in patients with COPD than in the general population (Livermore, 2010). Panic disorder consists of recurring, unforeseen panic attacks. This is followed by persistent worry about having further attacks. Panic attacks develop suddenly, are associated with intense fear, anxiety and physical arousal and are relatively short lived (David, 2006). In patients with COPD, worsening breathlessness is often interpreted in a catastrophic way: patients commonly think they cannot breathe and death is imminent. Symptoms of increased physical arousal follow leading to an escalating cycle, which results in panic (Livermore et al., 2010). Patients become anxious about becoming breathless and avoid exertion that may trigger unpleasant symptoms occurring. This leads to physical deconditioning and exacerbates the panic cycle.

DEPRESSION

Depression is an important public health problem and one of the leading causes of disease burden worldwide (Moussavi et al., 2007). National Institute of Health and Care Excellence (NICE) (2009) state that depression is two to three times more common in patients with chronic physical health conditions. Symptoms of depression include persistent low mood, loss of interest and enjoyment in usual activities and fatigue. Other symptoms involve appetite changes, negative thoughts, sleep problems and reduced ability to concentrate (David, 2006). Symptoms must be present for at least two weeks and be associated with marked impairment of daily functioning. Increasingly, it is recognised that minor symptoms of depression can cause distress and become disabling if persistent (NICE, 2009). Treating symptoms early is important.

COPD can cause and exacerbate depression (NICE, 2009). As a result of breathlessness, patients may not be able to participate in normal activities of daily living. This reduced activity leads to feelings of hopelessness, which ultimately affects mood. In a large prospective cohort study, Ng et al. (2007) found that co-morbid depressive symptoms in patients with COPD are associated with poorer survival, longer hospital stay, persistent smoking, increased symptom burden and poorer physical functioning. The authors found that patients commonly feel hopeless and helpless about changing their life circumstances; lack the drive and motivation to seek help and may succumb to early death instead.

SCREENING FOR ANXIETY AND DEPRESSION

Detecting symptoms of anxiety and depression is the first step in providing effective support for patients. There is evidence that the presence of physical illness makes detection of mental health problems more difficult (Naylor et al., 2012). Symptoms often overlap, e.g. breathlessness can occur as a consequence of COPD and anxiety. Within the National Health Service (NHS) there has been a major focus on pharmacological treatment of physical and psychological problems. Qualitative evidence suggests that both patients and healthcare professionals focus on physical symptoms (Coventry et al., 2011).

Screening is recommended in the National Guidelines for the Management of COPD (NICE, 2010). In clinical practice screening of psychological symptoms in COPD patients remains extremely poor and is not done to a consistently high level (Naylor et al., 2012). Four simple questions can be used to begin screening for anxiety and depression (Table 20.2).

A formal psychometric questionnaire should be completed if the patient has reported any symptoms of anxiety and depression in the initial screening. There are many psychometric questionnaires that can be used to identify symptoms of anxiety and depression and the most common questionnaire used in medical outpatient settings is the Hospital Anxiety and Depression Scale (HADS). This questionnaire has been validated for the use of COPD patients (Snaith and Zigmond, 1994). Seven questions relate to symptoms of anxiety and seven questions relate to symptoms of depression. The scores are added for each domain (anxiety and depression). Scores range from 0 to 21, and high scores indicate more symptoms. The interpretation of the scores can be found in Table 20.3.

Table 20.2 Basic screening questions for anxiety and depression

Anxiety	Depression
Over the last 2 weeks have you been bothered by feeling nervous, anxious or on edge?	During the last month have you been bothered by feeling down, depressed or hopeless?
During the last 2 weeks have worrying thoughts gone through your mind?	During the last month, have you been bothered by having little interest or pleasure in doing things?

Table 20.3 Interpretation of HAD scores

Score	Interpretation
0–7	Within normal range
8–10	Mild symptoms
11–14	Moderate symptoms
15–21	Severe symptoms

Source: Adapted from Snaith, R.P. and Zigmond, A.S. 1994. *The Hospital Anxiety and Depression Scale Manual.* NFER Nelson, Windsor.

If the patient's HADS scores are eight or above for either domain, then written information about anxiety and/or depression should be offered to the patient or alternatively the patient could be referred for CBT.

COGNITIVE BEHAVIOURAL THERAPY

CBT is a short-term treatment that has a very practical approach. In many cases CBT focusses on the patient's current difficulties rather than addressing issues from the past. However, sometimes experiences from the past can affect the present so may need to be tackled with more in-depth CBT. CBT is increasingly being used to help people manage chronic illnesses and help them cope with the difficulties they may encounter on a regular basis.

Put simply, the term 'cognitive' relates to our thoughts, images, dreams and memories. Behaviour relates to what we do or avoid doing and therapy is a term commonly used for a treatment. CBT was first developed by Dr Aaron Beck in the 1960s. Briers (2009) stated that Beck was frustrated with Freudian psychoanalysis which emphasised the importance of unpacking repressed conflicts of the past. Beck became convinced that for many of his patients the crux of their problems lay more in what they thought about the present (Briers, 2009). Beck and his colleagues undertook rigorous research into the efficacy of CBT and CBT is now one of the most evidence-based psychotherapies in the world (Briers, 2009). CBT is recommended by NICE for many psychological problems including anxiety and depression (NICE, 2009, 2011).

CBT explores the current situation, thoughts, emotions, behaviour and physical symptoms and the links between them. The current situation or events can affect the patient's thoughts, the way they feel and what they do to cope in situations. Often a vicious cycle develops which maintains the sequence (see Figure 20.1). CBT helps people make sense of their situation or difficulties identifying vicious cycles and ways to overcome these problems.

One of the key principles of CBT is that it is not the events or experiences that happen to us that are important but our interpretation of events and the way we react to them (Briers, 2009). For example, two patients with very similar lung disease may experience the same lung condition but can cope very differently. One person may respond by developing coping strategies that help manage their difficulties better such as planning and pacing their activities. Another person may make things worse by not planning or pacing activities or avoiding them altogether. When using CBT skills, the healthcare professional

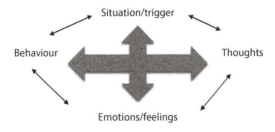

Figure 20.1 The CBT five-part model. (Adapted with permission from Padesky, C.A. and Mooney, K.A. 1990. Presenting the cognitive model to clients. *International Cognitive Therapy Newsletter*, 6: 13–14. Retrieved from www.padesky.com)

works collaboratively to understand the patient's difficulties and identify strategies that may be helpful.

CBT is rooted in an educational approach (Briers, 2009). By developing new skills, unhelpful thoughts and behaviour can be challenged and changed. Once skills are acquired patients can then become their own therapist and use the techniques they have learnt in similar situations. This can empower patients and help them learn to solve their own problems or difficulties rather than being fixed by an expert (Briers, 2009).

An example of a well-established specialist CBT service has been running for over ten years in Newcastle upon Tyne NHS Hospitals Foundation Trust and involves between two and six sessions of CBT. Respiratory nurses within the clinic have been trained in CBT skills and techniques. The aim of the treatment is to help identify ways of managing the impact of chest problems on patient's day-to-day life. There are huge benefits of nurses with respiratory expertise training in CBT skills. Firstly, respiratory nurses work at the front line with respiratory patients. Patients may be reluctant to be referred to mental health services but would be happy to discuss the impact of their lung problem with a respiratory nurse. Secondly, dual physical and psychological skills provide a better understanding and assessment of the cause of symptoms such as breathlessness and thirdly, CBT skills can help provide holistic care to patients with respiratory problems.

CBT TRAINING

Emotional distress is commonly encountered in the physical health setting as patients struggle to cope with ongoing adversity as a result of their physical health problem. Traditionally, nurses have used counselling skills to provide support for patients. However, these skills may be sufficient to facilitate emotional expression and relief for transient emotional distress but may not produce lasting emotional support in the face of continuing ill health when patients feel anxiety or depressed (Mannix et al., 2006). There is evidence that nurses working within the physical health setting can learn basic CBT techniques, successfully providing more structured psychological support for patients (Mannix et al., 2006; Heslop and Foley, 2009). Training can help healthcare professionals such as nurses and physiotherapists recognise emotional distress, select and use appropriate techniques that can help patients change their thinking or behaviour and regain control. A key component of CBT training is ongoing clinical supervision. Supervision has been shown to consolidate and build CBT skills following training (Mannix et al., 2006).

CASE STUDY

Mr Roberts was referred to the Chest Clinic Nurse Led CBT Clinic for assessment of his mood by his general practitioner. Mr Roberts is a 67 year old retired gentleman who lives with his wife in a detached house. Mr Roberts has previously been diagnosed with very severe COPD with an FEV_1 of 0.86 (23% of predicted). He also had evidence of emphysema with a transfer factor (T_{LCO}) of 48% predicted (see Chapter 3), his Medical Research Council (MRC) breathlessness score was 4 and his oxygen saturation levels were 96% on room air, falling to a nadir of 90% on exertion. It was probable that there was an asthmatic component to Mr Roberts' respiratory disease and also minor bronchiectasis which was awaiting confirmation from a high resolution computed tomography scan (HRCT). Mr Roberts had a productive cough; he could produce up to 1/2 egg cupful of sputum per day ordinarily with greater volumes during infections. Mr Roberts stopped smoking 18 months ago, though prior to that was a very heavy smoker of 60 cigarettes per day. His BMI was 28 and he was being treated for hypertension.

Mr Roberts had previously been self-employed in the jewellery trade. In his work he does not recall any significant flux exposure, although did work with sulphuric acid. He was not aware of any impact on his respiratory symptoms in relation to work. Mr Roberts drinks a little but within the recommended safe limits at around 14 units per week. Mr Roberts has a pet dog at home, has no regular contact with birds and is not aware of any significant asbestos exposure. There is a family history of asthma; his youngest son suffered from childhood asthma but now seems untroubled by it. Mr Roberts' brother also suffered from asthma. Mr Roberts was not aware of any childhood respiratory symptoms.

Medications include Mucodyne 750 mgs twice daily, Symbicort 200 two puffs twice daily, Tiotropium 18 ugm once daily, Salbutamol 200 ugm as required, Amlodipine 10 mg once daily, Candesartan 32 mg once daily and Citalopram 20 mg once daily.

Currently Mr Roberts' main symptom was breathlessness, which he had noted started approximately 20 years ago. The breathlessness had clearly progressed substantially since then. He estimated that he could walk approximately 50 yards on the flat now and was very limited indeed on hills or stairs. His breathlessness does display some diurnal variability, being worse in the morning and waking him from sleep, perhaps 3 times per week. He noted that he did feel anxious about his breathing, particularly when he exerted himself.

CASE STUDY DISCUSSION

Routine care within the chest clinic involves screening for symptoms of anxiety and depression. A Hospital Anxiety and Depression Scale (HADS) was completed. Mr Roberts' HADS score was 15 for anxiety and 8 for depression suggesting clinically significant symptoms. Mr Roberts was experiencing symptoms of anxiety as a result of his breathlessness. The presentation of his current difficulties and symptoms are illustrated in Figure 20.2.

The first session of CBT involved getting to know Mr Roberts and exploring his main difficulties. Once his current situation had been discussed and documented, a treatment plan was agreed. Mr Roberts was given some self-help leaflets on panic and depression and the Self-Help Toolkit to reinforce the discussion (Moore and Cole, 2009; Northumberland Tyne and Wear, 2013). The techniques used can be seen in Table 20.4.

Mr Roberts was also referred to pulmonary rehabilitation (PR), which is an exercise-based intervention rather than a psychological intervention (see Chapter 19). While the benefits of PR may well affect psychological well-being, its primary focus is improving exercise capacity. CBT can be used with other pharmacological and non-pharmacological therapies such as anti-depressants and pulmonary rehabilitation.

Mr Roberts made excellent progress during therapy, his HADS scores reduced to six for anxiety and five for depression which were both within the normal range. As expected Mr Roberts' lung function had not changed at all as a result of CBT. However, using CBT techniques helped Mr Roberts identify ways to improve self-management of his symptoms, which helped him cope with anxiety and depression more effectively.

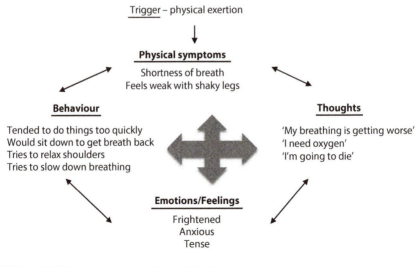

Figure 20.2 The CBT five-part model applied to Mr Roberts.

Table 20.4 CBT techniques used for Mr Roberts

Technique	Rationale
Education about COPD, anxiety and depression	Explaining what the illnesses are can help patients understand what is happening to them and how to manage their own health.
Goal setting	Setting small manageable goals that the patient feels are important to them is an integral part of CBT. Goals should be reviewed during therapy and new goals set when achieved.
Pacing activities	It is very tempting for patients to rush to complete tasks such as getting dressed or exerting themselves undertaking other activities. Rushing can exacerbate breathlessness. It is important for patient to pace themselves so they don't become so breathless it becomes very uncomfortable.
Relaxation	When people are anxious muscles can become tense. Relaxation helps breathing, heart and muscles. Learning to relax can take some practice but finding something that helps patients relax can help their breathing, reduce tension and help deal with the stresses and strains of life more easily.
Breathing control	Many patients hyperventilate when they are breathless. Explaining breathing control exercise can help patients take control of their breathing. Slow deep breathing should be encouraged. Ideally, breathing out should be longer than the breath in, e.g. breathe in for three seconds and out slowly for four seconds. This can take some practice when patients are feeling breathless but it works.
Distraction	Helping patients use an alternative focus rather than their breathing which can cause distressing feelings of anxiety and breathlessness (Booth et al., 2014). There are lots of ways distraction can be used. Some patients may find the following examples helpful, e.g. counting backwards from 100 in sevens, counting how many ornaments they have, think about a football team, places they have visited or imagine they are on a beautiful beach. The list is endless. If patients do not focus on their breathing it settles down much quicker. If distraction does not work well, it may be that the patient will need to practice when they are not anxious, try another technique instead or it may be they were too anxious at the time. It is easier for distraction to work if it is started early.
Increasing activity levels (behavioural activation)	Respiratory patients commonly avoid activities or exercise, which leads to deconditioning of muscles. Behavioural activation is a useful technique to increase levels of activity and provide patients with a sense of achievement or pleasure.
Stop and gain control	Encouraging patients to stop when they get breathless rather than pushing themselves too hard can help them gain control of their breathing. Once they gain control of the breathing they can carry on.
Exploring negative thinking	It is easy for patients to focus on negative things in life which can impact greatly on feelings of anxiety and depression (Booth et al., 2014). Encouraging patients to identify negative thinking and giving themselves credit for what they can do, rather than what they cannot do can help reduce negative thinking and increase confidence.
Hand-held cool air fan	Hand-held cool air fans can help the perception of breathing. The fan will need to be held about 6 inches away from the patient's face. It is important to point the fan at the nose and mouth as it will stimulate the nerves in the face which helps patients feel less breathless (Booth et al., 2014).

SUMMARY

Respiratory diseases such as COPD and interstitial lung disease have a massive impact on people's physical and psychological well-being. Identifying symptoms of anxiety and depression is the first step to help address patient's psychological distress. There are a growing number of studies evaluating the efficacy of psychological interventions to improve the psychological well-being of patients with COPD and most of the studies published in the last 20 years have used CBT. In a comprehensive systematic review, Baraniak and Sheffield (2011) concluded that there is some evidence that psychological interventions such as CBT impact on anxiety. Larger studies have been conducted recently and the results will hopefully provide useful guidance on the treatment of anxiety and depression for patients with respiratory problems (Heslop et al., 2013). Training in CBT skills can provide healthcare professionals with additional skills to address psychological difficulties as a result of respiratory problems.

REFERENCES

Aydin, I.O. and Ulusahin, A. 2001. Depression, anxiety comorbidity, and disability in tuberculosis and chronic obstructive pulmonary disease patients: Applicability of GHQ-12. *General Hospital Psychiatry* 23 (2): 77–83.

Baraniak, A. and Sheffield, D. 2011. The efficacy of psychologically based interventions to improve anxiety, depression and quality of life in COPD: A systematic review and meta-analysis. *Patient Education and Counseling* 83 (1): 29–36.

Booth, S., Burkin, J., Moffat, C. and Spathis, A. 2014. *Managing Breathless in Clinical Practice*. Springer-Verlag, London.

Briers, S. 2009. *Brilliant Cognitive Behavioural Therapy*. Pearson Prentice Hall Publications, Harlow.

British Lung Foundation (BLF). 2006. *Invisible Lives*. BLF, London.

Buck, D. 2014. How Healthy are We? A high-level guide. The Kings Fund.

Coventry, P.A., Hays, R., Dickens, C., Bundy, C., Garrett, C., Cherrington, A. and Chew-Graham, C. 2011. Talking about depression: A qualitative study of barriers to managing depression in people with long term conditions in primary care. *BMC Family Practice* 12 (10).

David, L. 2006. *Using CBT in General Practice. The 10 Minute Consultation*. Scion Publishing Limit, Bloxham.

Department of Health (DH) 2011. *An Outcomes Strategy for Chronic Obstructive Pulmonary Disease (COPD) and Asthma in England*. DH, London.

Giardino, N.D., Curtis, J.L., Abelson, J.L., King, A.P., Pamp, B., Liberzon, I. and Martinez, F.J. 2010. The impact of panic disorder on interoception and dyspnea reports in chronic obstructive pulmonary disease. *Biological Psychology* 84 (1): 142–146.

Global Strategy for the Diagnosis, management and prevention of COPD. 2015. Global Initiative for Chronic Obstructive Lung Disease Inc.

Heslop, K. and Foley, T. 2009. Using cognitive behavioural therapy to address the psychological needs of patients with COPD. *Nursing Times* 105 (38): 18–19.

Heslop, K., Newton, J., Baker, C., Carrick-Sen, D., Burns, G.P. and De Soyza, A. 2013. Effectiveness of cognitive behavioural therapy (CBT) interventions for anxiety and depression in patients with chronic obstructive pulmonary disease (COPD) undertaken by respiratory nurses. The COPD CBT CARE Study'. *BMC Pulmonary Medicine* 13 (1): 62–68.

Heslop-Marshall, K. and De Soyza, A. 2014. Are we missing anxiety in people with chronic obstructive pulmonary disease (COPD)? *Annals of Depression and Anxiety* 1 (5): 1023.

Livermore, N., Sharpe, L. and McKenzie, D. 2010. Prevention of panic attacks and panic disorder in COPD. *European Respiratory Journal* 35: 557–563.

Mannix, K., Blackburn, I.M., Garland, A., Gracie, J., Moorey, S., Reid, B., Standart, S. and Scott, J. 2006. Effectiveness of brief training in cognitive behaviour therapy techniques for palliative care practitioners. *Palliative Medicine* 20 (6): 579–584.

Maurer, J., Rebbapragada, V., Borson, S., Goldstein, R., Kunik, M.E., Yohannes, A.M. and Hanania, N.A. 2008. Anxiety and depression in COPD: Current understanding, unanswered questions, and research needs. *Chest* 134 (4 Suppl): 43S–56S.

Moore, P. and Cole, F. 2009. *The Self-Care Toolkit.* DH, London.

Moussavi, S., Chatterji, S., Verdes, E., Tandon, A., Patel, V. and Ustun, B. 2007. Depression, chronic diseases, and decrements in health: Results from the World Health Surveys. *Lancet* 370 (9590): 851–858.

National Institute of Health and Care Excellence (NICE). 2009. *Depression in Adults with a Chronic Physical Health Problem. Treatment and Management. Clinical Guidelines 91.* NICE, London.

National Institute of Health and Care Excellence (NICE). 2010. *COPD Management of Chronic Obstructive Pulmonary Disease in Adults in Primary and Secondary Care. Clinical Guidelines 101.* NICE, London.

National Institute of Health and Care Excellence (NICE). 2011. *Generalised Anxiety Disorder and Panic Disorder (with or without Agrophobia) in Adults. Guideline on Management in Primary, Secondary and Community Care. Clinical Guidelines 113.* NICE, London.

Naylor, C., Parsonage, M., McDaid, D., Knapp, M., Fossey, M. and Galea, A. 2012. *Long-Term Conditions and Mental Health. The Cost of Co-Morbidities.* The King's Fund and Centre for Mental Health, London.

Ng, T.P., Niti, M., Tan, W.C., Cao, Z., Ong, K.C. and Eng, P. 2007. Depressive symptoms and chronic obstructive pulmonary disease: Effect on mortality, hospital readmission, symptom burden, functional status, and quality of life. *Archives of Internal Medicine* 167 (1): 60–67.

Northumberland Tyne and Wear. 2013. Mental Health Trust Leaflets. https://www.ntw.nhs.uk/pic/selfhelp/

Padesky, C.A. and Mooney, K.A. 1990. Presenting the cognitive model to clients. *International Cognitive Therapy Newsletter,* 6: 13–14. Retrieved from www.padesky.com

Pooler, A. and Beech, R. 2014. Examining the relationship between anxiety and depression and exacerbations of COPD which result in hospital admission: A systematic review. *International Journal of Chronic Obstructive Pulmonary Disease* 9: 315–330.

Snaith, R.P. and Zigmond, A.S. 1994. *The Hospital Anxiety and Depression Scale Manual.* NFER Nelson, Windsor.

Weaver, T.E., Richmond, T.S. and Narsavage, G.L. 1997. An explanatory model of functional status in chronic obstructive pulmonary disease. *Nurse Researcher* 46 (1): 26–31.

Yohannes, A.M., Baldwin, R.C. and Connolly, M.J. 2006. Depression and anxiety in elderly patients with chronic obstructive pulmonary disease. *Age Ageing* 35 (5): 457–459.

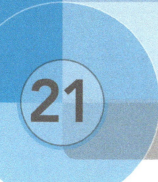

End-of-life care in relation to respiratory conditions

21

JOANNE ATKINSON AND ISABEL QUINN

LEARNING OBJECTIVES

Upon completion of this chapter the reader should be able to:

- Appreciate the importance of patient-focussed, end-of-life care
- Demonstrate understanding of the complexity of end-of-life care in chronic respiratory disease with particular reference to chronic obstructive pulmonary disease (COPD)
- Identify the principles of symptom control for common symptoms patients with COPD may experience at the end of life
- Understand the importance of communication as the foundation of good end-of-life care

INTRODUCTION

It is estimated that there are three million people living with chronic obstructive pulmonary disease (COPD) in England (Department of Health [DH], 2012). However, only 900,000 will have received a clear and accurate diagnosis and are getting appropriate treatment to improve their quality of life and clinical outcomes. It is also recognised that premature mortality from COPD in the United Kingdom (UK) is almost double the European average. The outcomes strategy for COPD and asthma produced by the Department of Health (2012) indicates that current UK incidence figures are not always accurate due to lack of confirmed diagnosis, but that COPD is a major cause of death and many people experience severe symptoms often with poorer outcomes than European counterparts.

The National End of Life Care Intelligence Network (NEoLCIN, 2011) produced a report which indicates that 14% of all deaths in England are from respiratory disease (as a primary cause) and if lung cancer deaths are incorporated, this figure rises to 20% of all deaths. Respiratory disease is also considered to be a contributory cause of 34%–39% of deaths from other primary causes. This report highlights that there are significant increased rates of respiratory deaths in areas where deprivation is most prevalent. There is also evidence that the proportion of deaths due to respiratory disease increases with age.

This chapter aims to provide an overview of the complex problems patients with a respiratory disease such as COPD may encounter at the end of life and will include a definition of end-of-life care and palliative care: an overview of the importance of full integration of end-of-life care into the patient journey. Patient and family support, major symptoms encountered by patients with COPD at the end of life, management of symptoms and challenges for practice will all be considered. A case study will be presented which illustrates the challenges that arise when caring for a patient with a respiratory disease, such as COPD, at the end of their life.

CHRONIC DISEASE

Chronic disease is the greatest challenge facing the NHS as the demography of living and dying is changing (DH, 2014; Taylor et al. 2003). Palliative care historically has emerged from the hospice setting being focussed on patients with incurable cancer (Traue and Ross, 2005). However, it is now integrated into practice throughout all spheres of care delivery and in all disease trajectories to varying degrees. Palliative care is the active total care of a patient with advanced disease, based on the principles of quality of life, good symptom control, support for the patient and their family, person centredness, respect, sensitive communication and choice (Addington-Hall and Higginson, 2006). It is important to make the distinction between palliative care and end-of-life care as the terms are often used interchangeably. Clarity regarding the definition and philosophy of end-of-life care was first given in 2008 when the Department of Health published the first End of Life Care Strategy.

End-of-life care is a term that has many varied interpretations; it includes physical, emotional, social and spiritual care that is required at any time in a person's life when their death or fear of death is an issue (Froggatt et al., 2006). Palliative care is an approach that is focussed on the improvement of quality of life for patients and their families when they have a life-threatening illness and is applicable early in the disease trajectory (Payne et al., 2008). There is often confusion around the terms palliative care and end-of-life care and they are not mutually exclusive. It is imperative to recognise that patients have the right to access high-quality palliative care and end-of-life care services and should be enabled to exercise choice about their preferred place of care at the end of their life (National Council of Palliative Care, 2010). End-of-life care services should support people approaching the end of their life to live as well

as possible until their death. Despite driving forces to improve the quality of care at the end of life articulated in successive policy documents, there are still significant inequalities in how and where people die (DH, 2007, 2008, 2010, 2011; NHS England, 2014).

Respiratory patients and their families have the same complex needs as many other patients who live with a chronic, life-limiting disease such as cardiac disease and renal disease. COPD is the commonest non-malignant respiratory disease and is a term that encompasses chronic bronchitis and emphysema: the principles of management and symptom control at the end of life are applicable to other respiratory disease (Higginson et al., 2014) (see Chapter 5 for further details on COPD).

Severe COPD and lung cancer patients are often cared for by the same professional teams. It is therefore important to recognise that COPD patients suffer from multiple complex symptoms at the end of life; those with severe COPD having worse physical symptoms, anxiety and depression than patients with inoperable non-small cell lung cancer (Gardiner et al., 2010). There still appears to be a disconnect between the needs of the patient and their family and access to palliative care services, despite guidance to start palliative care earlier alongside the curative care required to recover from acute exacerbations (Carlucci et al., 2012). Barriers to accessing palliative care services in COPD can be complex and there appears to be a misapprehension of palliative care being the same as end-of-life care (Hardin et al., 2008). This, alongside the difficulty in providing a prognosis for advancing disease, variable guidelines and practices for referral, lack of resources and importantly the poor patient and doctor/nurse communication about advanced care planning, all compound the difficulty in accessing palliative care (Janssen et al., 2010). Patients with respiratory disease and their families need good palliative care in order to reach the end of life with their needs addressed. Specifically, they require information about COPD and their prognosis, symptom control and access to specialist palliative care if required. Of equal importance is support for carers and for patients and carers to communicate their wishes and plan for their end-of-life care in advance (Cartwright and Booth, 2010). Further statistics relating to mortality from COPD are listed in Table 21.1.

Table 21.1 Statistics relating to COPD mortality

One person dies from COPD every 20 minutes in England – around 23,000 deaths a year.

15% of those admitted to hospital with COPD die within three months and around 25% die within a year of admission.

One in eight people over 35 has COPD that has not been properly identified or diagnosed, and over 15% are only diagnosed when they present to hospital as an emergency.

COPD is the second most common cause of emergency admissions to hospital and one of the costliest in-patient conditions to be treated by the NHS.

Source: Adapted from Department of Health 2012. *The Outcomes Strategy for COPD and Asthma.* Stationary Office, London.

UNPREDICTABILITY OF THE DISEASE TRAJECTORY OF COPD AND DIFFICULTY IN PROGNOSTICATION

As someone approaches the end of life there is usually a decline in their physical health. This can be quite apparent in people with a cancer diagnosis where there is an obvious decline in function over time. Using guidance from the End of Life Care Strategy (DH, 2008), this period usually refers to the last 6–12 months of someone's life. When end of life is less clear, the End of Life Care Strategy advocates that the surprise question should be used as part of the assessment process.

The surprise question asks *would you be surprised if this person died in the next 6–12 months?*

If the answer is no, then it should be considered that the individual is approaching the end of their life. However, the determination of someone's life expectancy is variable and unpredictable and healthcare professionals often look for other signs or factors to inform a timescale or prognosis. Many of these individuals may already be recognised as having advanced disease and if the answer to the surprise question above indicates that healthcare professionals would not be surprised if the person died in the next 6–12 months, then those individuals should be recorded

on a GP Practice Palliative Care Register. This would ensure regular discussions and review at Practice Multidisciplinary Team (MDT) meetings. This follows the recommendations of the Gold Standards Framework (GSF) (2005) for primary care. GP practices are allocated Quality Outcomes Framework (QOF) points to incentivise keeping palliative care registers and having regular meetings to discuss the patients on the register. It is estimated that in each GP practice of around 2000 patients, 20 patients would be expected to die from long-term conditions. Therefore, each Palliative Care Register would be expected to have around 1% of the practice population on this register if there was improved recognition. Of course another challenge is that many people are living with multiple long-term conditions. Intelligence data suggest that 80% of people with COPD have at least one other long-term condition (NEoLCIN, 2011).

There are a range of other recognised prognostication tools available to assist in identifying which patients may be in the last 6–12 months of life (GSF, 2005). Some of these are quite generic across a range of conditions such as gradually needing help with personal care activities. In addition to the surprise question and generic indicators mentioned previously, NHS Lothian (2010) cite some specific indicators of advanced respiratory disease that may alert health and social care professionals to the fact that someone may be approaching the end of their life. These are listed in Table 21.2. These correlate with

Table 21.2 Specific indicators of advanced lung disease

Poor or deteriorating performance status which may also be accompanied by low body mass index or cachexia

Severe or prolonged airway obstruction (FEV < 30%)

Severe restrictive defect (vital capacity < 60%, transfer factor < 40%)

Meeting the criteria for long-term oxygen therapy; persistent hypoxia (PaO2 < 7.3 kPa)

Persistent severe symptoms despite optimum tolerated treatment

Breathlessness limiting daily activities at rest

Source: Adapted from NHS Lothian 2010. *Palliative Care in Advanced Lung Disease.* NHS Lothian Palliative Care Guidelines. Available at http://www.lothianrespirator-ymcn.scot.nhs.uk/wp-content/uploads/2010/11/Respiratory-Palliative-Care-Guidelies_October-2010.pdf

the recommendations of a systematic review undertaken by Coventry et al. (2005).

There is often lack of acknowledgement that COPD is a life-threatening condition by healthcare professionals, and consequently many patients are unaware that the chronic disease they have is a life-threatening condition and as a result they have unmet communication and information needs in relation to end-of-life care issues (Spathis and Booth, 2008).

A range of disease trajectories devised by Murray et al. (2005) are used to assist clinicians to diagnose advanced disease and these are routinely included in prognostication guidance such as GSF (2005). This helps demonstrate that despite a gradual decline in functional status there are often acute exacerbations of symptoms secondary to complications of the underlying COPD. Such prognostication guidance generally considers functional status over a period of time. Despite the range of prognostic indicators, Crawford (2010) considers that these alone are not always useful as triggers for discussions related to deteriorating quality of life and advancing disease.

Patients who have COPD may present with a gradual decline in their functional status accompanied by acute episodes of poor health with marked deterioration, which they may or may not recover from (Dean, 2008). The case study demonstrates that acute episodes are often triggered by a chest infection. Further complications can actually lead to death such as respiratory depression or unresponsive pneumonia. This further complicates the issue of being able to accurately predict end of life in patients with COPD. Crawford (2010) advises that estimating life expectancy and predicting terminal disease is more challenging at the most severe end of the COPD spectrum.

Increased acute hospital admissions are a common occurrence in COPD patients in the last year of their life. Preventing avoidable readmissions to hospital has the potential to profoundly improve both the quality-of-life for patients and the financial impact on healthcare systems. There is evidence to support the fact that a significant number of readmissions are likely to be preventable (van Walraven et al., 2011).

There is still a large gap between where people say they would prefer to die (at home) and where they actually die, as 58% of people die in hospital (DH, 2008; Gomes et al., 2011). At the beginning of the twentieth century, 90% of deaths occurred as a result of acute illnesses; now conversely 90% of patients die from a chronic disease with about half receiving treatment for at least 30 months before they die. Therefore, most people, given the opportunity, have time to plan for their care at the end of life (Gadoud and Johnson, 2011).

CASE STUDY

Mr Jim Scott was a 68-year-old man when he was admitted to the ward. He was accompanied by his wife, who had called an ambulance as Jim was struggling with his breathing at home. He had required assistance with personal care tasks over recent days. On arrival at hospital, Jim was found to be acutely breathless and appeared cyanosed. Jim reported increased breathlessness on minimal exertion over the past few days and had had a cough with productive sputum noted to be green in colour; he was warm and sweating. Jim was tachycardic, his breathing was rapid and shallow and he appeared very anxious.

Chest examination indicated bilateral lower lobe crackles, palpation indicated reduced air entry and percussion sounded dull over both lower lung fields. Jim's respiratory rate was 28 bpm, pulse 109 bpm, temperature was 38.1°C and blood pressure 140/91 mmHg. His oxygen saturation was 89% on room air, he was given 2 litres of oxygen via nasal cannula and his oxygen saturation rose to 94%. Urinalysis was negative and chest X-ray showed consolidation in the lower lobes of both lungs suggestive of an infection.

Jim was diagnosed with COPD by his GP 18 years ago. He initially used to see the practice nurse at the GP surgery and took regular inhalers. Over the past 2 years he had become increasingly breathless even on minimal exertion, and found it too difficult to go out and was not attending follow-up clinics because of this. Over the past 6 months he had been admitted to hospital five times following acute exacerbations of his COPD. On two of these occasions this was triggered by a chest infection and during his previous admission he was in respiratory distress and was transferred to the Critical Care Unit for non-invasive ventilation. He found this experience distressing as he considered the pressurised airflow was out of sequence with his breathing and this caused increased panic. Jim was diagnosed with angina 5 years ago and also had high blood pressure.

Jim was an industrial painter but is now retired and lives in a second floor flat with his wife. He has two grown-up daughters who are both married and live nearby. He has smoked 20 cigarettes a day since he was 17 but stopped 5 years ago. He used to drink alcohol regularly but can no longer get out to his local club. He stated that he missed the company of his mates and felt very isolated at home.

Jim was taking a salbutamol inhaler four times daily, tiotropium inhaler twice daily, fluticasone (Flixatide) inhaler as required, isosorbide mononitrate 20 mg and GTN spray for angina, Bendroflumethiazide 5 mg for his blood pressure as he was unable to tolerate beta blockers due to persistent cough, co-codamol 8/500 mg two tablets, four times daily for back pain and Senna for constipation. Jim was prescribed oral morphine solution 2.5 mgs as required for breathlessness, which was prescribed at the last hospital visit, but Jim had not been taking this in case he got addicted to the morphine. Jim was also on oxygen therapy and had no known allergies.

Jim was admitted to the respiratory ward for treatment of his acute chest infection and was commenced on antibiotics and steroids and given nebulised salbutamol. He was also commenced on 2 litres of continuous oxygen. The consultant on the ward explained that Jim's COPD was more progressive and due to recent regular admissions he needed to be followed up more closely at home by the community matron for respiratory disorders. Jim was given 2.5 mgs of oral morphine solution for his breathlessness and this helped reduce his respiratory rate. Jim responded well to the antibiotics and was discharged home. He still required intermittent oxygen in the ward and an assessment was made for home oxygen. He also had a referral to community occupational therapy for assessment of equipment to prevent exertion at home and he was given a special elevator under his mattress that allowed him to sit higher in bed and also get up from a lying position. On discharge Jim declined a care package to provide personal care.

The community matron explained that she could work with Jim and his wife to help them deal with acute episodes of breathlessness more effectively. She encouraged Jim to use the oral morphine for acute breathlessness and explained that many people may have concerns about using oral morphine, but that in low doses it is beneficial for people who are very breathless and addiction is not a problem. Jim was advised to increase his Senna and his fibre and fluid intake to reduce the risk of constipation. The community matron also prescribed antibiotics and steroids to keep at home which can be started at the early stages of any further chest infections.

Jim agreed to attend a day hospice one day per week where he met a range of other people with respiratory and cardiac problems. He was surprised as he thought that hospice care was only for people with cancer. There was a specialist nurse who taught relaxation techniques and also offered cognitive behavioural therapy (CBT) to help people manage breathlessness.

Jim deteriorated over the next few months and was unable to attend the day hospice. The GP called to visit him and suggested that someone from the community palliative care team could come and assess him. Jim asked if that meant the doctor thought he was 'on his last legs.' The GP stated it was just to help with symptom advice. Jim also agreed to have carers to help with his personal care.

The community Macmillan nurse met Jim and he identified he was most concerned about going back into hospital in case he was given ventilator support. She explained that he could complete an advance care plan to record his future wishes and preferences, in relation to his care. She acknowledged how distressed he was about the prospect of having non-invasive ventilation and advised that he could complete an Advance Decision to Refuse Treatment (ADRT). This would allow him to specify that if he was in respiratory distress he did not want to be given assistance with his ventilation. Jim was aware that without this treatment he may not survive and said he thought he hadn't got long to live, and that no one had discussed this with him and, when asked, his wife and family always say 'oh he will be fine.'

Exploration of this indicated that Jim was worried that he was now dying and no one had told him. This made him increasingly anxious. The Macmillan nurse had an open discussion about his poor prognosis and that there has been significant deterioration but due to the unpredictability of his condition it is not possible to give him an exact indication of how long he had to live. She stated that the priority was to make sure that Jim felt supported and that his symptoms are well managed. She commenced him on a low dose of lorazepam to take when he felt really panicked and breathless. Further discussion about Jim's ADRT confirmed that the details and circumstances identified were still correct. He also indicated that he would not want to be given cardiopulmonary resuscitation and after discussion with the GP, a Do Not Attempt Resuscitation (DNAR) form was completed.

Over the next few weeks Jim deteriorated further and spent longer periods in bed. The Macmillan nurse arranged a pressure relief mattress for him. The GP and community matron observed that Jim appeared to be sleepier, less alert and was no longer able to eat or drink. An examination concluded that there was no underlying infection or other reversible cause. They recognised that Jim may be approaching the last days of his life and had a discussion with Jim's family. They advised the family that Jim's breathing may become more irregular and gave him some medication to reduce bronchial secretions. These secretions can be very noisy and distressing especially to family members. His morphine was converted from an oral to subcutaneous route via a syringe driver and the community nursing team visited regularly to monitor and assess Jim's condition. The family wished to assist in provision of mouth care as Jim had a very dry mouth.

Jim died at home the following day with his family present.

MANAGING SYMPTOMS

The following discussion that focuses on symptom management will be applied to the case-study above.

BREATHLESSNESS

Breathlessness is a common and distressing symptom in patients with advanced disease (Kamal et al., 2011, 2012). Breathlessness has a significant impact on quality of life and, owing to its diverse aetiology, can present a great management challenge for healthcare professionals and a great burden for patients, especially after having lived with the symptom for years (Kamal et al., 2011, 2012). Patients may describe breathlessness in many ways and the sensation is very subjective; the experience does not always correlate with physiological measurements such as oxygen saturation or respiratory rate (Kamal et al., 2011). It is important to listen to the patient's voice and appreciate the concept of total breathlessness and the impact it has on the patient's quality of life; the physical, social, psychological and existential effects interact to form the overall experience of breathlessness (Abernethy and Wheeler, 2008). This can be a real challenge to manage as patients reach the end of their lives and, as with all symptoms, the

aim should be careful assessment, good communication and review, with an acknowledgement that it is often difficult to address symptoms with neat solutions (Payne et al., 2008).

The use of opioid medication in the treatment of breathlessness has a large evidence base acting on both the physiological mechanism of action and offering symptomatic benefit in patient populations from varied disease groups (Johnson et al., 2012). Despite good evidence for efficacy, it appears that there are still barriers to the use of opiates for intractable breathlessness: some clinicians may be reluctant to administer opiates in chronic respiratory disease, either death may be hastened, respiratory depression may occur or addiction may develop in the patient (Johnson et al., 2012; Young et al., 2012). Such anxiety can reflect on patients and their family despite the fact that opiates reduce respiratory distress.

In Jim's case he had been given oral morphine; this should be administered regularly and titrated according to response. As Jim's ability to tolerate oral medication declined, he should have been given his opiates by syringe driver.

Benzodiazepines are used to manage breathlessness; anxiety is linked both as a cause and a consequence of breathlessness. Psychological support and interventions are required to support the patient and certainly benzodiazepines help cope with panic and anxiety (Gysels and Higginson, 2012). In Jim's case he was prescribed lorazepam by the Macmillan nurse, and as his condition deteriorated there was a need to continue with his benzodiazepines in conjunction with opioids in his syringe driver. Midazolam would be the drug of choice and has been evaluated both as a single agent and in combination with morphine. Midazolam in combination with morphine has a moderately beneficial effect compared with either drug given alone at the end of life (Navigante et al., 2006)

NOISY BREATHING

Noisy breathing or bubbly secretions causing laboured breathing sound like a rattle and occur because the patient is unable to cough or swallow properly in order to clear their airways of secretions. While the sound of this would suggest otherwise, this often does not cause the patient any distress. However, the noise does cause distress for the relatives and carers of the patient (Faull and de Caestecker, 2012). Anticholinergic drugs may help in reducing pharyngeal secretions. Hyoscine hydrobromide can be given subcutaneously or transdermally as in Jim's case (Watson et al., 2009).

MOUTH CARE

This is an essential component of care at the end of life. Saliva keeps the mouth clean and healthy; a dry mouth (xerostomia) is common in patients at the end of life. As in Jim's case, opioids, anticholinergics, anxiety and mouth breathing all contributed to a dry mouth, which in turn can become dirty and infected. The main principles should be to keep the oral mucosa clean, soft and moist with the frequency of mouth care being more important than the products used (Faull and de Caestecker, 2012).

OXYGEN

While Jim was given domiciliary oxygen in his own home, the decision to use oxygen should be made on a case-by-case basis. In terminal illness there is evidence to suggest that some patients benefit from this (Kamal et al., 2012). Equally, there is also an argument to suggest that fresh air or a fan and the movement of air around the patient has a similar beneficial effect (Abernethy et al., 2010).

COMMUNICATING SENSITIVELY AND SUPPORTING THE PATIENT AND THEIR FAMILY

It can be seen from Jim's case as his disease advanced that his anxiety and fear severely impacted upon his quality of life. Contact with healthcare professionals increases significantly as disease progresses (Crawford, 2010). Recognition that a patient has now entered the advanced stage of illness enables appropriate communication about expectations and the opportunity to formulate an advance care plan which is centred on the preferences of the patient and their carers (Gadoud and Johnson, 2011). Policy drivers and evidence highlights the need to provide an opportunity for patients and their carers to have end-of-life care discussions (DH, 2008, 2011, 2012); such opportunities can make the patient feel liberated, relieved and reassured (National Council of Palliative Care, 2010). There can be problems related to such open and honest conversations related to end-of-life care. Payne et al. (2008) discusses the dominance of symptom management and pharmacological approaches to the patient's care at a time when support, guidance and the consideration of psychological issues can offer reassurance and allay anxiety. Healthcare professionals involved in respiratory care need to grasp this nettle; although many are committed to assuring that patients have an advance care plan in place, there is still some reticence (Smith et al., 2014).

CARERS

COPD has a profound impact not only on the patient with the physical and psychological burden of living with a chronic disease, but also on families and carers (Gardiner et al., 2010). Family/carer support should be central to care delivery in COPD with special consideration being given to the burden of care, stress, social isolation, fatigue and anxiety (Janssen et al., 2010). Jim had the opportunity to plan for his death, and his family had been involved in the decision making as they had been included in his care throughout. Such an approach can offer the family reassurance that all has been done to care for the patient up to their death and can also prevent potential problems in bereavement.

SUMMARY

The need for end-of-life care in chronic disease such as COPD is clear; patients need to have their physical, social, psychological and spiritual care addressed. There is an increasing drive for care to be delivered in the community. If the patient's experience is to be enhanced then there is a need to make sure that clinical specialities work together, that palliative care is everybody's business and that quality end-of-life care is not denied because there is lack of communication or fragmentation of services (Gott et al., 2012). While symptom control is a key component of the palliative care service, equally so is the concept of patient autonomy and choice (Randall and Downie, 2006). At the cornerstone of all of the aforementioned is good communication.

REFERENCES

Abernethy, A.P. and Wheeler, J.L. 2008. Total dyspnoea. *Current Opinion in Supportive Palliative Care* 2 (2): 110–113.

Abernethy, A.P., McDonald, C.F., Frith, P.A. et al. 2010. Effect of palliative oxygen versus room air in relief of breathlessness in patients with refractory dyspnoea: A double-blind, randomised controlled trial. *Lancet* 376 (9743): 784–793.

Addington-Hall, J. and Higginson, I. 2006. *Palliative Care for Non-Cancer Patients.* Oxford University Press, Oxford.

Carlucci, A., Guerrieri, A. and Stefano, N. 2012. Palliative care in COPD patients: Is it only an end of life issue? *European Respiratory Review* 21 (126): 347–354.

Cartwright, Y. and Booth, S. 2010. Extending palliative care to patients with respiratory disease. *British Journal of Hospital Medicine* 71 (1): 16–20.

Coventry, P.S., Grande, G.E., Richards, D.A. and Todd, C.J. 2005. Predictors of appropriate timing of palliative care for older adults with a non-malignant life threatening disease: A systematic review. *Age and Ageing* 34 (3): 218–227.

Crawford, A. 2010. Respiratory practitioners experience of end of life care discussions in COPD. *British Journal of Nursing* 19 (18): 1164–1169.

Dean, M. 2008. End of life care for COPD patients. *Primary care Respiratory Journal* 17 (1): 46–50.

Department of Health 2007. *The Cancer Reform Strategy.* Stationary Office, London.

Department of Health 2008. *End of Life Care Strategy: Promoting High Quality Care for All Adults at the End of Life.* Stationary Office, London.

Department of Health 2010. *Delivering the Cancer Reform Strategy.* National Audit Office.

Department of Health 2011. *Third Annual Report on the End of Life Care Strategy.* Stationary Office, London, London.

Department of Health 2012. *The Outcomes Strategy for COPD and Asthma.* Stationary Office, London.

Department of Health 2014. *Government Response to the House of Commons Health Select Committee Report into Long Term Conditions.* Stationary Office, London.

Faull, C. and de Caestecker, S. 2012. *Handbook of Palliative Care.* Wiley Blackwell, Oxford.

Froggatt, K.A., Wilson, D., Justice, C., Macadam, M., Leibovici, K., Kinch, J., Thomas, R. and Choi, J. 2006. End of life care in long term care settings for older people: A literature review. *International Journal of Older People Nursing* 1 (1): 45–50.

Gadoud, A. and Johnson, M. 2011. Palliative care in non-malignant disease. *Medicine* 39 (11): 664–667.

Gardiner, C., Gott, M. and Payne, S. 2010. Exploring the care needs of patients with advanced COPD: An overview of the literature. *Respiratory Medicine* 104 (2): 159–165.

Gold Standard Framework 2005. Prognostic indicator Guidance. GSF available from http://www.goldstandardsframework.org.uk

Gomes, B., Calanzani, N. and Higginson, I.J. 2011. Reversal of the British trend in place of death: Time series analysis 2004–2010. *Palliative Medicine* 26 (2): 102–107.

Gott, M., Seymour, J., Ingleton, C., Gardiner, C. and Bellamy, G. 2012. 'That's part of everybody's job': The perspectives of health care staff in England and New Zealand on the meaning and remit of palliative care. *Palliative Medicine* 26 (3): 232–241.

Gysels, I. and Higginson, I. 2008. Caring for a person in advanced illness and suffering from breathlessness at home: Threats and resources. *Palliative and Supportive Care* 7 (2):153–162.

Hardin, K.A., Meyers, F. and Louie, S. 2008. Integrating palliative care in severe chronic obstructive lung disease. *Journal of Chronic Obstructive Pulmonary Disease* 5 (4): 207–220.

Higginson, I., Bausewein, C. and Reilly, C. 2014. An integrated palliative and respiratory care service for patients with advanced disease and refractory breathlessness: A randomised controlled trial. *The Lancet* 2 (12): 979–987.

Janssen, D.J.A., Spruit, M., Alsengeest, T.P.G., Does, J.D., Schols, J.M. and Wouters, E.F. 2010. A patient-centred interdisciplinary palliative care programme for end-stage chronic respiratory diseases. *International Journal of Palliative Nursing* 16 (4): 189–194.

Johnson, M.J., Abernethy, A.P. and Currow, D.C. 2012. Gaps in the evidence base of opioids for refractory breathlessness. A future work plan? *Journal of Pain and Symptom Management* 43 (3): 614–624.

Kamal, A.H., Maguire, J.M., Wheeler, J.L., Currow, D.C. and Abernethy, A.P. 2011. Dyspnea review for the palliative care professional: Assessment, burdens and aetiologies. *Journal of Palliative Care* 14 (10): 1167–1172.

Kamal, A.H., Maguire, J.M., Wheeler, J.L., Currow, D.C. and Abernethy, A.P. 2012. Dyspnoea review for the palliative care professional: Treatment goals and therapeutic options. *Journal of Palliative Care* 15 (1): 106–114.

Murray, S.A.M., Kendall, M., Boyd, K. and Sheikh, A. 2005. Illness trajectories and palliative care. *British Medical Journal* 330: 1007–1011.

National Council of Palliative Care 2010. *The End of Life Care Manifesto 2010*. NCPC, London.

Navigante, A.H., Cerchietti, L.C.A., Castro, M.A., Lutteral, M.A. and Cabalar, M.E. 2006. Midazolam as adjunct therapy to morphine in the alleviation of severe dyspnoea perception in patients with advanced cancer. *Journal of Pain and Symptom Management* 31 (1): 38–47.

NHS England 2014. *Actions for End of Life Care: 2014–2016*. Stationary Office, London.

NHS England 2014. *Five Year Forward View*. Stationary Office, London.

NHS Lothian 2010. *Palliative Care in Advanced Lung Disease*. NHS Lothian Palliative Care Guidelines. Available at http://www.lothian-respiratorymcn.scot.nhs.uk/wp-content/uploads/2010/11/Respiratory-Palliative-Care-Guidelies_October-2010.pdf

Payne, S., Seymour, J. and Ingleton, C. 2008. *Palliative Care Nursing Principles and Evidence for Practice*. Open University Press, Berkshire.

Randall, F. and Downie, R.S. 2006. *The Philosophy of Palliative Care*. Oxford University Press, Oxford.

Smith, T.A., Myong, K., Piza, M., Davidson, P.M., Clayton, J.M., Jenkins, C.R. and Ingham, J.M. 2014. Specialist respiratory physicians' attitudes to and practice of advance care planning in COPD. A pilot study. *Respiratory Medicine* 108 (6): 935–939.

Spathis, A. and Booth, S. 2008. End of life care in chronic obstructive pulmonary disease: In search of a good death. *International Journal of Chronic Obstructive Pulmonary Disease* 3 (1): 11–29.

Taylor, G.J. and Kurent, J.E. 2003. *A Clinician's Guide to Palliative Care*. Blackwell Science, Oxford.

The National End of Life Care Intelligence Network 2011. *Deaths from Respiratory Diseases: Implications for End of Life Care in England*. Stationary Office, London.

Traue, D.C. and Ross, J.R. 2005. Palliative care in non-malignant disease. *Journal of the Royal Society of Medicine* 98 (11): 503–506.

van Walraven, C., Bennett, C., Jennings, A., Austin, P.C. and Forster, A.J. 2011. Proportion of hospital readmissions deemed avoidable: A systematic review. *Canadian Medical Association Journal* 183 (7): E391–E402.

Watson, M., Lucas, C., Hoy, A. and Wells, J. 2009. *Oxford Handbook of Palliative Care*. Oxford University Press, Oxford.

Young, J., Donahue, M., Farquhar, M., Simpson, C. and Rocker, G. 2012. Using opioids to treat dyspnoea in advanced COPD. Attitudes and experiences of family physicians and respiratory therapists. *Canadian Family Physician* 58 (7): e401–e407.

Index